NURSE CASE MANAGEMENT
in the 21st Century

ELAINE L. COHEN, EdD, RN

Vice President of Patient Care
Dakota Heartland Health System
Fargo, North Dakota
Former Assistant Vice President for Nursing
The General Hospital Center at Passaic
Passaic, New Jersey

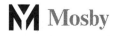 Mosby

St. Louis Baltimore Boston Carlsbad Chicago Naples New York Philadelphia Portland
London Madrid Mexico City Singapore Sydney Tokyo Toronto Wiesbaden

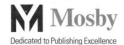

A Times Mirror
Company

Publisher: Nancy L. Coon
Editor: N. Darlene Como
Developmental Editor: Dana L. Knighten
Project Manager: Patricia Tannian
Senior Production Coordinator: Ann E. Rogers
Production by Shepherd, Inc.
Book Design Manager: Gail Morey Hudson
Cover Designer: Teresa Breckwoldt
Manufacturing Supervisor: Karen Lewis

RT
89
.N744
1996

Printed in the United States of America
Composition by Shepherd, Inc.
Printing/binding by Maple-Vail Book Mfg Group

Mosby–Year Book, Inc.
11830 Westline Industrial Drive
St. Louis, MO 63146

Library of Congress Cataloging in Publication Data

Nurse case management in the 21st century/[edited by] Elaine L. Cohen.
    p. cm.
    Includes bibliographical references and index.
    ISBN 0-8151-1518-0 (hard cover)
    1. Nursing services—United States—Administration. 2. Continuum of care. 3. Nursing care plans.
    4. Health care reform—United States. I. Cohen, Elaine L. (Elaine Liebman)
    [DNLM: 1. Nursing Care—organization & administration. 2. Nursing Care—trends. 3. Patient Care
    Planning—organization & administration. 4. Nurse-Patient Relations. WY 100 N9712 1996]
    RT89.N744 1996
    362.1′73′068—dc20
    DNLM/DLC
    for Library of Congress
                            96-41096
                            CIP

95 96 97 98 99 / 9 8 7 6 5 4 3 2 1

To

The La Paz Group
a think tank for case management.
Your focus, perspective, and leadership will
sustain the unfolding process of nurse case management.

Anne Marie Djupe
who dedicated her life to advance Parish Nursing.
She will be remembered forever as a pioneer in the field
and for the wonderful legacy she left.

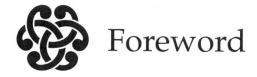

Foreword

Although any man or woman of good conscience who is responsible for client service delivery would agree that trying to improve client care while focusing on the bottom line is akin to trying to win a tennis match by watching the scoreboard, few would argue that fiscal accountability is unimportant. As managed care entities move rapidly from discounted contracts to capitation, the managers of health-service delivery systems seek solutions to the limits and demands this entails. Understanding the fiscal problem is one thing; coping with the practical everyday implications for providers and clients is quite another.

No longer paid retrospectively a fee-for-service or even a contracted capped amount, but rather paid a specific amount for each person covered in the managed care contract (capitation), providers know that every dime expended on service delivery comes off the bottom line. Therefore, for the first time in recent memory, preventing illness in the primary population has become profitable. Moreover, efforts to maintain an optimal level of health among the chronically ill are crucial to any provider's financial viability.

About 5% to 10% of clients account for about 80% of cost overruns. With capitation on the doorstep, the difference between success and failure rests on how well the organization manages that crucial 5% to 10%. In the last 10 years, payors have tried to contain their costs using the following measures:

- Limiting access to inservice care only to medically necessary conditions (usually accomplished by having panels of physicians develop criteria, requiring second opinions, and/or having a "gatekeeper physician" employed by the managed care entity give approval for the admission), with some success.
- Controlling the content of care, primarily through limiting the length of stay, again with some success.
- Tracking the outcomes of care (recidivism, cost per case, return to work, number of deaths per procedure, average length of stay, and the like) and contracting only with providers whose outcomes are acceptable, with limited success.

- Hiring a professional person (usually a nurse) to review client records, usually retrospectively but occasionally concurrently, to investigate the appropriateness of a care regimen, again with limited success.

None of these strategies improved the quality of care, although each contributed to decreasing the cost of care. Nonetheless, in terms of priorities, one of the first major studies to evaluate managed care plans found that employers were more interested in the quality of a plan's services than in the nature of a plan's financial controls. In July 1995, the Chicago Business Group on Health, a not-for-profit coalition of more than 60 private and public employers in the Chicago metropolitan area, released this study, which encompassed 14 Chicago companies, 7 health care plans, and 22,000 surveyed employees. It focused on the key areas of cost, access, and quality. Among its many findings is that "all managed care is not equal."

There were dramatic variations in cost performance from plan to plan and employer to employer. The study showed "one employer's plan was 142% of the community average cost, while another employer's plan was 72%." It is fair to say that the plans performed better on operational measures (e.g., access to physicians, responsiveness of member services) than on the clinical measures incorporating HEDIS (Health Plan Employer Data and Information Set) information. Specifically, "operationally all plans achieved a 4.0 rating on a 5.0 scale. On the clinical measures, however, the average score was 2.5."

The purpose of all this is to demonstrate that further cost savings and quality improvements are probably going to have to be realized on the clinical end. What is needed is a breakthrough strategy that genuinely improves the care clients receive, most especially for that crucial 5% to 10% whose complex, usually chronic needs drive up the cost of care. That breakthrough strategy is *professional nurse case management*. Although hardly new, it has not been disseminated nearly as widely as one might suspect—*primarily because it works.* That is, it slashes the number of inpatient days, dramatically reduces costs, and significantly improves the quality of care clients receive. Unfortunately, until the majority of people are covered by capitated contracts, cutting inpatient days reduces hospital revenue, which has a decidedly negative impact on institutions that are not operating in a capitated environment (i.e., almost all of the hospitals in the United States). As the nation moves toward capitated managed care, interest in professional nurse case management is booming.

The editor and authors of *Nurse Case Management in the 21st Century* are among the most experienced and prestigious pioneers in the field. They provide the reader with a blueprint for action as they share the practical techniques and outcomes they achieved when they integrated case management across the continuum of care.

Leah L. Curtin, Editor
Nursing Management

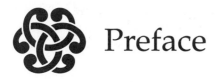

Preface

The imposing challenges and shifts in public policy and priorities have rocked the very foundation upon which health-care delivery has evolved. Almost Darwinistic in nature, the change process has required a force of near cataclysmic proportions to move forward in a system that for decades has been wallowing in a quagmire of fragmented, inefficient, and misappropriated care. Whether or not the influences of natural selection are at play, the dynamic changes embraced by a movement to reduce government spending and entitlements and at the same time create healthier communities promises to transform the traditional practice of health-care delivery and management.

Because it is not "business as usual," health-care consumers have become more receptive to alternative interventions outside conventional boundaries. The increased tolerance for change has compelled private as well as local, state, and federal agencies to become more flexible in exploring various options in the process of reinventing health care.

Integrated delivery systems, coordinated, comprehensive health-care networks, and community health-care programs and coalitions are examples of innovative approaches that portend future changes. Spurred on by the national reform movement, efforts such as these demonstrate an increased responsiveness to health-care needs of consumers, the development of collaborative partnerships with the recipients and providers of health care, innovative contracting arrangements and alliances across health-care settings, and the restructuring of professional practice to ensure productivity, efficiency, affordability, and quality of care delivered.

By encompassing innovation, versatility, and openness to client involvement in addressing the health-care requirements of diverse populations, nurse case management offers a framework to provide care and manage services in the new care system.

Nurse Case Management in the 21st Century provides the next steps in the transition by describing contemporary approaches to nurse case management and the different points of the process being experienced by innovators. It focuses on the conceptual, practical, and "how-to" applications of nurse case management as a system for coordinating care across providers, practice environments, and the health-illness continuum. This book delivers two powerful messages. The first is to the consumer by emphasizing the nursing services available to enhance an individual's health and well-being. The second is a message to nurses to advocate politically for consumers and to work in partnership with clients to enhance health-care delivery across services. The newness of the concepts and implementation of nurse case management in acute and long-term institutions and community agencies, the speed of the evolutionary process of health care and its anticipated changes, and the importance of the nurse's role in restructuring health care all point to the need for this book.

Through the methods of storytelling and relating individual experiences, the reader will be given a richer and more in-depth view of the specific functional components, processes, and clinical applications within the model's framework. Particular attention is paid to the nurse's role, the client's response, and the community's involvement in meeting the health-care needs of its members.

The special concerns and challenges of clients in a variety of settings are highlighted. Couched in the underlying values and elements of case management, integrated approaches are explored from an academic and service delivery perspective.

The contributors to this book are leading national experts who provide the reader a unique opportunity to learn from their experiences. As designers of their systems, these professionals represent the major force and conscience behind linking nurse case management with health-care redesign.

This book offers a view of the whole phenomenon of nurse case management by describing all components of the process such as development, planning, implementation, cost effectiveness, and outcome evaluation. By using the "hands-on" material, readers will be able to adapt and apply the principles and interventions from the models illustrated in the text to their own individual practice or education settings. Even the visual design of this book reinforces the underlying theme of interconnectedness. The interwoven symbol that is featured at the top of this page, on the book's cover, and at the beginning of every chapter captures and conveys the integration and openness that characterize case management.

Nurse professionals in the academic and service realm will find this book useful. It will also benefit all decision makers for nursing practice and model design, such as executive level management, nurse managers, educators, and faculty.

Other targeted audiences include clinical specialists, utilization and discharge planners, clinicians, and primary health-care providers in both acute and community-based settings, health-care planners, community leaders, and payors.

Graduate nursing schools will also find this book useful for the case management content of their curricula. It is of special importance as universities prepare advance practice nurses to address society's current health-care needs by applying new models of care delivery.

A book for people in the process of making change, *Nurse Case Management in the 21st Century* becomes a unique resource and benefit to professionals and consumers of health-care services in a multitude of settings.

Elaine L. Cohen

Acknowledgments

The concept for this book was conceived at the Fifth Annual Nurse Case Management Exchange in La Paz, Mexico. A dream come true, the idea became a reality as the group embraced and shared in the book's creation and development.

It was also the first time that a community of leaders had come together in a creative partnership to share their experiences, stories, and ideas. Their collective spirit, wisdom, and voice frame the power and purpose behind the book.

As with any undertaking there are those individuals who are deserving of special gratitude. I wish to express my deepest appreciation to Drs. Vivien DeBack and Cathy Michaels for their unswaying dedication and commitment as reviewers. Their gifts of friendship and nurturing are truly life affirming. To Darlene Como, for providing the literary freedom and guidance so I may continue to mature as a writer. Dana Knighten, for her tireless editorial efforts and fabulous sense of humor. Thank you for keeping me laughing! Mary Ellen Rauner, for providing the professional latitude and support to complete this project. To Lori Caravella, for her expert typing and manuscript preparation. Thanks for putting up with me. And to my husband, Allan, for his patience, friendship, and love.

My deepest thanks to the contributors for sharing their innovations and thereby shaping health care's new direction. I am humbly privileged by their enthusiasm and generosity.

The universal themes of "Freedom, Trust, and Caring" so eloquently expressed in the chapter by Annette McBeth and Alice Weydt was evident throughout this project and freely given by all members of the La Paz Group—the individuals of which portray what is the most extraordinary demonstration of connectedness. Thank you for gracing my life and nourishing a dream.

ELC

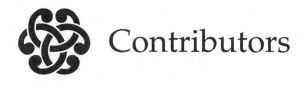

Contributors

GINA ASTORINO, MS, RN

Clinical Nurse Specialist
Senior Instructor
Denver Nursing Project in Human Caring
University of Colorado School of Nursing
Denver, Colorado

KENNETH D. BOPP, PhD

Director, Health Services Management Group
Graduate Program in Health Services Management
University of Missouri—Columbia
Columbia, Missouri

KATHLEEN A. BOWER, DNSc, RN

Principal and Co-Owner
The Center for Case Management, Inc.
South Natick, Massachusetts

ARLENE CARLSON, MA, LPN

Pre-Hospice Specialist
Carondelet Hospice
Carondelet Health Care Corporation
Tucson, Arizona

JOANN CLOUGH, MAOM, RN

Director, Outcomes Management
Birmingham Health Connection/Brookwood Medical Center
Birmingham, Alabama

VIRGINIA DAVIS, MSN, RN

Senior Manager
Ernst & Young, LLP
Dallas, Texas

VIVIEN DeBACK, PhD, RN, FAAN

Nurse Consultant
Empowering Change
Franklin, Wisconsin

ANNE MARIE DJUPE, MA, RNC

Director, Parish Nursing Services
Lutheran General Health Systems/Advocate Health Care
Park Ridge, Illinois

PHYLLIS ETHRIDGE, MSN, RN, CNAA, FAAN

Vice President, Community Health Services
Carondelet Health Care Corporation
Tucson, Arizona

CAROL D. FALK, MS, RN

Professional Nurse Case Manager
President, Carondelet St. Mary's Nursing Enterprise
Carondelet Health Care Corporation
Tucson, Arizona

BARBARA FRIEDBACHER, MS, RN

Director, Silver Spring Community Nursing Center
University of Wisconsin
Milwaukee School of Nursing
Milwaukee, Wisconsin

S. JO GIBSON, MS, RN, CCM

Director, Center for Case Management
Sioux Valley Hospital
Sioux Falls, South Dakota

JOYCE A. HOSPODAR, BS, MPA

Associate Site Director
Carondelet Community Nursing Organization
Tucson, Arizona

SUNNY R. HOWE, MS, RN, CNAA

Director of Nursing
Alexian Village of Milwaukee
Milwaukee, Wisconsin

MARJORIE K. JAMIESON, MS, RN, FAAN

Executive Director
The Living at Home/Block Nurse Program, Inc.
St. Paul, Minnesota

SHARON JEHLE, MSN, RN

Associate Vice President
Holy Family Memorial Medical Center
Manitowoc, Wisconsin

SUZANNE JOHNSON

Financial Officer/Cost Accounting Coordinator
Community Consultant
Carondelet Health Care Corporation
Tucson, Arizona

JoELLEN GOERTZ KOERNER, PhD, RN, CNAA, FAAN

Vice President, Patient Services
Sioux Valley Hospital
Sioux Falls, South Dakota

GERRI S. LAMB, PhD, RN, FAAN

Clinical Director for Research
Director, Carondelet Community Nursing Organization
Carondelet Health Care Corporation
Tucson, Arizona

SALLY PECK LUNDEEN, PhD, RN, FAAN

Associate Dean for Practice
Associate Professor
University of Wisconsin
Milwaukee School of Nursing
Milwaukee, Wisconsin

ANNETTE McBETH, MS, RN

Vice President
Immanuel St. Joseph's Hospital
Mankato, Minnesota

CATHY MICHAELS, PhD, RN

Professional Nurse Case Manager & Nurse Researcher
Associate Director, Community Health Services
Carondelet Health Care Corporation
Tucson, Arizona

MARY H. MUNDT, PhD, RN

Associate Dean for Academic Affairs
University of Wisconsin
Milwaukee School of Nursing
Milwaukee, Wisconsin

MARGARET MURPHY, PhD, RN

Nurse Consultant
Empowering Change
Wauwatosa, Wisconsin

MARGARET NEWMAN, PhD, RN, FAAN

Professor
School of Nursing
University of Minnesota
Minneapolis, Minnesota

JUDITH LYNN PAPENHAUSEN, PhD, RN

Professor & Associate Chair
Department of Nursing
California State University
Los Angeles, California

TIM PORTER-O'GRADY, EdD, PhD, RN, CNAA, FAAN

Senior Partner, Timothy Porter-O'Grady Assoc., Inc.
Senior Consultant, Affiliated Dynamics, Inc.
Assistant Professor, Emory University
Atlanta, Georgia

MARILYN RANTZ, PhD, RN

Assistant Professor, School of Nursing
University Hospital Professor of Nursing
University of Missouri—Columbia
Columbia, Missouri

SHEILA A. RYAN, PhD, RN, FAAN

Dean and Professor
Director, Medical Center Nursing
University of Rochester School of Nursing
Rochester, New York

MARITA SCHIFALAQUA, MSN, RN

Nursing Systems Consultants
Milwaukee, Wisconsin

CAROLE SCHROEDER, PhD, RN

Assistant Professor
University of Washington
Seattle, Washington

MARY SINNEN, MSN, RN

Nursing Systems Consultants
Milwaukee, Wisconsin

JOAN STEMPEL, MS, RN, CCM

Professional Nurse Case Manager
Community Health Services
Carondelet Health Care Corporation
Tucson, Arizona

GAIL TERRY, BSN, RN

Nurse Educator
Holy Family Memorial Medical Center
Manitowoc, Wisconsin

BECKY TRELLA, MSN, RN

Manager, Senior Services
Lutheran General Health Plan
Mt. Prospect, Illinois

ALICE WEYDT, MS, RN

Director, Patient Care Services
Immanuel St. Joseph's Hospital
Mankato, Minnesota

DONNA ZAZWORSKY, MSN, RN, CCM

Professional Nurse Case Manager
Carondelet Health Care Corporation
Tucson, Arizona

LISA ZERULL, MSN, RN

Program Director, Case Management
Winchester Regional Health Systems
Winchester, Virginia

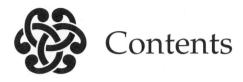 Contents

Part One   **NURSING'S CONTRIBUTION TO RESTRUCTURING HEALTH CARE**

     1   **The New Practice Environment,** 3
        Vivien DeBack and Elaine Cohen

     2   **Nurses as Advanced Practitioners and Primary Care Providers,** 10
        Tim Porter-O'Grady

     3   **Grass Roots Efforts: Nurses Involved in the Political Process,** 21
        Marjorie Jamieson

     4   **Nursing's Response to Health-Care Transformation:
        A Nurse Executive's View,** 28
        JoEllen Goertz Koerner

Part Two   **CREATING A FOUNDATION FOR CHANGE**

     5   **Academia's Involvement in Health-Care Redesign,** 43
        Sheila Ryan

     6   **Key Elements of Nurse Case Management in Curricula,** 48
        Mary H. Mundt

     7   **The Education of Nurses: Nurse Case Managers' View,** 55
        Mary Sinnen and Martia Schifalaqua

     8   **The Denver Nursing Education Project:
        Promoting the Health of Persons Living with HIV/AIDS,** 63
        Carole Schroeder and Gina Astorino

     9   **Academic Nursing Centers and Community-Based
        Nursing Information Systems,** 68
        Sally Peck Lundeen and Barabara Friedbacher

    10   **Case Management in Community Nursing Centers,** 81
        Gerri S. Lamb

    11   **Integrating Services across the Continuum:
        The Challenge of Chronic Care,** 87
        Becky Trella

    12   **Innovative Delivery Systems: Freedom, Trust, Caring,** 105
        Annette McBeth and Alice Weydt

Part Three   **PARTNERS IN HEALTH: NURSES AND CLIENTS**

13   Theory of the Nurse-Client Partnership, 119
Margaret Newman

14   Working in Partnership, 124
Joan Stempel, Arlene Carlson, and Cathy Michaels

15   Nurse Case Management in a Rural Community, 133
Lisa Zerull

16   Parish Nursing, 140
Anne Marie Djupe

17   Nurse Case Management and Long-Term Care, 149
Sunny Howe

Part Four   **THE NURSE CASE MANAGEMENT PROCESS**

**18   Case Management as a Response to Quality,
Cost, and Access Imperatives,** 161
Kathleen A. Bower and Carol D. Falk

19   Risk Indentification: Management versus Avoidance, 168
Joann Clough

**20   Issues of Design and Implementation from Acute Care,
Long-Term Care, and Community-Based Settings,** 181
Marilyn J. Rantz and Kenneth D. Bopp

21   Staff Development for Nurse Case Management, 189
Virginia Davis

22   Marketing Nurse Case Management Services, 202
Donna Zazworsky and Joyce A. Hospodar

**23   Implementing Nurse Case Management
in a Rural Community Hospital,** 211
Sharon Jehle, Gail Terry, and Margaret Murphy

24   Differentiated Practice within and beyond the Hospital Walls, 222
S. Jo Gibson

**25   The Influence of Reimbursement on Nurse Case Management
Practice: Carondelet's Experience,** 245
Phyllis Ethridge and Suzanne Johnson

26   Discovering and Achieving Client Outcomes, 257
Judith Lynne Papenhausen

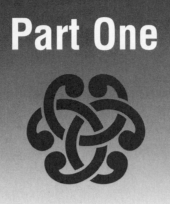

Part One

NURSING'S CONTRIBUTION TO RESTRUCTURING HEALTH CARE

Nurses must turn nursing's values into political priorities.
Marjorie Jamieson

Part One describes the global issues of health-care redesign and the complexity of engaging in such a process. Nursing's organizations, both national and local, are challenged to keep the momentum for change alive and moving forward. Chapters 1 through 4 describe restructuring issues at the institutional and unit levels and discuss the impact on nurses and their clients. Because nurses are found at all locations along the care continuum, the nurse's role in restructuring the system is defined as key to the process.

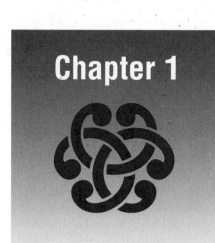

Chapter 1

The New Practice Environment

Vivien DeBack, PhD, RN, FAAN
Elaine Cohen, EdD, RN

OVERVIEW

*Nurses play a pivotal role in the complex activity
of social systems change.*

The changing political environment in the United States suggests that health-care reform will take some years to implement. Whether the reform movement receives substantial support at the national or state level is yet to be determined. What is clear, however, is the fact that any reform or shift in how health care is delivered will depend on the extent to which providers can demonstrate high-quality, cost-effective care provided to populations in community settings.

This chapter describes the complexity of attempting to make a major social system change. It discusses a new practice environment and the role nurses must play in creating and practicing in that environment.

HEALTH-CARE REFORM

Major health-care reform for America began in 1993 with the introduction of the *Health Security Act* (HR3600, 1993), a President Clinton initiative. For almost a year, the administration sought information about the existing health-care system through task forces, committees, and town meetings directed by the First Lady, Hillary Rodham Clinton. This data collection process stimulated discussions nationwide about the present and future health-care systems. The momentum created by a national discussion on health-care reform gave the change process a life of its own, separate from the administrative and legislative agendas. Health-care providers, health-care agencies, and state governmental agencies began to design new sys-

tems based on a shifting paradigm—even before federal laws were enacted. The basic premise of the new paradigm, which continues to unfold, is a focus on health and care replacing or augmenting the old paradigm of illness and cure.

PARADIGM SHIFT

A *paradigm* is a set of rules and regulations that defines boundaries and describes what must be done to be successful within those boundaries (Barker, 1989). The predominant paradigm of the *medical model,* defined as *diagnoses/treatment/cure,* no longer solves the health problems of today. Chronic disease, lifestyle-induced illness, and health and wellness are issues not amenable to the "cure" outcome of the *medical model.* As a result, an opportunity exists during this process of change to develop a new paradigm for the delivery of health care. The new paradigm is one of holism in which disease and the associated symptoms are seen as information rather than the focus of health care. The professional is partner with the client and decision making is shared. Self-care, self-reliance, and self-responsibility are key words. The emphasis is on human values, cooperation, and mutuality. The old paradigm focuses on "product." The new belief focuses on the "process." The old paradigm sees persons as machines in either a state of good or bad repair. The new approach sees persons as open systems of energy in constant exchange with the environment.

Shifting models and paradigms result when needs and demands create forces for change. Two of the major forces driving changes in the health-care system of the United States are (1) excessive costs to run the present system, and (2) lack of health care or access to care for millions of Americans. The nation spent $838 billion on health and illness care in 1993 and is expected to spend $939 billion in 1994. At the same time, it is estimated that there are over 37 million Americans who are uninsured (Conway, 1994). Force #1, cost of care, is an economic issue that has run unchecked for too many years. Force #2, the uninsured population, is a national disgrace that must be addressed. However, in spite of these and other forces demanding change and the determination of many individuals and groups to redesign a failing health-care system, there is no assurance that a new system will be the ultimate outcome of the reform movement. National and state laws will be needed over time to create a different health-care delivery environment, but laws alone cannot effect the major system change that is needed.

CONSUMER INVOLVEMENT

Consumers themselves must take part in the redesign of health care. Community involvement in improving the health-care system is not a new idea. Dr. Stanley Wohl (1984) described the public's role in creating a future system in his book, *The Medical Industrial Complex.* He encouraged the American public to become more knowledgeable concerning the health-care system and spoke of the need for a massive shift of resources from the curative side to prevention. He also described the behaviors needed for this country to make the paradigm shift. For example, he stated, "If Americans would eat, drink, and smoke less while exercising more, billions of dollars could be saved. . . . In short, we must work toward the goal of converting every American from a wasteful spender to a prudent buyer" (Wohl, 1984, p. 192). Over a decade later, it is still appropriate to recommend that all these issues be addressed by providers of services in partnership with community members to assure the success of health-care systems change.

SOCIAL SYSTEM CHANGE

Health-care reform as a social system change is a mammoth undertaking, as well as a long-term process. Social systems are the result of society's need to provide structure and rationale for addressing the public's most important issues. Education, health care, and human rights are examples of issues around which complex American social structures have been developed. Because social systems are created over time and affect all of society, they become integral to daily life and reflect the community's values and beliefs. It is both the integration of health care (19% GNP) and the deeply held values about the health-care system that mitigate against substantive change in this social structure without considerable time and effort.

Change in the American health-care system related to integration means that jobs in the old system will be lost (e.g., fewer medical subspecialities needed) and jobs for the new system will be created (e.g., larger numbers of primary care providers needed). Change in the system related to deeply held values means educating to place a higher value on health promotion and disease prevention than on technological interventions after disease and accidents occur.

The complexity of health-systems change can be better understood by comparing it with the civil rights movement in America. In 1954, the U.S. Supreme Court ruled on *Brown vs. The Board of Education* that "racial discrimination in public education is unconstitutional" (Wexler, 1993, p. 276). Three years later a commission on civil rights was established by Congress in the *Civil Rights Act of 1957* (Wexler, 1993, p. 280). The *Civil Rights Act of 1964* addressed voting rights, discrimination in places of public accommodation, and nondiscrimination in federally assisted programs (Wexler, 1993, p. 289). These actions by courts and legislators over a 10-year period signaled a change in the way the country would do its business, initially the business of education. Neither the Supreme Court ruling nor the 1950s and 1960s legislation resulted in immediate change in every city in America. However, these acts did signal the *beginning* of a process of major social system change. After civil rights bills were passed, the work to change the system began. Over time, new laws were enacted to assure all people of their rights in the electoral process, education, jobs, and business. Time was needed to assure that the educational system itself was a different entity than it was before. Time was also needed to educate the public to a new set of values related to human rights. Civil rights as a system change continues to unfold as the "system of rights" is redesigned over time.

Health-care reform, like the civil rights movement, is a major social-systems change. The idea for system change usually originates from unmet needs in the environment. Often just the discussion of change will have an immediate impact on an existing system such as those seen implemented in 1993 and 1994 by some hospitals, providers, and insurance agencies. Many hospitals have streamlined their organizations, reduced lengths of stay for clients, and eliminated costly or duplicative services. Health-care providers have joined HMOs, PPOs (Preferred Provider Organizations), and IPAs (Independent Practice Associations), and they have entered new group arrangements to reduce costs and increase effectiveness and efficiency. Insurance companies have designed an increasing array of products of health-care coverage and payment systems that include managed care, catastrophic or short-term insurance, deductibles, and copayments. These changes, however, are peripheral to the system, not system change itself because they tend to support continuance of the old paradigm.

Redesigning the massive system that includes all services and supplies that constitute the delivery of American health care will take years to accomplish. Health care provides jobs, creates new goods and services, and sells drugs and medical equipment. Health care also consumes one-seventh of the nation's resources. Because the system of health care permeates all of society and is so completely integrated throughout the country, new laws, new rules, and new behaviors of health-care professionals and consumers will be needed to assure a redesigned system. A new environment to deliver health care must be developed. The new paradigms need to be described, applied, and tested. Most importantly, health-care providers and members of the community need to understand and become involved partners in the long-term work of social-systems change. The health-care reform process has just begun. It will not end with a single health-care bill. Those who are willing to stay involved will, in the long term, be the final determiners of what the new system includes.

NEW ENVIRONMENT

The new paradigm of health is the building block for a new practice environment. When "health" is a focus of a delivery system, a shift is apparent in the location of services offered and in the types of services available. Healthy people reside in the community, in schools, in workplaces, and in places of worship. Therefore, health-promotion and health-maintenance services need to be available where people work, play, and pray. When health is the focus of delivery, illness, accidents, and injury become failures of the system and stimulate goals of care that are directed toward reattainment of health and well-being or movement toward the highest level of wellness. Because health is heavily dependent on individual behavior, services to maintain health or achieve a higher level of wellness can only be as effective as the partnership between provider and client. The environment for this partnership is significantly different from a delivery system in which the "expert" tells the "recipient" of care what to do.

The new environment for practice will have redesigned methods of determining costs and receiving payment for services and goods. A primary care, wellness focus precludes reimbursement through the current payment systems. As the service sector shifts to health-promotion strategies, surveillance, health maintenance and other care activities, a new criteria for payment will need to be developed. The present emphasis on fee for service will be replaced by population-based capitation, contracts for group services, and other innovative financial arrangements. All this suggests major changes in health-care policy in the way resources are allocated. For example, shifting the paradigm from illness to wellness and supporting that shift through financial incentives could provide payment for nursing case management of high-risk populations, nurse-directed teaching and counseling services, and monitoring interventions. It is important to note that simply covering the cost of some health strategies added to the old system will not be sufficient to assure the paradigm shift and will, instead, perpetuate old practice patterns.

The PEW Health Professions Commission (1993) analyzed trends shaping the future of health care. From this work, the Commission predicted a future health-care landscape fundamentally different from what exists now. The evolving system is expected to take on a new set of characteristics driven by empirical realities such as disease, demography, and costs.

The Commission's ten characteristics of an emerging health-care system are found in Box 1-1. This new environment, as envisioned by the PEW Health Professions Commission and described as community based, is more than a geographic shift of service providers. It includes interdisciplinary teams of health-care providers who practice in holistic organizations that emphasize wellness, wholeness, and prevention strategies. The new environment of primary health-care is described as continuous and comprehensive and includes identification of problems, management, and referral. It incorporates all the services necessary to prevent disease and maintain and promote health including rehabilitation (Anderson, 1988, p. 377).

BOX 1-1
CHARACTERISTICS OF THE EMERGING HEALTH-CARE SYSTEM

- Orientation toward health—greater emphasis on prevention and wellness, and greater expectation for individual responsibility for healthy behaviors.
- Population perspective—new attention to risk factors affecting substantial segments of the community, including issues of access and the physical and social environment.
- Intensive use of information—reliance on information systems to provide complete, easily assimilated patient information, as well as ready access to relevant information on current practice.
- Focus on the consumer—expectation and encouragement of patient partnerships in decisions related to treatment, facilitated by the availability of complete information on outcomes and evaluated in part by patient satisfaction.
- Knowledge of treatment outcomes—emphasis on the determination of the most effective treatment under different conditions and the dissemination of this information to those involved in treatment decisions.

- Constrained resources—a pervasive concern over increasing costs, coupled with expanded use of mechanisms to control or limit available expenditures.
- Coordination of services—increased integration of providers with a concomitant emphasis on teams to improve efficiency and effectiveness across all settings.
- Reconsideration of human values—careful assessment of the balance between the expanding capability of technology and the need for humane treatment.
- Expectations of accountability—growing scrutiny by a larger variety of payers, consumers, and regulators, coupled with more formally defined performance expectations.
- Growing interdependence—further integration of domestic issues of health, education, and public safety, combined with a growing awareness of the importance of U.S. health care in a global context.

From PEW Health Professions Commission: Health Professions Education for the Future: Schools in Service to the Nation, San Francisco, 1993.

Descriptors of the new environment of community primary health care reflect a set of beliefs held by others far beyond the U.S. health-care system. They are consistent with the World Health Organization's definition of *primary care:* "Essential health care made universally accessible to individuals and families in the community by means acceptable to them, through their full participation and at a cost that community and country can afford" (Anderson, 1988, p. 378).

The new environment for health-care delivery will support community-based primary health services (as opposed to illness services) and will, in the long run, reduce the nation's expenditure on costly, invasive procedures for preventable illnesses. Responsiveness to the health-care needs of consumers and the development of interdisciplinary and collaborative partnerships with both the recipients and providers of health care will assist in responding to the two forces driving health-care reform thus reducing cost and assuring access.

NEW ROLES FOR NURSES

Both organized nursing and individual nurses are positioned to support the reform process. Increasing numbers of nurses are actively involved in the development of public policy at local, state, and national levels. Through political activism, and by participation on committees and boards, these nurses have the opportunity to influence legislation that will shape the new system of health care. In addition, a growing number of nurses have been elected to public office where another dimension of influence is possible through drafting and voting on bills created for the new system. In 1994, the American Nurses Association reported 63 nurses serving in state legislatures and one nurse from Texas serving in the U.S. House of Representatives (American Nurses Association, PAC, 1993). These numbers may not seem impressive for a group that counts two million among its members. This record number of legislator nurses, however, signals a new commitment on the part of American

---

BOX 1-2

ELEMENTS FOR SUCCESSFUL ALLIANCES IN COMMUNITY-BASED HEALTH-CARE PROGRAMS

1. *Respect for Individual and Community Values*
   The goals and objectives of effective partnerships are to enhance and maintain quality of life while preserving the individual's worthiness within the community. Consequently, respect for a community's history and involvement of its members ensures the success, in most situations, of community-based primary health-care programs.

2. *Emphasis on Issues That Are Important to the Community*
   The strength of community coalitions is in targeting those issues and concerns that are of primary importance while simultaneously promoting cooperative goals and collaboration.

3. *Continuous Leadership Development*
   Ongoing, practical education and training in strategic planning and management are essential to ensure achievement of community programs and long-range goals.

4. *Community Celebration*
   Engaging in community social events and celebrating accomplishments help build trust among community members and aid in instilling a spirit of cooperation and group participation (Farley, 1994).

---

nurses to become actively involved in the political process.

Nursing's Agenda for Health Care Reform (American Nurses Association, 1992), developed by organized nursing, has been a key document for nurses to articulate the essential components of a new system as envisioned by the profession. The agenda supports:

- New design strategies for reimbursement of *non-physician providers* of health care such as nurses;
- Assesses and evaluates intervention and treatments through *medical effectiveness testing* and research;
- Promotes access to needed services and availability of resources by endorsing innovative *managed care options* such as community nursing centers; and
- Mandates a mechanism that promotes an informed and educated public by disseminating outcome and quality related data through general *disclosure of vital health information* (NLN & ANA, 1991).

Overall, the agenda describes a health-care system that is dramatically different, focuses on primary care, and is economically feasible. It calls for a new approach to delivery by taking health care to the consumer in community-based settings. Although hospitals and other institutions will still be significant components of the health-care system, they will no longer be either the central focus or dominant influence. The thrust will be on community health care, with the consumer taking on a more pivotal role. In fact, consumers of health-care services are described in Nursing's Agenda as informed participants in decisions affecting their care.

A new environment providing different services to informed consumers will require increased numbers of advanced practice nurses. In community primary-care settings, advanced practice nurses provide and coordinate care, case manage, advise and council clients on health behaviors, triage and monitor, advocate for families, help clients to choose health services wisely, and evaluate outcomes of care and services. Nurses' education, practice, and research must prepare them for these new roles along with additional skills of administration, management, and expertise in primary care delivery. To build effective community coalition and partnership arrangements, professional nurses will also need to develop expertise associated with trust, collaboration, and mutual goal setting. Farley (1994) outlined four essential elements needed for establishing successful alliances when developing community-based health-care programs (Box 1-2).

The new roles for nurses will call for adjustments in relationships with other health-care providers and may change the scope of professional practice. Words that describe professionals in a new practice arena include: responsive to clients' needs, accountable, interdependent, collaborative, and outcome focused.

The nursing profession's increased emphasis on the community as client will reconfirm its professional commitment to society. In addition to caring for individual clients, nurses will be involved in the improvement of whole communities. This involvement will entail the coordination of care across providers, practice environments, and the health-illness continuum. The inevitable change in practice will require new skills for providers and the involvement of people themselves in their own health care: better diet, proper exercise, and an understanding of the role they play in their own health status. There are compelling reasons to expect that nurses can and will play a leading role in the creation of a new health-care delivery system. Nurses have the support of the community to take the lead in contracting with community alliances and creating comprehensive health-care networks. An American Nurses Association survey (American Nurses Association, 1993) demonstrated that the vast majority of Americans (86%) are willing to receive everyday health-care services from an advanced practice registered nurse. Many policymakers admit that nurses can do a great deal, if not most, of the direct delivery of preventive services (Griffith, 1993).

To firmly establish the nurse's position in the new environment, however, leadership is needed in the development of public policy and the direct delivery of community health services. Nursing leadership intervention revolves around four determinants of community health practice (Salmon, 1994; White, 1982):

1. *Social factors*—targeting social forces and those effects on the community, such as the growing emphasis on health promotion and illness prevention, changing demographic trends (i.e., increase in an aging and homeless population), and the emergence of a global economy;

2. *Medical/technological/organizational factors*—recognizing the need for accessibility to care and availability of resources to deliver cost-effective, quality health-care services;

3. *Environmental factors*—addressing and educating the community about environmental issues. Leadership also includes maintaining active involvement and collaboration in implementing effective public policies and regulations; and

4. *Human and biological factors*—developing strategies and meeting the challenges faced by chronic and disabling illnesses, the resurgence in infectious diseases, the future of genetic engineering, and facilitating others in maintaining and recognizing the importance of good health practices and improved well-being.

As emphasized by Salmon (1994), understanding and implementing these elements are critical to nursing in framing a proactive stance and ensuring planned, effective interventions. For example, nursing has demonstrated leadership in effecting public policy in the new health-care environment in which there are now a myriad of roles nurses have and are playing in appointed, elected, and staff positions in the executive and legislative branches of government. For example, in 1994 a nurse was Director of the National Institute of Nursing Research at NIH; a nurse was National AIDS Policy Coordinator for the White House; a nurse was Commissioner of the Social Security Administration; a nurse was Administrator of Region IV for the Department of Health and Human Services; a nurse is the chief of staff and top health aide for the senate minority and GOP leader, and the President of the American Nurses Association has made frequent invitational visits to Congress and the White House to advise on health-care reform.

CHALLENGES

Health system restructuring of the size and dimension now being considered in America offers both opportunities and challenges to change agents. Creating a new environment in which costs are a primary consideration can result in adverse consequences to the quality of care. For this reason, nurses involved in creating a new system must focus their attention on *both* cost and quality as major design criteria.

A number of untoward effects of change are already surfacing. For example, some hospitals have changed the nursing skill mix, lowering costs by replacing RNs with lower paid ancillary staff. Yet, well-documented research indicates that a higher proportion of RNs in the skill mix is directly linked to fewer client deaths, decreased complications, shorter lengths of stay, and increased consumer satisfaction (American Nurses Association, 1994). In fact, a recent study demonstrating reduced Medicare mortality rates indicated that organizational factors associated with enhanced professional nursing practice, autonomy, and competence can improve client outcomes (Morrissey, 1994).

Another example of potential negative effects of change was reported in the *Washington Post* (May 8, 1994). Local hospitals in Washington, D.C., had invested in capital improvements, new technology, and advertising to compete in a changing marketplace, yet simultaneously reduced staff. There was no mention of how this trend would affect the quality of client care.

The challenge of long-term reform is to address not only methods of financing the system, but also, concomitantly, ways to improve how care is delivered. Subsequently, one of the greatest opportunities exists in making changes in systems associated with the delivery of client care. The focus is on integrated approaches that allow movement and provision of care across acute, long-term, and community settings. The goals of these new systems are improved clinical quality, lowered costs, efficient operations, and valued outcomes of care.

To meet the challenges of a reformed health-care environment, nurses must take an active role in redesigning care delivery and managing client-care services. This can be accomplished through leadership interventions in the following: restructuring the client's care environment by differentiating the skills of the caregivers and reorganizing the resources around a continuous, comprehensive, and integrated plan that maximizes efficiency and coordination of services; confronting and meeting the economic opportunities presented by managed care by identifying, measuring, and marketing nursing's contribution to cost-effective client care through timely, appropriate interventions; and actively engage in implementing mechanisms to track and evaluate outcomes of client care that have implications to both the financial integrity and the quality of health care delivered at the institution (Buerhaus, 1994 a,b; Curran, 1994; Davis, 1994; Joel, 1994). American Nurses Association President G. Betts summed up the work ahead: "Cost containment effort without consideration for quality and safety are a poor investment for the nation" (American Nurses Association, 1994).

CONCLUSION

As the change process continues to unfold, health-care providers will be challenged to adapt to new practice realities. Just what these different approaches will entail and the resources needed will depend upon the service and practice environment. Nursing practice is positioning itself as an evolving process responding to client needs, clinical research, and clinical experience. Innovative nursing leaders, many of whom are featured in subsequent chapters, are taking advantage of the change process and designing new systems of care and a new environment. Their work and the work of other nurses committed to long-term involvement as major players in health-system reform will create a new, cost-effective, accessible, and high-quality health-care system for all Americans—perhaps a system for the world to emulate.

REFERENCES

American Nurses Association. (1992). *Nursing's agenda for health care reform.* Washington, DC: Author.

American Nurses Association. (1993, December 9). News Release. Washington, DC: Author.

American Nurses Association. (1994, May 16). News Release. Washington, DC: Author.

American Nurses Association PAC. (1993). *Nurses elected to state and federal legislatures.* Unpublished survey of State Nurses Associations. Washington DC: Author.

Anderson, E. T., & McFarlane, J. M. (1988). *Community as client: application of the nursing process.* Philadelphia: JB Lippincott.

Barker, J. A. (1987). *Discovering the future: the business of paradigms.* St. Paul: ILI Press.

Buerhaus, P. I. (1994a). Managed competition and critical issues facing nurses. *Nursing & Health Care* 15 (1):22-26.

Buerhaus, P. I. (1994b). Economics of managed competition and consequences to nurses: part II. *Nursing Economics* 12 (2):75-80, 106.

Conway, A. E. (1994). Legislative matters. *Nursing Matters* 5 (4):5.

Curran, C. R. (1994). Work redesign: the key to true health care reform. In McCloskey, J. & Grace, H. K. (Eds.). *Current issues in nursing.* St Louis: Mosby.

Davis, C. K. (1994). Financing of health care and its impact on nursing. In McCloskey, J. & Grace, H. K. (Eds.). *Current issues in nursing.* St Louis: Mosby.

Farley, S. (1994). Developing community partnerships: Shifting power from health professionals to citizens. In McCloskey, J. & Grace, H. K. (Eds.). *Current issues in nursing.* St Louis: Mosby.

Griffith, H. M. (1993). Needed, a strong nursing position on preventive service. *IMAGE: Journal of Nursing Scholarship* 24 (4):272.

H.R. 3600. (1993). Health Security Act, 103rd Congress, Washington, DC: House of Representatives Document Room.

Joel, L. A. (1994). Changes in the hospital as a place of practice. In McCloskey, J. & Grace, H. K. (Eds.). *Current issues in nursing,* St Louis: Mosby.

Morrissey, J. (1994). Reorganizing nurses may reduce hospitals' mortality rates-study. *Modern Healthcare* 24 (43):66.

PEW Health Professions Commission. (1993). San Francisco: PEW Memorial Trust.

Salmon, M. E. (1994). Leadership for change in public and community health nursing. In McCloskey, J. & Grace, H. K. (Eds.). *Current issues in nursing,* St Louis: Mosby.

Wexler, S. (1993). The Civil Rights Movement. New York: Facts on File, Inc.

White, M. S. (1982). Construct for public nursing. *Nursing Outlook* 30 (9):527-530.

Wohl, S. (1984). *The Medical Industrial Complex.* New York: Harmony Books.

Chapter 2

Nurses as Advanced Practitioners and Primary Care Providers

Tim Porter-O'Grady, EdD, PhD, RN, CNAA, FAAN

OVERVIEW

A new type of advanced practice nurse is needed to coordinate care for people as they move through the health-care continuum.

The new framework for health care requires radically new approaches to health-care services. There are three factors influencing the future of health care: subscriber-based models, capitation of the costs of health care, and a stronger focus on the continuum of care. It is this context within which the future of the practice of nursing will unfold. Understanding the relationship among these factors and the role of the nurse along the continuum forms the foundation for the emerging practice of nursing. Integration, coordination, and facilitation of the health-care team in a new set of partnered relationships will require insight, energy, and commitment to make the new framework successful in meeting the health needs of the community.

We are watching the end of health care as we know it. In context, we are also seeing the end of nursing as we know it. Stimulated by the desire for true health reform, but driven by a broad-based transformational process at work on our globe, the process of major change is well under way. In fact, what comes out of the public sector and the political processes related to health reform has a much smaller impact on the delivery of services than that which is already under way at the center of health-care delivery and is transforming the very way in which we provide service (Anderson, 1993).

The financial constraints and evidence of unobtained outcomes in American health care have forced the system to look at itself anew and to raise some challenging questions. Can we afford what we spend on health care? What do we get for what we spend on health-care services? Are we efficient and effective in the way in which we provide health services? How can we assure that all Americans can pay for health care and that they get what they pay for (Bogdanich, 1991)? These and a host of related questions drive the current thrust toward retooling the system. The restructuring of the American workplace is also having a serious impact on health care. The move to worker empowerment, continuous quality initiatives, and integrative delivery systems are strategies that are influencing how the reformatted delivery system looks and operates (Clouten & Weber, 1994).

Leadership in nursing is struggling both to keep up with these myriad changes and to plan an organized and effective response to the changes that are affecting the profession. The response to the economic constraints through the layoffs of large numbers of nurses and the reconfiguring of the workplace is creating great concern in some leadership circles in nursing (Bryne, 1994). For the first time in many years, there seems to be a sustainable reduction in the number of nurses needed to provide client care services. Besides downsizing the hospitals because of a reduction in the number of occupied beds, there is the move to more outpatient and noninstitutionalized services not requiring hospitalization. As a result, the discipline is producing far more basically prepared nurses than it will ever use, and many of them, if not most, are today unable to find work in the places where work was always plentiful (Porter-O'Grady, 1994).

One of the critical changes in focus in health-care services is the move toward primary health services. This move is not driven by a sudden discovery of society's moral urge to see that Americans are healthy. It is, instead, a product of the economically driven move toward a managed care and capitated payment environment for the delivery of health-care services (Reinhardt, 1992). The overwhelming move into subscriber-based, competitive health systems has changed all the rules for health-care delivery. In a capitated, subscriber-driven system, control of the dollars becomes critical to the health of the system. Because price cannot be controlled, the only option is to manage cost well and to maximize the volume of healthy people in a way that reduces the resource demands on the health-service system (Buerhaus, 1994).

The problem with this approach, however, brings two considerations for nursing. The cost of nursing care is one of the highest expenses in the delivery of hospital services. Secondly, the majority of nurses are employed in the very sector of health care where the greatest impact of reconfiguring service will be felt. The temptation for organized nursing will be to lament the dramatic change that this will create and the subsequent losses this will imply for nurses. Indeed, the whole process of "downsizing" hospitals creates a substantive shift away from the kind and character of services historically offered there. As the client population shifts from the hospital setting, to maintain the same number and kind of resources there is simply financially untenable.

The problem of maintaining resources is compounded by the fact that little evidence suggests that the outcome of professional nursing care is somehow significantly different from that provided by other kinds of caregivers (Lathrop, 1991). When this suggestion is made, there is great hue and cry from the professional nursing sectors that such assumptions are dangerous and untrue. Unfortunately, there is more evidence to suggest that other less-expensive and less-educated caregivers are as manually dexterous and functionally proficient in hospital services as are registered nurses and can do the same activities for significantly less cost (Neubauer, 1993). Some suggest that the outcomes could or would be different. If these outcomes had been measured with any degree of proficiency in the past few decades, perhaps that assumption could be validated. Because that measurement never occurred to any great degree, the assumption cannot be validated and, as a result, the argument is not very persuasive.

We should not suggest that there is not a major contribution that nurses make in the delivery of hospital services. Most of that contribution is not in providing functional service but more in planning, evaluating, and adjusting care services as the need for them shifts (Dienemann & Gessner, 1992). Although nurses provide an excellent service in this regard, clearly, the hospital does not need them in the same numbers it once did in the cost-based payment system. Therefore, as institutional care services decline in the hospital, the need for registered nurses will continue to decline as well in that setting.

In many ways, the dramatic change in health-care institutions, driven by economic constraint, is really a blessing for the nursing profession. Nurses have historically been underused in hospitals. They have been prepared at every level far beyond their level of use within the hospital. The very medical model of service structures in hospitals only allowed nurses to function at a fraction of their capacity because anything beyond functional proficiency was considered the turf of the physician. Extreme medical direction and subordinacy have been the *modus operandi* for generations in hospitals throughout the country. Historically, any effort at intelligent, independent behavior on the part of nurses was immediately suspect and in time had to be diminished if the integrity and viability of the organization was to be maintained (Ashley, 1976).

In most ways, nurses should be happy that the hospital centric age is passing. Although most nurses have adapted to past diminished expectations and have become proficient at their rituals and routines, it is less safe or successful to remain complacent and accepting of this passing reality. Health-care service is changing in ways that will demand a different set of roles and characteristics for the nurse. Indeed, the opportunity to make significant change in the role of the nurse has never been stronger in the history of American nursing. The challenge to accept new roles and accountabilities in the emerging system now calls for all the skill and political wisdom of nurses as the system is reconfigured to provide different services in an entirely different context (Guild, Ledwin, Sanford, & Winter, 1994).

THE EMERGENCE OF THE CONTINUUM OF CARE

In a subscriber-based system, the goal is different from a cost-based, illness event-paid health system. The old, medical model system paid for intervention event by event. The procedure, task, test, and action is what generated payment for many years in the health-care system. Because most functions were both ordered and provided by physicians, the doctors were paid directly for those services. Indeed, no service is paid for unless it is ordered by a physician in the vast majority of circumstances. The more a physician ordered or did, the more he or she got paid for it. Even in times of great cost control, this framework for structuring service provision and payment did not measurably shift (Eckhart, 1993).

Emerging structures are challenging this whole approach. It is clear that addressing illness and the related interventions as the core of health service is the single most expensive circumstance in the delivery system. The system simply waits until someone is sick enough to access it and then does whatever is necessary to address the condition as it is presented. There is no effort to deal with the illness in any other context or earlier in its course. Instead, the system simply waits for the condition to become so notable that it eventually requires response because the ability of the person to function has been severely compromised. Embedded in this approach is the highest level of service cost possible in providing health care.

The goal of a capitated, subscriber-based system is 180° different from that of the prevailing approach. Because price is generally fixed, it cannot be adjusted. The goal of the capitated delivery system is to meet the needs of subscribers at the lowest possible cost to the provider. Indeed, the primary financial guideline, is *not to spend money unnecessarily for its subscribers*, because the only way the system can save dollars is not to spend them. The means to the goal are, therefore, to prevent, reduce, or eliminate the need for expensive care services.

In subscriber-based systems, the focus on not spending money or avoiding the use of resources calls the organization to focus on different priorities. The challenge for the health-care system now is not to provide services that are not needed and clearly not to generate activities that will cost the organization whatever margin it can glean from the difference between what is paid and what it costs the system to offer service and care for its subscribers. Indeed, the focus on preventing use of the system at a level of high intensity becomes a major goal of organized health systems.

This challenge confronts the current configuration of health providers and other resources. In the United States, the health system is physician dominated and controlled. Because of the medical model focus on health services, physician action or approval is central to the activity of every provider (Johnson, 1992). Furthermore, the emphasis on intervention facilitates physician activities and has created the focus on heavy specialization in medical practice. The problem that has resulted is the proliferation of specialty physicians so that they now account for about 80% of medical practitioners. At a time when primary services are becoming the foundation for the future of health services, too many physicians have inadequate background for the work of primary care (Goldsmith, 1993).

Furthermore, it may even be appropriate to suggest that much of the work that emerges in a primary point of care approach is best not done by physicians. Indeed, the physician may not be the best prepared provider to render specified services along the continuum of care. The medical component of such services may be a small part of the work necessary to take care of the needs of an essentially healthy consumer. Not only would medical resources not be best directed to such activities, but also the activities themselves may actually lie outside of the competence of physicians. To ensure that the subscriber gets the best fit between services needed and the most beneficial practitioner, it may be necessary to look elsewhere to find that person. Increasingly, that person's focus must be on the continuum of care—the linkages between the providers now being more critical than would be the unilateral skills of any one provider. There is no paramount provider, no individual whose skill base circumscribes all others. There is only a team of providers with a variety of skills all somehow directed to meeting the needs of those they serve. In a continuum of care approach, there is no one person who can meet all the needs of the subscriber, nor can that person assume responsibility for the consumer to determine for him or her what services will or will not be accessed (Newman, Lamb & Michaels, 1991).

The emerging critical role in this new health system belongs to the person who integrates the roles, follows the client, and helps the consumer access the specific resource needed at the time and in the manner in which it is beneficial to the user. This primary role belongs to the person who not only provides specific clinical services, but also accesses on the client's behalf those other resources they might not otherwise know about or use. The move to primary-care systems bodes many changes in the way in which health-care services are provided. These changes are:

- Physicians are a part of a much larger partnership than previously accommodated. This partnership includes all the members of the health-service team and will strongly demand a more collegial relationship between them.

- The primary service arena will not be institutional but will instead be community based. The overwhelming movement to outpatient services is only the first stage in a journey away from hospital-based health-care services.
- Control of the variables affecting health service will shift out of the provider's hands. No matter how much there is a desire to return care to the doctor, the real control of what happens will be in the consumer's hands in a subscriber-based approach. The client will have to respond to health initiatives and practices or the cost of illness-care services will simply continue to incline.
- Services must be integrated along the continuum. This means that the continuum includes all providers at some level of seamless service. The relationship between providers becomes critical to the quality of the service they provide.
- The "protection" to the employee that comes from being a part of such institutions as hospitals is fast disappearing when one considers that most of the work of health will occur outside hospital walls. There is a greater requisite for decision making and independence not previously experienced in institutional models. The policy and procedural approach to work simply will not succeed in this new context, thus raising the risk of service accountability for each practitioner.
- Functioning along the continuum means that someone must coordinate, integrate, and facilitate the players along the continuum. The client will interact with a range of players in the effort to maintain health; coordinating that arrangement will assume much of the role of one of the players. It is not unlikely that the player will be the nurse because it is an extension of the role component with which she or he is already familiar.
- There will be much negotiation of the roles and functions of the providers as the system becomes more focused on health than on care. Providing for health is a much different equation in the service arena than caring for the sick. This is a new experience for health-care providers and will demand a new set of skills and an altered approach to the delivery of services. There must be an openness to the relationships that emerge as the roles and functions are enumerated in the new service configurations.

BUILDING THE CONTINUUM OF CARE

Constructing a new framework for the delivery of health services in a primary-care environment will be considerably different from that unfolded for sickness care. First, there should be no assumption that the need for illness care will decline. The issue is not whether there will continue to be a need for complex illness-care services. Rather, it is a matter of how much of the aggregate of services provided will be devoted to such services. As health care continues to move out of the illness model, illness service will actually increase in intensity, because clients who are treated in hospitals will require a higher level of intensity of service. Fewer clients, more care. The cost of this more acute care will also be quite high because the kind of service that could not be provided in any other setting will demand more resource use.

Nurses will continue to be used in great numbers in hospitals and other acute care settings. The likelihood however, is that it will require about 50% of all practitioners to staff these settings. That requirement is a far cry from the 68% of all nurses now practicing in such settings. The processes associated with downsizing organizations for the real number of occupied beds currently attests to the initial stages of reconfiguring that component of health care (Moffit, 1993).

The vast majority of new roles in health care will emerge in settings outside of the hospital. Preparation of new roles is already under way with a number of experimental models being explored in a range of settings across the country. Unfortunately, these new functional roles will demand fewer registered nurses than were used in the institutional settings. This shift creates some real challenges for the nursing profession (Box 2-1).

The challenge for nurses is to confront the ambiguous and those things over which they have limited control. The effort to control the events of life are universal. The problem with noninstitutional practice is that much of the control over the events of life that affect what nurses do is in the hands of those whom nurses serve. The ability to control those variables is limited. Furthermore, practice must be an accommodation to the situations and practices of the consumer *within the context of the consumer's values and culture,* and thus these can never be fully subjected to the knowledge of the provider as was more often the case in hospital, medical, and institutional practice approaches. This shift will create a huge demand for retraining and reformatting the skill and knowledge base of a whole range of nurses.

Nursing case management has begun to do this for a limited number of nurses whose primary role is to manage the adaptation between health system and consumer. The impact at this stage, however, is still limited because only about 15% of all clients receive continuous case management services. The model, however, is very adaptive to the emerging system of health services. Indeed, case management has imbedded within its processes the very elements of the

---

BOX 2-1
CHALLENGES FOR THE NURSING PROFESSION

- We are preparing large numbers of associate degree graduates who will never find jobs in the current and future health-care marketplace based on their current preparation and skills.
- Nurses currently in diminishing or expendable roles are unable to find work in other settings because the demand for their skill base is simply no longer present, leading to larger unemployment for registered nurses than has been experienced in the recent past.
- There is increasing demand for community-based nurses with the attendant clinical skills. That demand, however, requires a different focus on the preparation of nurses suitable to assume these roles. Currently, there is a deficit in appropriately prepared nurses for these new clinical roles.
- The move to primary-care health models increases the demand for advanced practice nurses in the primary-care arenas of family, children, women, gerontology, and adult health services. Demand will grow at a rate beyond the ability of either medicine or nursing to respond adequately.
- Nurses will be central to the success of any continuum of care approach if only because of the sheer numbers of nurses at the point-of-service. Almost

60% of all point-of-service providers in the health-care system are nurses. It is simply untenable for nurses not to be the major providers of services in the emerging subscriber-based and capitated health system.
- There is a perception of nurses by other health professionals that is constraining and disconcerting. Either there is a notion that nurses are further up the hierarchy than the others or that nurses are obstructive and problematic in their relationship with other providers. There seems to be major uncertainty and distrust in the relationships between nurses and in nurses' relationships with others.
- Although nurses are relatively creative in their responses to client situations and events, they have a reputation of being less responsive to process and content changes in nursing practice. Most change is viewed within the context of loss rather than with a view to enhancement of practice. Often it seems that nurses would keep activities and situations that are dysfunctional but well known rather than take on challenge and opportunity that would improve practice or relationships simply because it involves uncertainty (Porter-O'Grady, 1990).

---

majority of health services that are provided in a continuum of care approach. Those nurses whose primary practice is nursing in the community or hospice services or in Planetree model approaches are already operating within the context of the emerging paradigm for health services. It is as Russell Coile has suggested: there will be a need for more health services and less care services (Coile, 1989).

Advanced Practice and Primary Care

Regardless of how we have prepared nurses in advanced practice, the majority have been used to support the medical model of care services. This has nothing to do with the desirability of this scenario or nurses' own desire to practice in a much different way than they ultimately do. The health system as currently configured really does not let any provider do much differently because almost everything is a subset of medical approaches to health service. State legal requirements bow to the ascendancy of the physician's role; referral patterns lead ultimately to physician approval for them or to medical intervention. Payment

for services is always medically controlled. Just to survive, the prevailing system nurses have had to accommodate the prevailing medical oligarchy (Diers, 1993).

In a subscriber-based approach, as currently driven by both reform and managed care processes, these mechanisms begin to break down. Point-of-service structures simply do not allow individuated control over the activities requiring judgment and action along the continuum of care. Present exclusionary models do not get supported well because the goal for service is not based on who gets paid but what service is provided; it is the service that does or does not get paid for. In this set of circumstances in a subscriber-based approach, it is in *not* spending money that the value stream depends on (Womack & Jones, 1994). Facilitating this is the clear understanding that medical intervention is resource intense. The intent of an effective system is to ensure that resource use does not occur in whatever situations they are not needed. How do we gatekeep, yet assure that the client receives what he or she needs along a continuum that addresses each client's own health requirements?

In this kind of system there is a refocus on the processes related to health giving and keeping activities that would prevent or delay the need for high-intensity medical intervention. It is in this arena that the focus of primary care takes form. There is much conflict over current definitions of primary care. However, there will be less uncertainty about what it is when it no longer is subjugated to the medical context within which the definition becomes practice. It is precisely for this reason that the primary role of the nurse will become increasingly critical.

Coordinating the continuum of care will require a different focus on the client and service provision than that present in the practices of almost all health providers other than nurses. In concept, the role of the nurse is not based on any particular intervention or activity; rather, *it is the relationship between all clinical events and activities and their impact on the client's journey through the health continuum that defines the role of the nurse.* The nurse's function relates to the client's journey not the clinical events. It is precisely this role that will be of central value in the unfolding of a subscriber-based and capitated continuum-of-care framework for health services (Madden & Prescott, 1994).

This reality will require considerable changes in focus, preparation, and use of nursing resources in the unfolding health system.

- Preparation of the professional nurse and for advanced practice will require a health focus that is culturally sensitive, continuum-based, and emphasizes life management rather than diagnosis and intervention.
- The role of the clinical specialist and the nurse practitioner will have to merge to provide a nurse whose skill base includes the performance expectations of both areas in relationship to clients and other providers along the service continuum. There simply is no rationale for segmenting the role of the advanced practice nurse in an integrated continuum-of-care system. Increasingly, the skill sets found in each role are necessary for the health-based approach to managing the continuum of care.
- The role of the professional nurse cannot be defined by simply enumerating function and activity. State boards of nursing that are struggling to establish the parameters of practice by elucidating levels of function (surreptitiously called "domains of practice") are missing the point in an effort to make it easy on themselves in distinguishing between what is allowable and that which is not. Understanding a continuum of process indicates that the fundamental obligation of the nurse is to see that the client moves through service events safely and appropriately regardless of who does what along the way. The nurse's focus is on the

journey and its outcome, not on any single or series of events along the way.

- Advanced practice means just that. It means deepening the client's understanding of his or her health needs and obtaining whatever services for the client are necessary, until the client can do that independently. It means, at times, that the nurse directly provides a variety of services within the nurse's competence. At other times, it means identifying others who will provide service within their areas of expertise. Advanced practice indicates that the understanding of the relationships between provider and client is broader and deeper and that whatever occurs in the continuum of health care will best meet the health needs of clients.
- In a predominantly primary care model, *all nursing roles* will be radically altered from an institutional complex of structured care services to a predominantly community-health-prescribed set of services. These services will be influenced and moderated by culture, location, understanding, and availability. It is the nurse who will adjust, accommodate, modify in the interests of the client rather than the reverse as has been the case in hospital-based practice that has employed 68% of the nursing resource. A large learning curve on the part of nurses is required to respond to this paradigm shift.
- Configuring nurses in single-discipline service structures is now coming quickly to an end. Nursing service structures are no longer a viable format for organizing client care services. Integration of the disciplines (all of them, including physicians) is, for the foreseeable future, the method of choice for constructing clinical relationships. Nurses will find that they have more colleagues from other disciplines in their immediate work group than other nurses. This approach will require an ability to articulate the nurse role, to negotiate the clinical relationship, to enumerate the economic and outcome contribution to the team's effort provided by nursing, and to dialogue with the team at a level and with a proficiency that ensures confidence of all the members. There is some evidence that this may be a major problem for many nurses.

Higher Expectations

There are higher expectations in the emerging delivery system. Competence and confidence are requisites of leadership on the clinical team. The team approach to managing the continuum of care lies at the core of the effectiveness of subscriber-based approaches to the continuum of care. Ambiguity and uncertainty about the competence and contribution of the members of the clinical team is simply unacceptable. As clinical protocols and pathways become the framework for service delivery and outcome evaluation, it is becoming less possible to hide in the ambiguity of clinical process. If process is not specifically tied to outcome and the relationship is not viable, process must be moderated or adjusted until it achieves the expected outcome of both provider and consumer.

Evaluation of care in the future is designed to identify the value of services clearly and compare them with the same set of measures in competing health plans. Because the buyer (or consumer) will have the right to make choices regarding which plan he or she will be a part, the consumer may change affiliation if the measures do not offer a reason to continue to participate. The financial and, thus, service health of the plan depends on the health and faithfulness of the subscriber. It is incumbent upon each clinical role to assure that value is facilitated, the essential outcomes are achieved, and high levels of satisfaction are maintained if the organization is to remain viable. Every member of the team will contribute to that end or will, quite simply, not be there.

As indicated previously, the focus of the future health plans necessarily will be health. Keeping the client on the continuum and away from the hospital is an essential obligation of health professionals. The advanced or primary care nurse will have that as her or his primary goal. There is high probability that that effort will consume a larger number of the resources of the system than were devoted to that activity in the past. Although there is great discussion about the physician's role in gatekeeping and primary care practice, there are neither sufficient medical resources nor adequate time to prepare them to assume that they can adequately play that role. It is increasingly evident that managing the continuum and guiding the client in the use of services along it will be the nurse who is already there and is more than adequately prepared to facilitate client choice and use of the system.

With every opportunity, there are challenges. There is a large number of nurses who cannot or will not make the shift to this much broader and significant role. Hospital compression driven by a reduction in bed use, reengineering, and managed care are driving nurses out of the hospital and will continue to do so for some time. However, it is not driving nurses away from the clients. Instead, it is calling nurses to move to where the clients are and design cost-effective, low-resource–intense services that keep the client well in the context of his or her own set of life circumstances. There will be an obligation to provide opportunity for more health, therefore requiring less care (Barger and Rosenfeld, 1993).

The advanced practice and primary care nurse will be required, in the new role, to assist the client in developing or enhancing life management skills.

Recent data suggest that many of the problems that clients present to primary care providers relate not so much to their illness but to the level of their personal life-management skills (Fagin, 1990). The ability to understand what personal health is, how to cope with limitations, how to adjust in the downside of family dynamics, what the triggers are that set off a descent into either behavioral or physical illness are all critical to good life management. Simple activities such as food selection and basic nutrition, good body mechanics, healthy personal relationships, and effective personal health-skills building all contribute to a much more sustainable notion of health and reduce the demand on the time and services of the primary care provider and, in reflection, to any other part of the health-care system.

Still, there are not unlimited resources to shift nurses into the primary-care arena where there is a preponderance of preventive care services. In subscriber-based approaches, no more money is provided simply because the patient required more resources. Shifting the same number of resources into primary services that have historically occupied acute care service positions will do nothing to facilitate essential cost control. There is a much lower demand for professional staff in the hospital system than at any time in the last two decades. Volume and economies of scale will require the more judicious use of highly educated nurse resources. The nursing discipline, however, will have to realize that opportunity does not wait for readiness. The demand for primary services will quickly outstrip the numbers prepared for the new roles. Getting ready for that time means encouraging advanced study now and altering advanced and undergraduate professional nurse curricula to get a foundation of competent nursing professionals as quickly as possible playing out roles that are already quickly emerging (Riley, 1994).

Furthermore, nurses will have to be assertive with regard to their presence, competence, and value in delivering primary-care services. The challenge for advanced practice nurses is they are often employed by the very people who mistrust their intent and hold their competence suspect. The circumstances of their employment contain the same elements that limit their use. Physician control of advanced nurse practice creates the circumstances that limit its value. Fulfilling the requirements of medical practice or physician performance expectation creates a milieu that results in performance that may not address real needs driving the symptoms or circumstances that bring the client to the physician in the first place. The continuum management role in a subscriber-based system is critical to both the value and the success of the role. Value is addressed in the effective location of the nurse to assess and decide the necessary level of service for the subscriber. Success is determined by how independent the nurse is in making decisions and how collateral and interdependent her or his relationship is with other key providers. Equity in this situation would demand a parallel consultant relationship with all other providers, including physicians (Mitty, 1991).

Advanced practice nurses will have to understand the business relationships in professional practice to assure that equity drives their location, value, and reward in the delivery system. Being contracted to health plans is different from being employed by them. Forming advanced nursing practice group arrangements for the purpose of plan contracting further changes the relationship and creates a stronger opportunity for equity and risk-sharing arrangements or other economic benefits. Furthermore, such arrangements give the practitioner increased opportunities for influencing protocol development and policy formation in a way that facilitates the value of nursing work in managing the continuum and contributing to cost effectiveness in the service structure (Bhide, 1994).

Enumerating the value contribution of individual practitioners will emerge as a central theme of accountability in the future. The value stream in health care will have to include the contribution to the health of the plan made by every kind of worker in the system. Every element of cost will be tied to outcomes. The success of the service will be directly related to how tight the relationship is between cost and outcome (Niven, 1993). Examination of the variables will include the assessment of the contribution of each member of the team and each process used to render patient services. When outcomes determine viability, the only real concern is how well they are achieved and at what level of cost effectiveness. Primary nurse providers must recognize that they have as "tight" a relationship to this reality as any player. Often it will be this recognition and the supporting data that will truly prove the value of primary and advanced practice nurses.

The continuum of care will also demand a set of relationships in the delivery of service that has not been previously expected. As health-care work redesign takes functional shape in an organization, it means breaking down as many walls to relationships as possible (Kanter, 1994). The clinical process is reevaluated, and the interactions between the players is redescribed to be more integrated and thus more functional.

The loss of compartmental and departmental structures that result from redesign forces the organization to reconstruct based on the centrality of its customers. Any configurations that do not support the work of the clinical providers, it is assumed, constrain their relationship. For the advanced practice nurse and other primary care nurses, this emerging structure implies the need to relate to, communicate with, and work effectively with a whole coterie of providers that had been insulated by departmental barriers. These people are now partners in the service arena and demand integration and inclusion in service processes, decision making, and evaluation of outcomes. The nurse must have a significant quality of interaction, communication, and leadership to integrate, coordinate, and facilitate the myriad functions and relationships in which a number of partners will participate along the continuum of care. Indeed, the major role of the nurse will be to ensure that the client has the services and relationships necessary to retain or regain the highest level of independent functioning. Any activity provided by all skilled practitioners contributes to that outcome. Therefore, the relationship between the nurse and other team players is critical to both process and outcome. Ultimately, this relationship has a dramatic impact on value.

A NEW REALITY FOR ADVANCED NURSE PRACTICE

The context for health-care services is driving the system into a new phase of creativity and innovation. Partnership principles are changing the hierarchy of relationships into a more equity-based set of associations that will be necessary to respond to new realities in health care. The nurse at every point along the continuum must be aware of the characteristics of the journey out of old models into newer frameworks for work and service provision in health care.

- Technology will continue to make health care less costly per unit of service and much more portable. Time spent on activities that keep the provider from client service will be reduced simply because the technology will provide the opportunity for it.
- Service simply cannot be focused around buildings and structures. Although there will be certain high-acuity services that will be fixed, most services will be mobile. It is essential that services be brought to the client, not clients brought to the service, as much as possible. The costs associated with the duplication, travel time, and provider costs well evidence the expense of fixed nonflexible services.
- The hospital is not the center of the service structure in the health plan. Instead, the hospital should be avoided as much as possible because it promulgates the highest resource use and the greatest cost along the continuum. The primary care provider has a major obligation to avoid having to use those services except when all options have been exhausted and the hospital services are required for the integrity of the client's care.

- For the first time in generations, it will be the obligation of the nurse to educate, to facilitate use of the client's resources, to reduce the need for task-based intervention, to assure that the client retains control over his or her life processes, and to truly create a partnership relationship with the client. This mutual relationship will not bear fruit consistently and certainly not overnight. The process, however, will result in a reduced demand on technology and intervention and a greater use of knowledge, life management skills, and noninstitutional processes to resolve health-related issues.

- The advanced practice nurse and other primary care nurses will provide a bridge between what the client needs and what he or she does not already have to make the right decisions and take the necessary action. This primary role of linkage to all resources that empower the client provides a different foundation for the nurse-client relationship and the relationship of the nurse with other involved providers. Equity is an outcome of this scenario, and the increased potential for client accountability is enhanced. Although this journey to client empowerment is somewhat long, there is little in the emerging framework for health that does not facilitate the journey. How quickly it happens depends in great measure on the degree of success of the role of the nurse in managing the continuum of care.

- The continuum of care demands that the primary and advanced practice nurse focus on the whole rather than the parts. As Drucker suggests, the work of leadership is now about wholes not parts (Drucker, 1993). Seeing the client within the social, cultural context for his or her life is as important as assessing and acting on the health needs the client presents to the provider. Sustainable response and health generation cannot result if the context within which they get addressed is not incorporated into the provider's role. This intimates a loss of control on the part of the provider because the outcome has more to do with the consumer than the nurse. It is in this set of circumstances that the role of the nurses takes on specific meaning. Perhaps the unique character of nursing, which focuses on the client's health experiences rather than illness events, will be especially meaningful.

There are a number of factors that will influence how the continuum of care unfolds and how advanced and primary practice operates over the next two decades. There are changes that will drive the context of health services and that will demand a different characterization of health services and an altered configuration of the service environment.

The multicultural environment of America is unique among all the democracies of the world. The wide variety of immigrants has changed the character of the nation and created a new context for health service. Language, health practices, familial relationships, and the social context within which various components of our society live create the milieu for health services in the future. The hospital cannot remain aloof or at a distance from the community in which it is a resident. Taking the service structure to the population served and moderating it to their needs in their own setting will be a common practice in the future of health care. Because health will be essential to the economic viability of the various plans, reducing the cost and intensity of service will be a primary initiative for the health system. This will require that the points of service be positioned as closely to the subscribers' life processes as possible—in the workplace, home, community center, church, and anywhere else the subscribers live their lives. The more that health care can look like a part of the life of the community and integrate with the subscriber's life experience, the more viable it will be and the greater the impact on cost and service outcome.

Leading the way in these settings is a provider whose focus is the life process and its integration with health services. The nurse in advanced practice is the appropriate player in this context prepared (it is hoped) to provide the kind of linkage between components of the system that reflect the sociological, physiological, and psychological relationships necessary to assure adequate health services.

This means that focus on the preparation of this advanced primary caregiver will have to be broad based and integrate a number of skills in the application of the role. Merging the content in the preparation of the clinical specialist with that of the nurse practitioner provides one solid step in broadening and deepening the emerging role in primary practice as the health system becomes more subscriber based. The old paradigm issues of diagnosis and treatment with some level of follow-up is simply not adequate for this role in primary care. Linking and integrating resources, systems, and players require a different set of skills apart from those associated with one-to-one intervention.

The same holds true for undergraduate preparation for primary nursing practice. At the baccalaureate level, at least, building on the continuum of care and the community experience for service is critical to the viability of nursing practice. Clinical experiences in a broader range of settings that include a fraction of the time currently spent in hospitals will be a requisite of the professional nurse. Reducing the number of associate degree and other nurses and increasing the number of advanced practice nurses will assure a better distribution of properly prepared primary nurses and assure that we do not prepare nurses for jobs that do not exist and roles that are no longer appropriate (Freeman, 1994).

CONCLUSION

It is evident that health care is experiencing a major transformation in both structure and service. The framework for the delivery of service increases the accountability of the system and calls its participants to make service health-based and cost-effective. All players in the system will have to reconfigure their roles to be consistent with the demand to keep subscribers healthy, not merely to treat illness (Murphy, Pearlman, Rea, & Boyce, 1994).

Every profession has to journey to new roles and expectations in the preparation and use of its members. Nursing has done much to build healthy foundations for the education of nurses, focusing on the whole person rather than on the events of illness. Although there are a variety of approaches used, foundational nursing principles are consonant with the move to a more health-based system. In the arena of primary service, case management, continuum of care, and culturally sensitive service, nursing is on the cutting edge of response. To compete with others to match consumer needs with adequate preparation, nurses in advanced practice will have to be both politically and economically astute and position themselves to continue both to serve and advocate for the public.

The times are exciting in their intensity and opportunity. Nurses are capable of responding to society's changing health-care needs. There is a lot of "noise" in the system that will challenge nursing leadership in the near future. There are many who do not see the continuum of care as an integrated system of linkages and relationships. Nursing's experience at linking and facilitating the many roles of health care bodes well for expanding roles along the continuum of care. Clinical case management and primary approaches to assuring health and maintaining consumers in the health continuum instead of illness events brings fulfillment to years of accommodation to the medical model of care. The glaring failure of that approach to improve the social circumstance while building an expensive monolithic sickness service system is testament to the need for change (Starr, 1992). And again it is nurses who will lead society to a more healthy future.

There is much work yet to be done. Political diligence regarding the desire of some to make no meaningful change in the sickness system, the commitment of others to keep the role of the nurse subsequent, and the desire of still others to deny the public access to a service provider whose competence in health care is well documented remain continuing challenges.

Models of whole system and continuum services exist and nurses are positioned to provide leadership to move the system to more health-based approaches (Lutz, 1991). The future is bright for advanced practice and primary roles for nurses. The transition in case management and the lead role of the nurse in moving toward the future is a sign that the best is yet to be.

REFERENCES

Anderson, R. (1993). Nursing leadership and healthcare reform. *Journal of Nursing Administration* 23 (12):8-9.

Ashley, J. A. (1976). *Hospitals, paternalism, and the role of the nurse.* New York: Teachers College Press.

Barger, S., & Rosenfeld, P. (1993). Models in community health: findings from a national study of community nursing centers. *National Study of Community Nursing Centers Report: National League for Nursing* 14 (8):426-429.

Bhide, A. (1994). How entrepreneurs craft strategies that work. *Harvard Business Review* 72 (2):150-161.

Bogdanich, W. (1991). *The great white lie: how America's hospitals betray our trust and endanger our lives.* New York: Simon & Schuster.

Bryne, J. (1994). The pain of downsizing. *Business Week* 3370 (May 9):60-69.

Buerhaus, P. (1994). Managed competition and critical issues facing nurses. *Nursing & Health Care* 15 (1):22-26.

Clouten, K., & Weber, R. (1994). Patient focused care . . . playing to win. *Nursing Management* 25 (2):34-36.

Coile, R. (1989). *The new medicine: reshaping medical practice and health care management.* Rockville, MD: Aspen Publishers, Inc.

Dienemann, J., & Gessner, T. (1992). Restructuring nursing care delivery systems. *Nursing Economics* 10 (4):253-256.

Diers, D. (1993). Advanced practice. *Health Management Quarterly* 15 (2):16-20.

Drucker, P. (1993). *Post-capitalist society.* New York: HarperCollins.

Eckhart, J. (1993). Costing out nursing service: examining the research. *Nursing Economics* 11 (2):91-98.

Fagin, C. (1994, Oct). Nursings value proves itself. *American Journal of Nursing,* 17-30.

Freeman, R. (1994). *Working under different rules.* New York: Russell Sage Foundation.

Goldsmith, J. (1993). Driving the nitroglycerin truck: the relationship between the hospital and physician. *Healthcare Forum Journal* 36 (2):36-40.

Guild, S. et al. (1994). Development of an innovative nursing care system. *Journal of Nursing Administration* 24 (3):23-29.

Johnson, R. (1992). The entrepreneurial physician. *Health Care Management Review* 17 (1):73-79.

Kanter, R. (1994). Collaborative advantage: the art of alliances. *Harvard Business Review* 72 (4):96-108.

Lathrop, P. (1991, July/August). The Patient Focused Hospital. *Healthcare Forum,* 17-20.

Lutz, S. (1991). Practitioners are filling in for scarce physicians. *Modern Healthcare* 21 (19):24-29.

Madden, M. J., & Prescott, P. (1994). Advanced practice roles in the managed care environment. *Journal of Nursing Administration* 24 (1):56-62.

Mitty, E. (1991). The nurse as advocate. *Nursing & Health Care* 12 (10):520-530.

Moffit, K. et al. (1993). Patient focused care: key principles in restructuring. *Hospitals and Health Service Administration* 38 (4):509-522.

Murphy, R. et al. (1994). Work redesign: a return to the basics. *Nursing Management 25* (2):37-39.

Neubauer, J. (1993). Redesign: managing role changes and building a new team. *Seminars for Nurse Managers 1* (1):26-32.

Newman, M., Lamb, G., & Michaels, K. (1991). Nursing case management: the coming together of theory and practice. *Nursing & Health Care 12* (8):404-408.

Niven, D. (1993). When times get tough, what happens to TQM? *Harvard Business Review 71* (3):20-34.

Porter-O'Grady, T. (1990). *The reorganization of nursing practice: creating the corporate venture.* Rockville, MD: Aspen Publishers.

Porter-O'Grady, T. (1994). The real value of partnership: preventing professional amorphism. *Journal of Nursing Administration 24* (2):11-15.

Reinhardt, U. (1992). Whither private health insurance: self destruction or rebirth? *Frontiers of Health Service Management 9* (1):5-31.

Riley, R. (1994). Educating the workforce of the future. *Harvard Business Review 72* (2):39-51.

Starr, P. (1992). *The logic of health care reform.* Knoxville, TN: Whittle Direct Books.

Womack, J., & Jones, D. (1994). From lean production to the lean enterprise. *Harvard Business Review 72* (2):93-103.

Chapter 3

Grass Roots Efforts: Nurses Involved in the Political Process

Marjorie Jamieson, MS, RN, FAAN

OVERVIEW

Nurses as political strategists can help to secure support for community nurse case management.

In the growing elderly population of the authors' community, it was found that many nursing home residents needed less skilled care and could have remained in their own homes if appropriate support services had been available. The Living at Home/Block Nurse Program (LAH/BNP) is a community program that utilizes professional and volunteer services of local residents to enable elderly neighbors to remain in their homes, where many prefer to be. This program came to fruition because of local citizens' willingness to take responsibility for the "public good." This chapter demonstrates how systems can change when people work cooperatively within the community setting. This case study is based on the authors' experience in obtaining city, county, state, and federal support for LAH/BNP in Minnesota.

If there is one certainty in health-care reform in the 1990s, it is change. Health Maintenance Organizations (HMOs), Diagnostic Related Groups (DRGs), Managed Care, Integrated Service Networks (ISNs), Capitation, and Community-Based Care are some of the concepts that are rapidly changing and being defined differently across the United States. Case management is mentioned when each of these concepts is discussed; in fact, most health-care reform proposals under development talk about the need to find effective ways to plan and coordinate the array of services needed as exemplified in case management. As continuity and comprehensive health delivery programs across acute and long-term care systems are discussed, consensus is emerging in support of case management. For example, as a policy issue, Minnesota has separated the roles of primary health-care provider and case manager for its publicly supported programs,

although it has not come to any conclusions about roles.

CASE MANAGEMENT CLIENT POPULATION

The burgeoning growth of the elderly population in the United States is well known. In 1935, when Social Security became part of the future of seniors in the United States, the average life expectancy was age 65 (Jazwiecki, 1986). Today it is 75 for men and 79 for women. People aged 85 and older are the fastest growing segment of the population. It is predicted that by the year 2000, up to 75% of a nurse's patients are going to be over the age of 65.

American families do a tremendous job in caring for their elderly relatives. Approximately 85% of seniors who need some type of care because of a chronic condition or because of an activities-of-daily-living deficit are cared for by their families. Of the 5% that are in nursing homes, about 30% would not need to be there if they could get some help in their homes (Eustis, 1984).

A COMMUNITY-BASED CASE MANAGEMENT PROGRAM

The Living at Home/Block Nurse Program (LAH/BNP) is a community program that draws upon the professional and volunteer services of local residents to provide service coordination/care management, information, social and support services, nursing and other services for their elderly neighbors to enable them to remain in their homes. The pilot community's success prompted replication in three socio-demographically diverse communities. Their success generated interest in other communities until there are now 15 Living at Home/Block Nurse Programs in Minnesota. A national demonstration, funded by the federal government, is expected to begin in late 1995.

The key to the success of the program is two-fold:
- The extent of neighborhood response and commitment, sharing of energy and provision of support (including in-kind contributions and donations) to help their older neighbors; and
- The identification of specific needs and the coordination and delivery of services in the person's home by neighborhood professionals and volunteers who use the informal resources of nearby family, neighbor, church, and service groups, and integrate them with the formal services.

As a result of the efforts of a board of directors composed of community residents who are responsible for the program, staff from within the community, and tremendous volunteer involvement with organizing and delivery of services, within 3 years, an external evaluation of the original community documents that 85% of the clients who received nursing services would have been in nursing homes without the program. The average cost of providing these services was less than $300 a month, whereas in nursing homes it was about $1500. Because of these findings, grants were received from the U.S. Department of Health and Human Services, Division of Nursing and the W.K. Kellogg Foundation for replicating the program in three socially and demographically diverse communities. After three years of replication, another external evaluation (done by a different evaluator) reports that 38% of the clients who received nursing services would have been in nursing homes. It was costing less than $500 a month living at home—where they wanted to be; however, it would have cost about $2000 a month in a nursing home—where they didn't want to be. Both evaluations reported a high level of client satisfaction and quality of service provision. Anecdotal evidence speaks to the savings of Medicare because of nursing case management, health education, and early intervention.

The success of the LAH/BNP is based on people—residents of communities who invest time, enthusiasm, and their skills and knowledge to make the program work. It is built on the capacity to care, best expressed in local communities where relationships and interdependencies naturally form. In his book, *CommonWealth: A Return to Citizen Politics,* (1989) Harry Boyte offers a reinterpretation of politics and power in which citizens, not experts, take center stage. He proposes that citizens take responsibility for the "public good," and that citizen initiatives demonstrate alternatives to what has been the purview of experts and professionals. This stance calls for a different definition of community. In the LAH/BNP, the term *community based* (done by and with people) as opposed to *community oriented* (done to and for people) is operative. It means more than token representation or citizen participation. It means real governance in which citizens make decisions and assume ownership of the program. The program is the combination of professionals living in the neighborhood with volunteers from the neighborhood who become lasting friends with clients. It links with organizations and agencies that provide services and designs new ones where they are not currently available.

BLOCK NURSE CASE MANAGEMENT

When one considers the diagnosis and treatment of acute episodes of illness, the management of chronic disease and disability, the deficits in activities of daily living and instrumental activities of daily living, failing cognition and social isolation, the argument for case management is self-evident, especially in light of the fragmented health-care and long-term care systems that exist.

Care (in fact, LAH/BNP prefers the term *care management* to *case management*) means almost anything needed that can be provided so that senior citizens can remain healthy: volunteers calling a client who is on a bladder training program every two hours to remind her to go to the toilet, helping a client who can function independently once out of bed to get up each morning, providing telephone reassurance for the "worried well," and organizing flu shots for the community.

The client and the family are at the very center of the care plan in which the block nurse is the pivotal person in arranging, coordinating, delivering services, and advocating with the client so that needs are met, regardless of entitlements or ability to pay. The nurse, during weekly care conferences (which often include the client's block volunteer) in the community, integrates the non-nursing community support, such as

Boy Scouts painting the inside of a house after the Rotary Club has patched falling plaster, cleaning the gutters, providing meals on weekends and holidays when Meals on Wheels does not deliver, addressing Christmas cards for a blind client, free grocery delivery by the local store, and transportation to church, with nursing interventions. The block nurse also serves as a resource for people who receive these services *before* requiring nursing care.

Money needs to be raised to pay for the services that entitlements do not cover, which the client cannot afford, but without which the client will not have needs met and will likely be accessing more expensive care delivery systems: emergency rooms, physician offices, 911 calls, ambulances, and nursing homes.

NEED FOR NURSING "POLITICAL" INVOLVEMENT

Consensus on who should be the case manager in any proposed health-care and long-term care system has not evolved. In home care for the elderly, for example, the Medicare (acute care services) case manager is a physician and the Medicaid (welfare custodial-maintenance care) case manager is a social worker in most states. Nurses become involved under the direction of the physician case manager. Yet nurses are "in the trenches" and are pivotal in coordinating all services and in meeting the illness and health needs of the client. They make care cost effective because they can manage comprehensive community-based care; physicians and social workers do not provide the primary components of community health care—health teaching, self-care, activities-of-daily-living adaptations, and convalescent care.

If we assume that developing more cost-effective ways of providing care is a major agenda for the government, nurses must be involved in changing the health-care delivery scene because nurses provide case management and many health- and disease-centered interventions less expensively.

This change is going to be difficult because there has been a shift to financial profit and away from social good in health and long-term care systems in the United States. Financial profit is the goal for both fee-for-service and for managed-care systems; both are showing increased profits. By making money providing services (fee for service) or by eliminating services (managed care), the emphasis is not where nurses have historically placed their values. Most nurses, to date, have entered the profession because of the social good to which they can contribute.

Turning nursing values into political priorities is essential. In addition, effecting change by becoming involved in a political process will be easier when it is based on values. When we act from our value base, we are energized, committed, and sometimes driven.

To effect change, nurses need to become involved politically. An immediate effect will materialize by starting locally. If the 1.3 million nurses in America, instead of passively accepting all the new changes in health care, would proactively become involved in shaping health policy, the entire health-care delivery system could be turned upside down. The question is whether nurses have the political will to make this happen.

POLITICAL STRATEGIES: A CASE STUDY

The idea that politics is "dirty," not ethical, of questionable integrity, and something professionals should avoid is not uncommon among nurses. Yet it is the very basis upon which democracy is founded. Sitting around complaining about what the government has done or not done is not logical because *we are the government.* It is disappointing to talk with nurses who do not know that each state has two senators and representatives based upon population, who do not know the names of their congressional delegation (their state's senators and representatives), have never written or telephoned their elected officials, do not know anything about their state, county, or city government. Yet laws are passed because somebody advocated for these laws. In the history of our country, many laws have been passed by *one* vote—and that one vote could be a result of the knowledge and influence of nurses. As citizens, it is our right to contact and influence our elected officials; they are elected to represent us. Change *does* come because of systematic societal action.

This action became more formalized for the LAH/BNP after the first evaluation and after replication to test the model became a strategy. The first LAH/BNP created a nonprofit corporation, the Living at Home/Block Nurse Program, Inc. (LAH/BNP, Inc.) whose mission is to assist local communities in developing and sustaining LAH/BNPs and to effect societal change that will encourage and support ongoing neighborhood-based, long-term home care systems.

The processes and functions used in case management are much the same as those used for effective political outcomes.

The book *Effective Political Action: Prescription for Nurses* (1990) by Goldwater & Lloyd-Zusy is a good primer about political strategy development and how to effect change. The book speaks to the more formal methodology for being a political change agent. However, this chapter will be more of a case study, or "how to" based on experience in getting city, county, state, and federal support for the LAH/BNP in Minnesota.

Importance of the Block Nurse

Pivotal to the program are the block nurses (called primary block nurses in the LAH/BNP) who live in the respective communities and who view the communities in which they live as their clients—quite different from viewing each person to whom the nurse delivers services as a client. The block nurse is not unlike the district nurse of the past who was responsible for the health of the people in her community. The district nurse could get things done politically because she knew the people of the community and the local elected officials and politicians.

The designers (four out of six were nurses) of the LAH/BNP included changing "the system" of long-term care delivery and case management as a goal from the beginning. There was a firm belief that changing "the system" happens when people band together because of a common cause and a belief that citizens have the power to change government through officials who are elected by them. Voters put these people in office and politicians, therefore, *do* respond to their constituents. The language of change and hope was always the message.

Building Relationships with Elected Officials

Building relationships with elected officials and their staff locally was a start with making appointments with county and city commissioners to first gain their interest, and their support over time. Whenever there was any public meeting, rally, or reason to wear the Living at Home/Block Nurse Program name tag and the opportunity to shake hands with the elected official, it was capitalized upon. This activity also provided incidental learning about other issues because *any* meeting that gave the impetus to shake hands with officials and talk about the program was attended.

Sharing information (stories) and data was done in other ways, too:

- Inviting elected officials to participate in meetings
- Including them in community activities (e.g., picnics, etc.)
- Meeting informally for lunch
- Keeping their staff informed

Relationships with elected officials were also built by:

- Including them in press conferences
- Asking for their advice; going *to* them
- Making our goals and theirs as congruent as possible
- Supporting; trying not to differ
- Recognizing them publicly
- Sharing copies of written support

Such opportunities soon made familiar the officials and their staff so that an appointment to discuss the LAH/BNP and its goals for the future could be made. Thank you notes were handwritten and personal. Letters followed when new information or data were available; sometimes copies of newspaper articles and published reports were mailed.

Importance of Community

Each LAH/BNP is managed by a board of directors composed of people from within the community. This community board determines the boundaries of the community and contracts with a local home health-care nursing agency that works as a partner with the community and hires the staff who live in the community and who provide services for their neighbors. Each community is committed to provide services based on *need;* all entitlements are accessed when possible, but the money for the services for those who fall through the cracks of the system and who cannot self-pay is raised by the community. The nursing agency, often a public health nursing agency with county financial support, bills the community for this uncompensated care but often will do it at a discounted rate; this amount of subsidy varies from program to program. In addition to county financial support, many of the programs also receive financial support from their cities or towns. This practice has occurred because the people in the communities have included their elected officials within the planning and implementation of the program and have asked them for support.

Evidence of this support of the county and city was included in a proposal to the "Innovations in State and Local Government" initiative of Harvard University and the Ford Foundation by the pilot community in 1986. When the LAH/BNP was one of the 10 winners out of 1400 applications, there was a celebration in New York City, to which the mayor of St. Paul and a Ramsey County commissioner were able to attend. The Ford Foundation sent the $80,000 award to the city and a call was received describing the process for receiving the money, the forms to fill out, and the amount of money the city would need to manage this process. Because of the ongoing relationship with the mayor, one phone call resulted in the entire amount being mailed directly to the LAH/BNP office.

The need to initiate relationships with state government through Minnesota state senators and representatives and with the Minnesota U.S. senators and representatives (the Minnesota congressional delegation) was recognized. Much the same procedure used with city and county elected officials was followed.

Pounding the sidewalks in Washington (it's surprising how open the doors are) has produced lasting relationships. A trip to Washington, after visiting with the congressional delegation members in their local offices, afforded the opportunity to speak with the Washington staff. Visits were also made to staff leaders in the House and Senate, especially those on committees who might be of assistance in the future. A nurse who is the chief staff person to one of the key congressional leaders in Washington has been an important contact. Periodic updates to these people and additional personal appointments when possible keep them in contact.

Recognizing Elected Officials

Giving credit to elected officials for their part in realizing LAH/BNP goals has paid dividends. During a local political campaign for city commissioner, a candidate distributed brochures in which she wrote that she supported the program (which she may indeed have done though unknown to LAH/BNP). Was the program being used for her political ends? Whatever the reason, it became a wonderful free advertisement! Credit can be given to elected officials by:

- Crediting them for success as much as possible
- Giving them awards for their contributions
- Recognizing their assistance in reports, publications
- Thanking them publicly for *any* help
- Asking them to speak, present awards on behalf of the program
- Including them when awards are given to us

An example of these strategies is the invitation of a U.S. senator from Minnesota to speak at a W.K. Kellogg Foundation funded conference. Consistent work with this senator has resulted in his authoring legislation for a national demonstration. Also, a St. Paul city commissioner was invited to the annual meeting of the LAH/BNP program in her district where she was able to speak to the people. She has been supportive of city funding for the program. Other examples include inviting representatives to community board meetings and strategic planning where they have spoken about their issues and, at the same time, have learned about the program. One city commissioner convened a task force of city and county commissioners and Minnesota senators and representatives to strategize for getting legislation passed for a statewide program. The three legislators present at the meeting became authors of a bill authorizing the program across the state. (When the bill was before the Senate committee where LAH/BNP, Inc. testified, the chairperson asked, "Who is going to vote for this creative, innovative program?") During the committee testimony in the House, a committee member objected to funding the program. However, another representative who had been kept informed rallied to support the program, even though she does not represent a community that has the program.

Establishing relationships with the staff of public elected officials has opened many doors. Much has been learned from them. Valuing the staff by asking their advice, thanking them, and following up on issues has led to their reminding elected officials to be sensitive to LAH/BNP concerns. Staff of these officials have urged support of the LAH/BNP and when issues have arisen, LAH/BNP, Inc. has dealt with the person directly. Staff have become advocates in many cases. The administrative assistant of a Ramsey County commissioner identified $10,000 in the County budget for the LAH/BNP, Inc.

Over time, government department personnel that operationalize laws and regulatory staff have been spoken to, educated, and kept up to date. They have been invited to planning meetings, asked for advice, and seen how our respective activities compliment each other. Because of these associations, participation has been invited in ad hoc committees and task forces before government budgets are set and goals are determined. Because state commissioners and deputy commissioners have been invited as members of task forces planning for the future, the program has become well known. Consequently, they were able to give support during the legislative process in Minnesota. Relationships with research staff at the capital resulted in being invited to write/critique the language in the bill that was passed. One of the state commissioners volunteered to peruse documents, critique them, and give us address lists. Government staff have helped to find alternatives and "loop holes" that work.

Importance of Volunteerism

LAH/BNP, Inc. has discovered how to become a member of government commissions, boards, task forces, and committees by volunteering and having influential people support this involvement. Because of interest shown in the concerns of officials and their staff, support has been generated and LAH/BNP, Inc. has been invited to participate in planning processes. Taking an active role, such as volunteer secretary, has brought knowledge about issues and has also made LAH/BNP visible participants. These activities have also led to invitations to join boards and task forces in the private sector and have subsequently widened LAH/BNP, Inc.'s base.

This strategy was particularly important when a Senior Agenda for Independent Living Program, a 20-year state strategy, was on the drawing board. One person, either staff or board member, volunteered for each of the planning subcommittees. As a result, the LAH/BNP was used as a basis for recommendations to the Department of Human Services and formed the foundation for state funding for the LAH/BNP and for LAH/BNP, Inc. Other examples have been invitations to be on the United Way planning task force and a Long-Term Care and Aging Work Group of the University of Minnesota Division of Health Services Research and Policy.

Importance of Good Public Relations

Attending public hearings that deal with any issue similar to or that affect LAH/BNP interests has been educational and has demonstrated interest in the larger picture. It has been most effective when community people have testified; their commitment is so obvious. Several local board chairpersons have had their pictures taken with their mayors, the governor, and other officials.

Attending community meetings, identifying ourselves, asking *appropriate* questions, networking, and identifying the movers and shakers have been learning experiences. By genuinely asking their advice, giving them information, and following up, they have become enrolled in our cause. Talking about our success yet being honest and listening to people's concerns without being defensive has seemed to dissipate potential opposition. Trying to understand and phrasing issues differently facilitate working with those who are skeptical.

Early on, support from agencies that might perceive the LAH/BNP as competition was garnered. Contacts were made through board members. Lunches were arranged with important individuals; groups were invited to brainstorm; and LAH/BNP goals that augment others were emphasized. Not only did board members make contacts, they became very involved. Coalition building became the answer!

When asking specific advice or needing the expertise of others, the most creditable person available was approached; he or she could say no but might say yes. For example, Michael Patton, a national expert on evaluation from the University of Minnesota, helped design the pilot evaluation; he then asked if he could be a candidate to do the evaluation. Just having his name on the evaluation has given us instant credibility. Lunch with the Director of Health Computer Services, University of Minnesota, developed into a graduate student project that recommended the LAH/BNP computer system.

Other university involvement came by bringing them money to do the evaluation component of our replication project. They have also been included in consultation, data analysis, and other projects. Such collaboration also brought credibility to the LAH/BNP, Inc., including participation in invitational conferences, panels, speaking opportunities, and testimony.

Watching requests for abstracts for presentations at national conventions and meetings and responding to them has resulted in opportunities to talk about the program across the nation. Publishing in professional journals has occurred almost annually, and through communities and press releases, the LAH/BNP has been written about in local newspapers and periodicals. Working with, and informing national organizations has resulted in people such as the president of the National Institute on Aging (NIH) using the term *block nurse* generically.

Directors of foundations have given helpful advice, sometimes about issues other than funding. Thanking them and keeping them informed (especially of outcomes) has resulted in several invitations to submit proposals. Reports and information back to foundations sometimes leads to an invitation for further funding; foundations like to hear what they are accomplishing through grantees.

The need for funding from county, city, state, and federal grants, though a wish of the electorate, has been substantiated with rigorous data analysis and evaluation outcomes to government entities. This support contributes to the rationale for funding from local foundations followed by national foundations.

Data analysis reports and external evaluation outcomes have been sent to insurance companies, public officials, and staff who are concerned about issues of health and human services. Follow-up visits have been opportunities for questions and answers.

In 1992, a U.S. senator from another state who was chair of the Senate Finance Committee and who was a member of the Medicare/Long-Term Care Subcommittee asked one of the Minnesota senators if he was aware of any programs with a community focus for managing the care of the elderly. We were immediately contacted and were invited to participate in writing language for inclusion in the reauthorization of the Older Americans Act that would include a demonstration of the LAH/BNP concept. LAH/BNP, Inc. worked closely with the senator's staff and the rest of the Minnesota congressional delegation to get the amendment passed.

Lobbying

It soon became clear that we needed the services of a lobbyist, although some of us were uncomfortable with such an approach. A nonprofit, tax-exempt organization is very limited in what it can spend on lobbying. We had only $10,000—a drop in the bucket when it comes to usual lobbyist fees. Through neighborhood contacts, an expert was found who taught us who to talk with and what to emphasize. He opened the doors, and LAH/BNP, Inc. presented its cause to everyone and anyone in Washington who might be able to influence passage of the amendment. The lobbyist became so enamored with the LAH/BNP that he now provides his expertise *pro bono.* The effort was a success; in October of 1992, the amendment passed.

It was then that reality hit; many laws get passed, but without a financial appropriation they cannot be implemented. Thus began a plan to get the money to make a demonstration happen with visits, letters, telephone calls, and general strategizing with the Minnesota congressional delegation's staff. Fortunately, one Minnesota representative holds key positions on the House Budget Committee, Appropriations Committee, and Subcommittee for Labor Health and Human Services Education. Although meetings had been held with him and his staff before, now a concerted effort was initiated with a well-thought-out message that was concise, had key points, and was conclusive. One page of information for reference was left with him. Data analyses and evaluation results were used heavily.

One of his staff persons became very involved and made a site visit to homes of clients. Telephone calls occurred almost weekly for a while as strategy was planned for getting the appropriation through the House—where all financial bills begin. A budget was put together. Questions from other representatives on the committee were anticipated; she knew the arguments and LAH/BNP, Inc. knew the answers. It seemed important to influence those who might not be supportive (e.g., with calls for help to the ANA lobbyist, to the president of AARP who had given us an award, to our *pro bono* lobbyist, etc.). At each stage, from subcommittee to full committee, letter writing and telephone calls to committee members made a phenomenal impact. Nursing colleagues from around the nation who had state representatives on the committees wrote letters. Letters were sent by relatives, friends, friends of friends, shirt-tail relatives—anyone who could influence the person who represented them in Washington. The letters were all hand written or typed personally, all were different, and stamps were licked. The staff person from Washington reported one day about all the mail coming into their office—they were beginning to tabulate it on the computer. Many followed up their letters with telephone calls. LAH/BNP, Inc. staff and community residents learned that bulk mail looks like bulk mail and that postage machines used with mass mailing look like mass mailings. However, personal messages from the electorate bring results.

The most important participants in the whole process of getting the appropriation passed for the amendment to the Older Americans Act, which calls for a national demonstration of the LAH/BNP, are the people in each respective LAH/BNP community. These residents, so committed to meeting the *needs* of their senior neighbors so that they can remain in their homes and communities, have made the difference. They have worked with their local county commissioners, mayors, their Minnesota senators and representatives, and their U.S. congressional delegation. They have been *politically active* in the true sense of the word. Also, they have discovered that the most convincing form of engaging a public official in their cause is a site visit to the homes of clients. All have become converts to the cause.

The day the appropriation was passed by the House floor after having survived three committees was indeed a time for celebration. Already work with the staff of the two U.S. senators had begun. The appropriation was doubled in the Senate, and was passed on the Senate floor. This was accomplished because of the political influence of a LAH/BNP in another state whose senator was in a key position on the Senate committee.

Work behind the scenes as the two appropriations were discussed in conference committee commenced immediately. Washington staff assured the lower amount but prepared strategies to get the doubled amount. Daily telephone calls between Washington and Minnesota occurred. In conference committee, there was a compromise, and Congress authorized $1.5 million for a national demonstration of the Living at Home/Block Nurse Program.

During this entire time, because the amendment is under the Older Americans Act and the appropriation will go to the Administration on Aging that administers the Older Americans Act, a relationship through visits, letters, and telephone calls with AoA staff as the appropriations have progressed has been nurtured. LAH/BNP, Inc. has begun working closely with them, offering assistance, the opportunity for a site visit, and access to resources such as handbooks and manuals.

Given what has been learned about the success of impacting government for implementing demonstrations of and funding for the LAH/BNP, efforts are now concentrated on how to use these experiences in permanently changing the way care for seniors is provided and financed. Although, tongue in cheek, it might be said that all good health and human services programs in the United States are demonstrations, there has to be a way to bring about lasting change. The data collected and used as rationale for a national change to community-based, nurse-managed care are going to make the difference.

Do we, as nurses, have the political will? The LAH/BNP believes it can happen!

CONCLUSION

Every nurse across the United States can participate in making nursing's agenda a reality in the context of cost-effective health and long-term care delivery. Even in counties and towns, elected people are making decisions about health care—especially about the dollars that will be spent. If nurses believe their practice and case management is cost effective, there are many opportunities to use their political clout on behalf of their profession—and ultimately, on behalf of the people they serve.

REFERENCES

Boyte, C. (1989). *CommonWealth: a return to citizen politics.* New York: Free Press.

Eustis, N., Greenberg, J., & Patten, S. (1984). *Long-term care for older persons: a policy perspective.* Brooks and Cole.

Goldwater, M., & Lloyd-Zusy, M. (1990). *Effective political action: prescription for nurses.* St Louis: Mosby.

Jazwiecki, T. (1986, April). Financing options for long-term care services. *Business Health,* 18-24.

Chapter 4

Nursing's Response to Health-Care Transformation: A Nurse Executive's View

JoEllen Goertz Koerner, PhD, RN, CNAA, FAAN

OVERVIEW

A nurse executive looks at the emerging global community and its implications for transforming health care.

This chapter examines futuristic trends that are laying the foundation for transforming health care in America today. A framework for change is presented based on two focal points: social change in the superstructure of society, along with a major shift in fundamental values and world view of health care by providers and consumers. A futuristic "learning society" model redefines work, technology, and the outcomes we are seeking in a postindustrial society. Strategies for change focus on the role of organized nursing in facilitating movement for the grassroots nurse, interdisciplinary teams, and the consumer. Finally, the restructuring of social policy must be accomplished if the change is to be sustained.

The winds of change are blowing across the universe. Patterns emerging in 1995 are grounded in situations that have been occurring and are now becoming manifest. For instance, patterns that connect nations, rather than separate them, have been displayed by an economic need for collaboration and cooperation as seen in the case of a united Europe. Similarly, we are coming to realize our ecological connections, as when the winds and tides showed Chernobyl and the Valdez oil spill to be international rather than local incidents.

When clients become ill they enter a microsystem consisting of a physician in charge of the client; a hospital with nurses, physician specialists, administrators and a host of other allied health professionals; diagnosis and treatment plans designed to return the client to good health; and follow-up visits to help the client through the process of recovery, advising him or her on healthy living.

In this scenario, no one is helping the clients manage their transitions through this complex system. It is inadequate and fragmented and is the root problem in American health care today. No amount of restructuring or refinancing at the macro level will correct it. Reform is not enough, but transformation is. However, transformative change can occur only when a new vision emerges for and within health professionals that radically alters their world view and their work. To sustain this change in health care, this same transformative shift must also occur within the global community with regard to the definition, expectations, and self-responsibility surrounding the phenomenon of health.

Futuristic professionals must be closer to the clients and their families. With 80% of all current illness lifestyle related, they need to develop a better understanding of why people behave the way they do, particularly under stress. The traditional model of medical education and its translation to other disciplines and practice, based largely on organ-specific illness and cure, are no longer adequate. The ultimate goal of the contemporary health professional must expand to provide cure for those diseases that are curable and contain those that are not in ways that allow individuals to function with a quality of life they determine for themselves.

A revolution of this nature will not be easy. Many educators and professionals believe that their system is adequate in its current form. Some accreditation and licensure requirements as well as reimbursement methods discourage new and innovative practices and approaches. Funding for pilot projects in education is inadequate. Nevertheless, health-care reform must proceed along two parallel paths: (1) reorganization and refinance of the system to contain costs and provide access for all citizens, and (2) reform of education and training to produce more effective and responsive professionals. One without the other will not reach the goal of Healthy America 2005 (PEW, 1991). It is within this ever-changing and complex arena that national nursing organizations are called to define and articulate the emerging role of the profession.

FUTURISTIC TRENDS: THE FOUNDATION FOR HEALTH-CARE TRANSFORMATION

Current economic, political, cultural, and technological realities define and direct health-care delivery in the United States, as well as the rest of the world. To bring about transformation, not just variations of the current system or even reform, a clear understanding of our present reality and awareness of future trends must be woven into a plan for social action to achieve effective and lasting results (Table 4-1). Organized nursing should play a role.

Trend #1: Everyday Experiences Will Be Increasingly Multinational

Today for various interacting reasons, the power and influence of any one postindustrial Western nation is increasingly a function of international connections— of a "global web." This connection can be seen in the world of business (NAFTA and other trade agreements), the military (Desert Storm, a war that united the power and energy of many nations), economics (the financial performance of any major industrialized nation has a powerful impact on the stockmarket in the United States), religion (in many regions of the

TABLE 4-1	Futuristic trends that shape health-care transformation
Trend	Implications
Increasing multinationality	Expanding markets Constricted access and increased regulation
Eclipse of biomedical paradigm	Reemergence of primary preventive care and decreasing demand for health professionals
Deconstruction of mediating social systems	Reconstruction of the health-care system

world a blend between Eastern and Western belief systems is emerging), and information and communication (Harman [1988] observed that the emerging information highway uniting the global village will be a legacy from this era in history as lasting as the pyramids of Egypt and the cathedrals of Europe).

Implications for health care: We are being enmeshed in our international relations. Increased multiculturalism has become so much a part of all our activities, including health care, that it is more the status quo than a trend. This diversity of ethnic origins is seen in the demographics of our country, our community, our client populations, and our providers. In health care, this increased multinationalism will show itself through expanded markets, constricted access, and increased regulations.

- Implication #1. Expanded markets: As in other business sectors, the health-care industry will continue to seek new markets for its existing products and services. The makers of the latest models of CAT scanners and MITs, and research innovators in the pharmaceutical companies are among those seeking to expand beyond U.S. shores. This trend will accelerate in proportion to our success in tightening our own cost control or moving U.S. health care into a preventive mode. Having shifted from an acute to a preventive focus, new markets may open. Organized nursing can influence this shift, as well as the markets. As health teachers and counselors, nurses could make a major contribution to preventive services that meet the needs of the individuals and communities, not the needs of the health-care system.

- Implication #2. Constricted access and increased regulation in an effort to control the inflow of migrant populations. Despite our history and tradition, the United States is gasping for air under the cloud of a scarce and diminishing resource mentality. In 1995, we are tightening the prerequisites for inclusion into our society and are constricting access to our systems through increased regulations. The health care of children of Mexico and Central America is a growing concern as they attend U.S. schools, seek health care in the emergency rooms of municipal hospitals, and their mothers give birth in U.S. hospitals without the benefit of prenatal care. We can anticipate quarantines by design and denial of access for non-U.S. citizens. Reasserting national boundaries is a band-aid solution at best.

Organized nursing must join forces and call for a broader examination of such issues as "illegal aliens," because these kinds of social issues are truly health-care issues. As caring professionals, we must raise the bigger question: *why* are migrant workers streaming into America in such great numbers in the first place? The answer reveals a bigger and more global problem—the misery and poverty in their own land. Over two million nurses could join forces and partner with the public, legislators, and lawmakers in fostering a global perspective on employment, unemployment, and poverty. Further, nursing colleagues throughout the world could partner with each other, local teachers, and others who minister to the social service needs of the global community in an effort to restore harmony and balance.

Trend #2: The Eclipse of the Biomedical Paradigm Is Occurring

Dominance and control are valued and preferred assumptions based on the biomedical paradigm around which Western health care is structured and organized. They represent an approach to our experiences that focus on separation and differences rather than connections and relationships. They support the values inherent in the physical sciences that posture a technological imperative over a human-oriented one.

This biomedical paradigm is flawed in that it supports the notion of the person as an individual, autonomous being. Given the reality of our relational nature, Albert Einstein viewed this autonomous perspective as an "optical delusion of consciousness."

Western medicine has built a health-care system on "scientific" realities. Despite the relational context of our clients' experiences, this paradigm has us isolate individuals from their societies as we search for linear and single cause-and-effect answers to their maladies. To wit, Shaw (1984) observed that "the art of healing could be summed up in the formula: Find the microbe and kill it."

Few involved in the current health-care system are satisfied. Recent polls (Blendon et al., 1990) showed that 89% of the U.S. public think that their health-care system needs either fundamental change or complete rebuilding (p. 188). In recent years, the payors—public

and private—have added their concerns. Yet the industry has grown and prospered. Why? And to what good?

Because, in addition to reinforcing the position of organized medicine and assuring profits of the surrounding industries, the biomedical paradigm has supported the state. It has reinforced, reproduced, and extended the dominant patriarchal influence. In the context of the emerging global web, however, this approach to health care is not only misaligned with the human experience, it is also unstable as an agent for the international corporations that have replaced nation states. As such, this paradigm is increasingly dysfunctional and problematic to both the theory and practice of the country's health system.

Implications for health care: The eclipse of the biomedical paradigm will allow other models for health care to emerge: primary care and nontraditional healing modalities as delivery models for health services, individual and community needs as a determining factor in what those services will be, and the educated lay worker, rather than the professional as a care provider.

- Implication #3. Primary, preventive care as the major delivery model. This shift will replace the current focus on diagnosis and treatment, calling for more family practice physicians. A shortage of primary care physicians (currently 17% of all physicians choose general medicine with the remaining 83% selecting careers in subspecialty medicine) will foster an increase in the role responsibilities given to advanced practice nurse practitioners and clinical nurse specialists.

   Current Western treatment modalities will be supplemented or replaced with an increasing number of "nontraditional" healing approaches. Chiropractors, acupuncturists, and others will be sought in increasing numbers as individuals make choices based on their healing and spiritual beliefs rather than simply the decision or dictate of a physician focused only on illness.

- Implication #4. Decreased demand for health professionals: New structures will be designed to allow the greatest community involvement in support of promoting health and preventing disease for the greatest numbers of people. The theory and practice of health will come together in community "care" centers where the "nurse" will be increasingly an educated lay worker.

Trend #3: The Deconstruction of Our Mediating Systems Such as Education, Penal, Legal, and Health Care Is Occurring

These structures are organized for their particular function, but also, and perhaps most significantly, to reflect, reproduce, and extend the authority of their respective group. These systems serve to sustain the hierarchical relationships between individuals and their governments; they sustain a country's power structure.

Our country's health-care system has been structured and organized to deliver health care to its citizens while extending a certain influence in which power relationships are maintained between professionals and the clients. These power relationships parallel the expected interactions between the state as ultimate authority and citizen as quintessential object. Here the doctor is the repository of expert knowledge, and all other health-care professionals and the client are supplicant and dependent upon his or her direction and control.

The process of deconstruction will be the most painful trend as the entire spectrum of mediating systems disintegrates. Increasing numbers of community members will experience their relationships with mediating systems as controlling and irrelevant to their lived reality. Communities will not stand by without resorting to violence as they watch their children grow up unfed, illiterate, without basic immunizations for health care, ill prepared for employment or the responsibilities of community participation. As the Los Angeles riot demonstrated, there will be an increase of incidents when city police fire on, gas, or push back angry crowds of disenfranchised and desperate individuals.

Implications for health care: In such disorder lies the potential for a dramatic turnaround through reconstruction. The connections between mediating systems will be made clearer as public discussion emerges about the need for a comprehensive integrated approach to health and human services. The press already carries stories that identify the relationship between a healthy child and literacy, literacy and a future, the future of individuals and the hope of a community.

- Implication #5. Reconstruction of the health-care system: The health-care industry is being offered an opportunity to transform a system that no longer works. The greatest potential lies within the relationships between our national and local communities. Here is where both the need and the possibilities are most immediate. We are being offered a chance to move the best of trends into structures and systems that reinforce and extend the health of our communities. As always, our choices as individuals and as a community will either contribute to the increasing clarity of our connections or sever them further. It is with this public debate that the role of nursing case management is emerging as a solution to the fragmentation that is the hallmark of our current system. Herein lies nursing's agenda for change.

ESTABLISHING A FRAMEWORK FOR CHANGE

Peter Drucker (1989) believes that the next century is already here, and we are well into it. Our current realities are different from the issues that politicians, economists, scholars, businessmen, and union leaders still address in their books and speeches. This is evident by the profound sense of unreality that characterizes much of today's politics and economics.

Some of the major challenges we face are those created by the successes of the past: the success of the welfare state (Walzer, 1990), the success of this century's invention of the fiscal state (Kassiola, 1990), and the success of the knowledge society (Dalton & Kuechler, 1990). Some of our greatest impediments to effectiveness are the slogans, commitments, and the issues of yesterday that still dominate public discourse, still confine our vision as we move forward.

Transformative social change occurs on two levels for success. The social superstructure must address politics and government, economy and economics, and social organizations such as health care and education. A second shift occurs at a more fundamental level—the work view and values that form a belief system and way of ordering the world for individuals, cultures, and societies.

Social Change

Social change in the superstructure of society is essential. The role of government is no longer the only power center in a nation. Local ownership of issues is demonstrated in new "mass movements" with small, highly organized minorities or single-cause units who are totally political. This is moving society from an era of omnipotent government to privatization, whether in Central Europe or the United States. By partnering with self-help and special-interest coalitions around their health-care needs, nursing can assume a powerful advocacy role on behalf of aggregates of clients in local, state, and national arenas where social policy is formulated.

In the economic domain, a shift is also occurring. The government has attempted to change income distribution through the tax system. The original goal was to redistribute income from the rich to the poor. In the twentieth century, we have been spending much larger sums of government money to change the social conditions of the poor with almost uniformly disappointing results. It is becoming clear the government cannot effectively change the distribution of incomes.

We must learn once again to limit the government's ability to raise taxes. We must budget with available resources, denying ourselves and others of some "entitled" goods and services. Unless politicians learn to make the hard decisions, even though they are risky, we are in a perilous economic state. This tension between health-care entitlements and business spending on health-care benefits is a **major** issue in the current health-care debate. The economics of health-care financing are driving much of the federal activity surrounding health-care reform. Thus it is imperative for nursing to demonstrate and articulate—with story and data—the fiscal impact of nursing case management on the efficient and effective use of health-care resources.

Special and business organizations are also at this critical juncture as we evaluate the concept of work and its place in society. Our present conceptions about work emerged in an era when one had a single job with one institution throughout one's career. The technological and information explosion has facilitated change of such magnitude that most professionals will hold several jobs throughout their careers. This requires a flexible world view and the capacity to learn new skills continuously to interface with this changing world. Displaced health-care workers will be a reality in the twenty-first century. It is imperative that nursing continue to develop community-based services while designing ways for nurses with a strong institutional focus to retool their skills and abilities to work effectively in these new settings. This change must include a stronger focus on health promotion and health maintenance competencies. Further, planning career strategies across the professional's lifespan in changing work environments must become part of every nurse's mindset.

There is growing admission in the U.S that the long-term future of an industrial society is characterized by chronic unemployment and underemployment (working less than full capacity). Two reasons for this possibility emerge: (1) economic growth may not generate enough jobs to encompass the growing work force; and (2) the quality of available jobs may not be compatible with the rising educational levels of the work force. This is a major source of alienation with resultant workplace problems. Increasingly sophisticated technology and economic constraints will facilitate the replacement of expensive professional workers with less skilled, highly trained technicians. This will comprise much of the health-care labor force in the twenty-first century. Nursing must learn to work with and through a changing mix of health-care providers in a way that maximizes both quality and productivity. Further, we must develop skills in empowering clients, multiskilled technicians and lay community members to assume a substantial role in health maintenance activities within their community. If we cannot move to this stance, others will replace us who can.

Shifts of Fundamental Values and World View

A second major shift in fundamental values and world view is essential if we are to move successfully into the twenty-first century. What if society advances technologically until all goods and services needed can be produced and offered with ease by using a small fraction of the population? In our current paradigm of "work to eat, the fortunate may work, whereas the remainder will be kept as pets—supported with little more demanded of them than that they be housebroken" (Roszak, 1978). The assumption that income distributions should be linked strongly to jobs in the mainline economy needs to be reassessed.

Based on new values that transcend consumption and competition, in a technologically advanced society where production of goods and services can be handled with ease, employment may exist primarily for self-development and is only secondarily concerned with production of goods and services. Nursing has always been focused on "quality-of-life" issues; therefore, it is appropriate that this profession enlarge the current debate on teaching-learning organizations to include the concept of a "learning society" (Table 4-2).

A "learning society" implies reversal of a number of aspects of the long-term industrialized trends. The occupational focus of most people is learning and developing in the broadest sense. Diverse activities would include formal education, exploration, self-discovery, reflective thinking, ecological stewardship, assuming various specialized roles, and participation in the community of concerned citizens to create a better future. These activities would contribute to human betterment and fulfillment, being humane, nonpolluting and nonstultifying.

This strategy would involve "intermediate technology" (Schumaker, 1974). The United States and, more specifically, the health profession would utilize technology that is resource conserving, environmentally benign, frugal in the use of energy, relatively labor-intensive and understandable, and usable at the individual or community level. Such technology would complement a strong ecological ethic; strong identifi-

TABLE 4-2   Attributes of a learning society

Role component	Technology	Outcomes
Formal education	Reflective thinking	Human fulfillment
Exploration/ discovery	Nature connection	Human betterment
Changing roles	Creative flexibility	Nonstultifying work
Ecological mindset	Voluntary frugality	Nonpolluting lifestyle
Community steward	Volunteerism/ activism	Being humane
Simple lifestyle	Healthy living	Honor future generations

cation with nature, fellow human beings, and future generations; a lifestyle characterized by voluntary frugality and adaptability, appreciation of the simple life and simple virtues; and the kind of work that fosters these attitudes.

These concepts are already emerging in some of the case management practices in our country. We must accentuate them in our work and name them in the dialogue that surrounds it. These elements must now become an intricate component in our redefinition of "health." We must expand beyond mere physical, psychological, and emotional health to a collective view of health as ecologically and socially based as well.

As a growing group of people perceive the interconnections among principles of ecological wisdom, sustainable peace, an economy with a future, and participatory democracy, a national and global health agenda may have a chance to come alive. Such an agenda includes emphasis on a holistic view, ecological awareness, ending the nuclear arms race, decentralization of power and control, human-scale technologies and enterprises, feminine perspective, transmaterialist beliefs, social responsibility, nonviolent change, and the empowerment of people. There is a keen awareness of the destructive aspects of patriarchal industrial society with its specialization and bureaucratization, as well as its masculine competitive, aggressive, and exploitative values. Global health will emerge only if economic and political activities embrace values with an emphasis on self-realization and inner growth leading to wisdom (Devall & Session, 1985).

We are most reluctant to recognize how powerfully the world's belief systems, including our own, lock us into a death march toward the future. Collectively held unconscious beliefs shape the world's institutions and are at the root of oppression and inequity. Nevertheless, by deliberately changing the internal image of reality, people can change the world.

STRATEGIES FOR CHANGE

Substantial and lasting change of this magnitude requires a coordinated, multilevel strategy with attention to the internal and external environments affected by the change. Skills in leadership and communication plus a compelling vision must be coupled with a comprehensive strategic plan to reach the desired results. These changes call for all professional nursing organizations to examine their work and the processes that support it. In a review of mission and goals, we must discern nursing's "common ground" to shape a unified response to opportunities and challenges posed by health-care reform.

The Tri-council represents organized nursing from a national perspective. It is comprised of the National League for Nursing (NLN) representing nursing education, the American Association of Colleges of Nursing (AACN) representing advanced nursing education, the American Organization of Nurse Executives (AONE) representing nursing administrative practice, and the American Nurses Association (ANA) representing professional nursing practice. These organizations are challenged to identify and express nursing's common ground from a global perspective to the various constituencies that nursing serves. Several core questions must be addressed if this common ground is to be established.

What Is Nursing?

The first task facing organized nursing is the redefinition of our work in a changing world. The ANA has revised the Social Policy Statement for Nursing which defines the scope of the work. AONE created a document entitled "Nursing's Role in a Restructured Environment" as a working document for nurse executives charged with responsibility for the redesign of care delivery systems. AACN is carefully examining the role and responsibilities of advanced practice nursing, while NLN is creating a curriculum revolution.

AONE has partnered with AACN in a project to define competencies across the continuum of care by studying the work of practicing nurses. Funded by a grant from the Robert Wood Johnson Foundation, a group representing leadership from across the continuum of care (acute, long term, community) and the collective nursing education spectrum (AD, BS, MS, PhD) has examined nursing resource needs in a changing health-care scene. Transcending the focus on one set of competencies for all practitioners, the concept of differentiated practice provided the foundation for this work. The roles and responsibilities of nurses with varying levels of education, placed at strategic positions on the care continuum, unified by a shared set of core values (nursing's common ground), are being lifted from the actual work of nurses within the field.

The role of advanced practice nursing in case management is a pivotal piece of the evolving profession. Reexamination of the traditional clinical nurse specialist (CNS) role as well as the current nurse practitioner (NP) role is part of the restructuring effort. Does the profession still need both, or is a hybrid composed of the best of both an evolutionary step in the profession's metamorphosis? How does advanced practice relate to the traditional AD and BS nursing roles? Where and how do the differing roles of nursing articulate to maximize the health outcomes for clients whom we are privileged to serve? A new definition of nursing must build on and celebrate our unique roles as well as our collective contribution. We must realign the "community of nursing" within the changing and increasingly complex and diverse communities we serve.

Who Are Nursing's Partners?

Nursing does not work in a vacuum, but rather, within a larger network of health-care professionals. We must also find our common ground with our professional colleagues in other fields, incorporating our shared agenda into nursing's total agenda. The PEW Foundation established an interdisciplinary commission to consider the competencies needed by health practitioners of the future. These competencies call for expanded skills and new attitudes appropriate for every health profession, allied health, dentistry, medicine, nursing, pharmacy, public health, and veterinary medicine (PEW 1991: 17-26).

The identified set of tasks and values reflects the agenda for health-care reform shared by all professional groups, including nursing. It is time for nursing—and all other disciplines—to transcend the notion of autonomy (thinking and acting for one's self in matters of opinion, conduct, etc. without being subject to external constraint or authority), moving to a higher level value of interdependence (seeing and acting on the awareness that personal and interinstitutional cooperation is always preferable to individual decision making)(Hall, 1986).

If true interdependence in health care is to be achieved, new education and practice patterns that are collaborative and integrative must be designed for current practitioners as well as those entering health education programs today. Change of this magnitude must include new visions and behaviors within leadership groups, redefinition and redesign of the work within the service industry, as well as curriculum and educational strategies within the schools. These changes must be supported by appropriate adjustments in policy at federal, state, institutional, and professional group levels. Most importantly, the public must be given more authority and accountability for their own health practices through appropriate education and partnership models.

To truly embrace the notion of interdependence requires the death of the old patriarchal mindset. Nowhere is this issue more prevalent than the nurse-physician interface. As nursing case management continues to evolve, the debate between physician and "mid-level practitioner" is escalating. Some nurses and some physicians confuse the issue by saying "I can do anything you can do . . ." in a competitive spirit. Professionals, however, who are clear on the unique contribution each role holds for the total needs of the client work in a *partnership model*. They clarify the specific role of medicine and nursing, create a middle-

ground for shared responsibilities designed and executed through collaboration, and evaluate outcomes with the consumer.⁴

Moving to interdependence is noisy business. As advanced practice models continue to evolve, the debate between nursing and medicine intensifies. The American Medical Association (AMA) created Report 35 (I-93) entitled "Economic and Quality of Care Issues with Implications on Scopes of Practice—Physicians and Nurses" to address the growing wave of advanced practice nurses. Rather than responding to accusations from the AMA with angry justification comments, AONE created a "talking points document" (Appendix A) that lifts up the major facts about advanced practice nurses. This document was sent to all nurse executives in the country to assist nurses in articulating the facts of the issue with one clear voice. Nurse managers and advanced practice nurses alike in many major health-care organizations received copies of this document and were encouraged to educate physician colleagues on the truth of advanced practice without engaging in the emotional accusations being lifted by some practitioners on either side of the issue.

This debate released medicine's concern and skepticism about the efficacy and legitimacy of advanced practice nursing. It also raised some of the "dark side" of the advanced practice issue. Nursing must address the formal education of advanced practice nurses and more clearly define the parameters of practice for this domain. We must join forces in legalizing (as in Nurse Practice Act language) this evolving role. Also, we must collaboratively formulate strategies for direct reimbursement. Finally, we must strive to establish our evolving case management models in a spirit of cooperation—with the client as central—rather than continue the competitive model of doctor versus nurse, with both controlling the client's care. We can, and must, use the energy generated by this current RN-MD debate as a wonderful vehicle to facilitate the work of healing with and on behalf of the public.

Dialogue and debate of this nature is not new, nor need it be destructive. Nursing must come to embrace the notion that conflict is the *key* to releasing intellectual capital. In fact, it is the root of a conflict that holds the prototype for new order. When we are able to equip ourselves with quality information and assist others to enlarge their understanding of an issue, an expanding answer to the root issue may be found. National nursing organizations must help professionals at the grassroots level engage in meaningful debate by providing accurate information to them in a timely fashion. When the same facts are raised by nurses throughout the country, a common voice will be heard . . . and the clarification of nursing's work will emerge.

What Systems Will Nursing Co-Design and Work In?

The current activities of finding common ground and building new delivery systems around the unique services various agencies offer are changing the health-care scene significantly for individuals and communities. These integrated system networks are based on commitment as a service organization, focusing on the emerging needs of a changing society. Another hallmark of the new systems is a creative focus on new partnerships—partnerships among service agencies, partnerships among clinical care providers, and partnerships with individual clients, families, and communities.

Professional schools are facing the same challenges within the services they provide. They must reexamine their core curriculum, looking at both content and context. The focus must shift from a process orientation to one based on outcomes; the introduction to outcomes-based practice and management is vitally needed in this new era. Finally, they must redesign the teaching-learning process in a manner that facilitates teamwork, partnership, and a collaborative mind set. This will assure the orientation and socialization of a health-care professional who possesses the competencies to facilitate interdependence with the client and community as core.

All providers must engage in a major shift from focusing only on the individual to identifying the aggregate—the community, the country, the world. We must redefine health to include ecological and social health as well as the traditional biopsychosocial and spiritual model. Further, we must include economic health indicators if a holistic, quality life is to be maintained by individuals, institutions, business, and the community.

Health care and education are increasingly being held accountable for outcomes achieved and resources utilized. Information-based decisions can only be achieved with adequate technological support from well-developed information systems. Nursing case management must demonstrate, through data and story, the quality and economic impact of its unique contribution to health care. Multiple sources of data should be developed, along with mechanisms that lead to creatively innovative responses for issues identified from the information obtained.

Although service and education are vital to the overall change process, public policies must be designed that encourage change and reinforce the changing focus on the public's health. Federal and state agencies have a unique opportunity to develop policy and funding sources for health education and health services. These policies must focus resources on plans and programs based on comprehensive, collaborative models between education, service, and the public sector. Nurses must facilitate the development of consumer coalitions and small self-help groups as effective ways to influence the direction that policy will take at the state and local levels. At a recent Consumer Summit held in Washington, D.C. (February, 1994), an articulate consumer stated:

> Nurses, for so long you have been standing at our bedside, advocating for us as individuals when the doctor would come by. You helped us frame questions, seek advice, present our concerns and demands relating to our needs. Where are you now . . . when will you stand with us in the halls of political debate? Why aren't you standing beside us, advocating for the collective with the same clear voice? We need you to explain to various funding sources that as a diabetic I can get reimbursed for the amputation of my leg, and yet I can't get reimbursed to acquire the education on how to prevent my leg from becoming diseased in the first place. . . . Come, stand along side us in the arenas of policy debate.

We must develop professional coalitions that consist of major nursing organizations at the state level to lobby locally as well as in Washington, D.C., on nursing and public health issues. Nurses need to become involved in policy efforts at all levels of government, based on our unified vision for health care, emerging from changing client and community needs.

What Values Will Guide Our Collective Work?

As we move forward with health-care reform, the work must be based on core values that maintain the integrity of our commitment to the public whom we are privileged to serve. Values are the priorities by which we live, through which we select our information, and from which we shape our consciousness. Specifically, they are the priorities upon which we act. Socialization is a process used to gain knowledge, skills, and behaviors to participate as a member of a particular group. Professional socialization is primarily a subconscious process through which an occupational identity is gained and values and norms of a profession are internalized (Pardue, 1987).

Professional socialization integrates personal and professional values into a unified whole, fostering the following outcomes pertinent to nursing (AACN, 1986; Rath, Harman & Simon, 1986):

1. A linkage between the individual's motivation for entering nursing and the development of professional behaviors;
2. A common nursing perspective and related critical-thinking and problem-solving skills;
3. A mastery of knowledge, skills, and competencies that are core to the profession;
4. An internalization of the values, traditions, and obligations of the profession; and

5. An identification with and commitment to the profession.

A multitude of factors affect the socialization outcome of nurses, including the educational institution they attend; beliefs, values, and role modeling of the faculty; classmates and professional colleagues; family and friends; other health care professionals; clients and the general public (Blatchley & Stephan, 1984; Whelan, 1984).

Core nursing values have been based on looking through the lens of the experience of being human. The physical, social, mental, and spiritual dimensions of existence are of equal value and interdependent. Values surrounding the physical dimension of being focus on continuity of life, balance of body functions, and fulfillment of physical needs (Rattikainen, 1989). Mental dimensions include values related to personality, human growth and development, and human dignity. These values are demonstrated through maintaining a unique perspective on the client and assisting the individual with the right of self-determination. Respect for human dignity, for religious conviction, and satisfaction of spiritual needs addresses the spiritual dimension of humankind (Bandman & Bandman, 1985). Valuable aspects of sociability include independence, community membership, ability to cope, close harmonious human relationships, and self-realization (Davis & Aroskar, 1983).

Nursing has a rich heritage based on these values of caring, sharing, wholeness, and actualization. Our focus has primarily been on the client and family. We are now being called—in the advanced practice role especially—to adapt our decision making and practice styles to work with and respond to an empowered client in an interdependent fashion with other disciplines. Further, our focus on a singular client must be enlarged to a larger aggregate—the community, the ecology, and global health issues.

One of the primary working values within the profession is on the "doing for" aspect of our work. We must increasingly shift our emphasis from the task to the valuing of the critical reflection aspect of our work. This requires us to strengthen our commitment to lifelong learning with a strong intent to deepen our capacity for innovation, analysis, and synthesis. As we learn to extract the "meaning" from experiences and situations, we transform our view of the world and our place in it. We must also strengthen our capacity for "doing with" the client/family/community as *they make informed decisions* regarding quality of life as defined by them from a stance of partnership and support, rather than as expert in control. This empowers *them* to lead their own health-care experience.

We must also learn to value new relationships with our professional nurse colleagues. No longer viewing ourselves as "the nurse," but rather as "a nurse within the nursing community," we mutually come to value and appreciate the unique contribution other nursing colleagues within the discipline bring to the unique client situation we face. Extended further into the field, we seek collaborative relationships with medicine, pharmacy, dietary, and therapy partners who bring a focus and depth in related areas we do not have. Only when we truly value the unique contribution of others to the "whole" of the situation, can we partner effectively in true interdependence around the complex health-care issues facing clients today.

Our traditional values surrounding health have fostered activities focused on efforts to eliminate physical disease processes. Evolving holistic values call for activities that assist clients in defining health as a way of life—the way in which they define quality of life for themselves. Thus, they can be "healthy" in the midst of a chronic or terminal illness. This redefinition of health extends into our relationship to and responsibility for nature and the ecology. It views social issues such as poverty, homelessness, and violence as health problems and reconnects us to the broader universe in substantial ways beyond eradicating physical manifestation of illness. Our social responsibility as healers becomes profoundly enlarged.

Finally, we must value the notion of change itself. Rather than viewing it as a destructive force, we must see and embrace the opportunity that lies in adversity and chaos as an invitation to creation of new order. It is in the wild ferment of ambivalence and uncertainty that the seeds for new growth and development lie. This era in history offers nursing the opportunity to rescript our reality, strengthening the things that are important to the profession while tossing aside patterns, attitudes, and behaviors that have not served us well in the past. We must move from patterns of victimization and distrust to those that truly value and embrace the risk-taker, innovator, and creator who lie hidden within each soul free to trust its own essence.

Nursing Leadership Is Essential

Strong, visionary, innovative leadership, speaking with a clear voice, is essential if radical, life-giving change is to be accomplished. Leadership is a responsibility for every administrator, department manager, faculty person, and professional within the evolving health systems. Employing organizations as well as professional organizations must assist currently practicing leaders to acquire the prerequisite skills needed in these changing times. Further, it is the responsibility of people in leadership positions aggressively to seek ways to acquire information, education, and experiences that will strengthen their capacity to lead into arenas yet to be developed. Such a professional commitment is essential if nursing is to be viewed as a major player in the health reform debate. To that end, professional associations must commit their time and energy to ensuring the facilitation and support of leadership development for all nursing professionals.

Professional associations play important roles in determining the unfolding of new systems, as well as how members, old and new, are responding to them. The leaders and working agenda of these organizations must be focused on contemporary issues from a futuristic stance with a collaborative focus to stretch the imagination and set of possibilities for the membership which is caught in its current, pressing reality.

Accreditation processes must fully embrace the competencies emerging in a changing health-care system. Advanced nursing practice must be assured its autonomy to act in response to changing needs of the public it serves if its place in health-care reform is to be assured. Certification programs must be designed in a way that ensures that current practitioners understand the emerging changes in the health-care system, developing required skill to remain competent.

It is **critical** that national leadership understands the issues and the context in which they are nested, so nursing's unique contribution to health care can be articulated clearly to all of the public involved in health-care reform. Information and strategies designed on behalf of the profession must be based on outcome data rather than individual opinion. Publications to the membership must contain accurate information so that the professionals within the group can make appropriate life-giving career decisions.

CONCLUSION

Finally, if nursing is going to speak with one voice, unifying tools for change must be made available to the membership. A shared agenda for action, talking points papers on specific issues sent to membership in a timely fashion, monographs, prototype models, accurate aggregate data on shared work of nursing, guidelines on regulations and professional standards are all mechanisms that can maintain quality while providing synergy to the collective work of nursing. Facilitating the rich work of transformation based on our common ground is the call for organized nursing's response to health-care reform.

REFERENCES

American Association of Colleges of Nursing. (1986). *Essentials of college and university education for professional nurses.* Washington, DC: Author.

American Medical Association (AMA). (1993). Report 35 (I-93) Economic and quality care issues with implications on scopes of practice-physicians and nurses. Report of the Board of the Trustees: Author.

Bandman, E., & Bandman, B. (1983). *Bioethics and human rights.* Boston: Little Brown.

Blatchley, M. E., & Stephan, E. (1984). RN students in generic programs: What to do with them? *Journal of Nursing Education,* 23 (8), 351-352.

Blendon, R., et al. (1990). DataWatch. Satisfaction with health systems in ten nations. *Health Affairs,* Summer:185-192.

Dalton, R., & Kuechler, M. (1990) *Challenging the political order: New social and political movements in Western democracies.* New York: Bantam Books.

Davis, A. J., & Aroskar, M. A. (1983). *Ethical dilemmas and nursing practice.* Norwalk, VA: Appleton-Century-Crofts.

Devall, B., & Sessions, G. (1985). *Deep ecology: Living as if nature mattered.* Boston: Peregrine Smity.

Drucker, P. (1989). *The new realities: In government and politics/in economics and business/in society and world view.* New York: Harper & Row.

Hall, B. P. (1986). *The Genesis effect: Personal and organizational transformation.* New York, NY: Paulist Press.

Hardison, O. B. (1989). *Disappearing through the skylight: Culture and technology in the twentieth century.* New York: Viking Press.

Harman, W. (1988). *Global mind change: The promises of the last years of the twentieth century.* Indianapolis, IN: Knowledge Systems, Inc.

Kassiola, J. J. (1990). *The depth of industrial civilization.* Ithaca, NY: State University of New York Press.

Lawday, D. (1991). Europe: My country, right or what? *The Atlantic,* 286 (1), 22-26.

Miligrand, R. (1990). *Divided societies: Struggles in contemporary capitalism.* New York: Oxford University Press.

Pardue, S. (1987). Decision making skills and critical thinking, ability among associate degree, diploma, baccalaureate and masters-prepared nurses. *Journal of Nursing Education,* 26 (9), 354-361.

PEW Health Professions Commission. (1991). *Healthy America: Practitioners for 2005.* Durham, NC: Duke University Medical Center.

Rath, L., Harman, M., & Simon, S. (1986). *Values and teaching.* Columbus, OH: Merrill.

Rattikainen, R. (1989). Values and ethical principles in nursing. *Journal of Advanced Nursing,* 14, 92-96.

Reich, R. (1987). *Tales of a new America.* New York: Time Books.

Roszak, T. (1978). *Person-planet: The creative disintegration of individual society.* New York: Anchor/Doubleday.

Schumaker, E. F. (1974). *Small is beautiful: Economics as if people mattered.* Boston: Abacus.

Shaw, G. B. (1984). *The doctor's dilemma.* Baltimore, MD: Penguin Books.

Walzer, M. (1990). *The company of critics: Social criticism and political commitment in the twentieth century.* New York: Basic Books.

Whelan, E. G. (1984). Role-orientation change among RNs in an upper division level baccalaureate program. *Journal of Nursing Education,* 23 (4), 151.

Talking Points Document Exemplar

American Organization of Nurse Executives

TALKING POINTS IN RESPONSE TO REPORT 35 (I-93) OF THE AMERICAN MEDICAL ASSOCIATION:"ECONOMIC AND QUALITY-OF-CARE ISSUES WITH IMPLICATIONS ON SCOPES OF PRACTICE—PHYSICIANS AND NURSES"

GENERAL FACTS ABOUT NURSING PRACTICE

- Nursing care has traditionally focused on a wellness, prevention-oriented, holistic model of care. In contrast, the medical model of care is one of disease treatment and symptom alleviation. Nursing's historical and continuing framework for health care is consistent with the goals of health-care reform.
- Nursing practice has three role components:
  1. A contingent component which requires physician authorization for treatment;
  2. An independent component which focuses on nursing interventions for health conditions;
  3. A role as integrator and coordinator of client care, across the lifespan of individuals, as well as across settings and among health-care providers.
- The majority of services performed by registered nurses are performed independent of physician supervision. In some instances, physician signature may be required to initiate or validate a service; yet the service itself is delivered separately from and without supervision of a physician.
- Nurses are independently licensed and accountable for their actions. Most of the services furnished by nurses are performed based on their own licensure and scope of practice.
- Nurses believe that collaboration among caregivers is a foundation of sound, responsible, and responsive client care. Nurses do collaborate with physicians and other health-care providers, as appropriate. However, collaboration does *not* mean supervision.
- Advanced practice nurses (APNs) are RNs with education and clinical experience beyond the two to four years of basic nursing education. The four types of APNs are nurse practitioners, certified nurse midwives, nurse anesthetists, and clinical nurse specialists.

EDUCATION AND PREPARATION OF APNS

- Since 1992, the American Nurses Credentialing Center of the American Nurses Association has required a master's degree in nursing for all nurse practitioner offers. Clinical nurse specialist certification has always required a master's degree.
- Although there are 26 certifying bodies for nursing, only three credential nurse practitioners. Since 1989, all 26 nurse certifying bodies have worked together to establish common grounds for credentialing, peer review, test development, and other aspects of certification.
- Fourteen (14) states currently allow nurse practitioners to write all prescriptions.
- Seven (7) states allow nurse practitioners to write most prescriptions, with the exception of narcotics and certain other controlled substances.
- Twenty-one (21) states allow nurse practitioners to write prescriptions only under the supervision of a physician.
- Eight (8) states do not allow any prescriptive authority for nurse practitioners.

QUALITY OF CARE

- According to the National Practitioner Data Bank and American Nurses Association claims data, APNs and nurses in general have a low rate of malpractice claims.
- As a matter of licensure and liability for their own services, APNs are held accountable for delivering care safely and responsibly, just as physicians are.

REIMBURSEMENT

- In rural areas, nurse practitioners and clinical nurse specialists are generally reimbursed for services at 85% of physician rates. These services need not be delivered "incident to" physician services. "Incident to" services are reimbursed by paying the physician at the rate of 100%.
- In all areas, certified nurse midwives are reimbursed at 65% of physician rate.
- Medical payment is determined state by state and is often at 100% of the physician rate.

CONSUMER CONFIDENCE

- An independent opinion survey by political pollster Peter Hart (1990) found that the general public respects nurses more than any other health care provider—70% for nurses and 12% for physicians.
- According to a recent Gallop poll, 86% of Americans are willing to receive their every day health-care services from an advanced practice nurse.
- Nurses believe that consumer satisfaction is a valid measure of quality of care.
- Consumer dissatisfaction with health care reflects consumer desire to have care that supports their needs, priorities, and expectations. AONE believes that it is essential for consumers to be involved in health-care planning and policy development, as well as to be responsible decision-making partners in the delivery of services.

Part Two

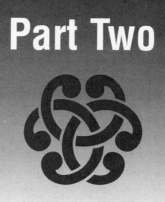

CREATING A FOUNDATION FOR CHANGE

Key elements of case management constitute a value-oriented approach to improving both health care and educational systems.

Mary Mundt

Part Two shifts attention from broad issues of systems change to the foundations or underpinnings for transformation. Several authors describe elements of education, practice, and research that form the supporting structures for change. Chapters 5 through 9 address the role of education in preparing practitioners to become part of a redesigned health-care system. These chapters question the readiness of educational institutions to change rapidly in response to the dramatic shifts in health-care structures. Elements of nurse case management that could be infused into today's curricula are identified.

Chapters 10 through 12 take the lessons learned in the previous chapters and apply the principles and values of nurse case management to developing community nursing centers, coordinating care across the health/illlness continuum, and creating innovative health-care delivery systems.

Chapter 5

Academia's Involvement in Health-Care Redesign

Sheila A. Ryan, PhD, RN, FAAN

OVERVIEW

Nurses in academic health centers are uniquely qualified to identify challenges and opportunities in a managed care environment.

Academic health centers' response to rapid and profound changes of health-care reform will succeed with strong leadership, advanced information systems, clinical integration with an integrated governance structure, and shared financial risks. Success will be measured with financial and clinical accountability for health outcomes for a defined population. Survival strategies include enhanced decision-making capacity, increasing primary-care capacity, reducing costs, participating in integrating care networks, and accepting as much financial risk as possible. Managed care is here to stay, as are the rapidity of change, the domination of local markets, and the important presence of the academic health center. Self-reliance and competition to be the first and the best will be replaced with determination for interdependence.

We are living in a watershed era in the history of humankind, in a period of renaissance and rebirth. We daily experience the irrelevance of current models and systems to the issues pressuring us. We are called to "let go" of our present reality to create a more relevant role in the emerging new order (Koerner & McWhinney, 1994). Such transformation of ourselves, our professions, our health delivery systems, and our academic health centers of higher education are based on unique collections of values and beliefs, attitudes or assumptions that create individual reality by the meaning we ascribe to our lived experience. Meaning exists within ourselves rather than in external forms such as books or experts (Adams, 1984). "However

sufficient the Academic Health Center's effort in the past, the world of academic health centers is so diverse, so poorly understood, under so much pressure to change, and so heavily criticized . . ." some assessment and codification is warranted (Association of Academic Health Center, 1994).

Many academic health centers are feeling imperiled by health-care reform. Growth of managed care threatens client bases, income, and even the teaching and research enterprises; however, opportunities abound. What does health-care reform mean to existing health-care organizations and providers? Although pressures to reduce costs and provide quality care continue, health-care reform will mean new and expanded services, care site expansion and compression, new competition and new partners, new methods for delivering and managing care, new clinical roles and relationships, and new decision support and information systems. The Institute of Medicine recently addressed three fundamental quality-of-care issues that must be addressed in a reformed health-care system: use of unnecessary or inappropriate care; underuse of needed, effective, and appropriate care; and shortcomings in technical and interpersonal care. Clearly, there is an urgent and timely opportunity for academic health centers to provide the leadership in preparing the future health professionals to practice in these reformed systems (IOM, 1994).

A system's performance depends on the quality of its parts, how well the parts fit and work together, and how well the system is aligned with its environment, as a subsystem of its community. The academic health center will be guided by a population-health perspective for research, education, and professional services that are community responsive within efficient, interdependent delivery systems.

Academic health centers must determine this preferred future, adopt an anticipatory management style, ensure customer satisfaction, foster an environment for risk-taking and develop a global outlook (Valberg et al., 1994). Strategic planning will involve mergers, practice plans, primary care, and information systems. In other words, purposes must evolve to include new emphasis on how to organize and work with communities to address the public health needs of their communities. Academic health centers must be concerned with reducing fragmentation and improving continuity of care systems. Reliable measures of quality and effective care outcomes should be the prerogative of health center scientists. Tertiary care centers must eliminate excess costs associated with teaching and research and high-tech, specialized practice to compete effectively with lower cost community-based managed care systems.

Further, academic health centers need organizational structures and mechanisms that encompass collegial, participatory governance, and management with clear lines of authority. Responsibility and accountability to promote an array of strategic alliances and partnerships with research institutes, health-care agencies and organizations in the private sector will be essential. Promoting economic development and systems' knowledge and understanding must be emphasized for all health professions working interdependently. Change will be insignificant until academic "preventive" professionals develop links to clinical practice to bridge the gap between population perspectives of public health and the individual orientation of traditional inpatient clinical

health care. Practice sites must also deliver large volume primary care, have a definable population with accountability for improving health status, and a delivery model that focuses on integration, efficiency, and outcomes. Academic health centers must have students participate in such settings, whether owned or not.

EDUCATION

Developing a population perspective requires reorientation and shifting emphasis from sickness to health, reducing illness, disability and premature death, while improving health status of the population. This development will require more attention to the determinants of health:

- Family
- Community
- Human biology
- Psychosocial, economic, and physical environment
- Work
- Behavior
- Lifestyle

Population perspectives must be taught through practice opportunities such as aggregate teen pregnancy prevention or group exercises for those with severe chronic multiple sclerosis. One-on-one interventions and assessments will reduce with more group work.

Future health professional roles will include advocate, learner, collaborator, coach, and resource manager of groups and other care providers. Boundaries of responsibility and role sharing will need to be clarified between health professionals and measured for outcome effectiveness. Establishing a population perspective in the curriculum will require experience for health professionals in the delivery of programs and services that will also require faculty development and interdisciplinary sites of practice and teaching.

Competencies required of all health professionals in the future include:

- Critical thinking
- Flexibility
- Relational skills for collaborative team practice and working with auxiliary personnel
- Resource utilization skills
- Information management skills
- Deep sensitivity for cultural diversity (O'Neil, 1993)

Community health and systems orientation will become the foundation for all curriculums. In general, curriculum content about diseases will be consolidated as efficiencies will be sought. Further, information systems will provide ready, rapid, and in-depth on-site information access to the knowledgeable workers that our future health professionals will become (Drucker, 1994).

Balancing clinical experiences in primary care, acute care, long-term care, and home care will be augmented by occupational health and risk management experiences. The basic placement sites for teaching ambulatory, preventive, and health-promotional care include:

- Clients' homes
- Physicians' offices
- School-based clinics
- Church basements
- Corporate health settings
- Health-service organizations
- Long-term care settings
- Nursing homes
- Home health agencies

Another important educational mission of the academic health center is continuing education to help professionals prepare for role and knowledge and skill transitions with these changes.

RESEARCH

Research is an integral role for the academic health center and should in no way be diminished. Nevertheless, shifts in goals and program objectives toward population health are necessary. Expansion of health-services research, population health, clinical epidemiology, quality and outcomes effectiveness research, cost-benefit analysis and information systems research (Genel, 1994) should not be at the expense of the bio-medical research enterprise. Academic centers have an opportunity, however, to become their community voice for the indices of quality, effectiveness, and status indicators.

Limited resources will necessitate managing the boundaries of the entire research enterprise, changing the conditions of faculty promotion, and protecting time for both aspects of research. It is crucial that critical inquiry—so essential for quality care and continuous improvement of both client and group services and professional education—not be compromised.

Systemic issues impede a natural growth in clinical research. Flat discretionary budgets are imposed with recent federal legislation. Increasing bioethical controversies add to the polarization of an already diminished public trust. Decaying infrastructures add internal pressures to compete for indirect cost recovery. Popular congressional mandates such as AIDS and gender-based research, although necessary, add to the micromanagement and increasing pressures on a diminishing resource base. Health-system reform emphasizes bottom-line efficiencies and cost controls. Cross-subsidization will be cau-

tiously and perhaps only specifically allowed. Pressure to produce increased faculty practice revenue further reduces the time and support for research. Faculty training especially for the health services and clinical outcomes research is in need of some bolstering.

PRACTICE

Providing professional services with the participation of students is an essential part of the educational mission. Developing multidisciplinary learning opportunities to enhance client and community care must be a top priority for academic health centers to prepare for the future. Integrated delivery system structures are the focus of much of today's strategic attention (Moore, et al., 1994). Affiliation agreements must extend beyond the traditional hospital settings and include consortium networks of many new partners from both public and private sectors. Such aggregate social contracts among institutions require common decision making, but authority remains with the home institution. Some authority and control must be ceded in this model and combined with generous mutual respect, trust, and desire to collaborate.

Several other models of governance evolving from the changes in health care include federation models, affiliation models, and corporate or holding company models. Regardless of the choice of the model, or its implementation, the integration of clients across settings, their services and their information, seeks to reveal the efficiencies sought by managed care corporations. The importance of any structural governance models must be rooted in relation to the community-based structures for management of services at the local and state levels.

Strengthening cooperations and collaboration among academic health centers at the regional and national levels can assist in the development of social contracts to meet societal needs while avoiding costly competition through shared resources. Use of information technology and new teaching pedagogies can allow for national and regional monitoring of learning requirements while providing students with realistic and valuable consultation from a distance. Instead of duplicating all faculty resources at each site, pools of the best qualified faculty in the areas of oncology, epidemiology or informatics, for example, could be made available by national networking.

BARRIERS

Barriers to change within academic health centers require examination of several internal and external factors. Academic institutions are limited with organizational inflexibility. Stability over time has been an academic value that now makes for difficulty in aligning with different organizations or employer goals. Such institutions demand many substantial non-value behaviors attached to inadequate systems of information, cost analysis, support, inadequate facilities and rigid compensation incentives, all at a time with limited resources, vision, and risk-taking ability.

Universities are concerned about innovation and enhancing recognition, yet their structures and systems have not allowed for much innovation within their own systems. This experience will be difficult to undo. It is safe to conclude that just as health delivery is engaging in managed care systems to reduce excess costs and produce targeted, effective outcomes of quality of care, so too will education and research enterprises need to be better managed in the future. Targeted areas of excellence (planned in concert with the needs and participation of local communities and customers) for both research priorities and educational endeavors will guide these changes for efficiency, cost controls, and quality outcomes responsive to our public's.

Success will be found with strong leadership, advanced information systems, clinical integration with an integrated governance structure, and shared financial risks. Success will be measured with financial and clinical accountability for health outcomes for a defined population. Survival strategies include:

- Enhanced decision-making capacity
- Increasing primary-care capacity
- Reducing costs
- Participating in integrating care networks
- Accepting as much financial risk as possible

Managed care is here to stay as is the rapidity of change, the domination of local markets, and the important presence of the academic health center. Self-reliance and competition to be the first and the best will be replaced with determination for interdependence.

CHANGE: EVOLUTION OR TRANSFORMATION

Transformation can follow two relevant paths in response to present world crises. One is a path of unfolding, of transcending limitations through practice to develop new patterns; the other is one of renaissance, of "letting go and taking up" requiring radical movements rather than the more quiet process of evolving. Transformation can follow a disciplined, clearly outlined journey toward a known by opening new views, new experiences, new patterns. Such boundary-breaking transcendence provides one with a broader world view with each spiral-like ascendance, from conservative to radical, from inner to outer, or from opposite sides of a perspective. The process is incremental with cumulative gain at each step along the way (Koerner & McWhinney, 1994).

The other path is experienced as abrupt and radical, an explosion in current reality with no clear new way (Prigogine & Stengers, 1994). Profound crises often reveal that old patterns no longer serve well. Such journeys are required in response to an evolving new reality. These challenges are painful callings to question deeply held values and beliefs that threaten our very sense of self. It involves difficult negotiation, compromise, stalling, backsliding, self-deception, and failure. More than intellectual understanding of the need to change, such transformation requires emotional strength and will to move forward over sustained periods of time. Often transformation begins with a flash; integrating new beliefs into established patterns of thinking and performing takes time (McWhinney, 1992).

Although seemingly different in nature, both paths require similar processes and reflect universal phenomena. Put simply, humanity has always existed in a state of transformation. To understand what is involved in managing change, one must grasp the level and complexity of the change desired. First-order change calls for pattern reformulation but no change in meaning or context. Second-order change calls for creation or change of the context. Reality and thought patterns are reconstructed, such as community as client, partnership versus competition. Third-order change requires thinking beyond current logic leading to a transcending world view where dichotomies are replaced with holistic unity to the system (Land, 1973). An example might be the redefinition of health as the quality of life as defined by clients who assume mutual accountability for their health status. Transformation results in the emergence of a new order such as a transformed view of health as the inclusion and merging of Eastern and Western belief systems regarding health. True transformation is a metaphysical shift of deep nature, with profound and life-long changes occurring which no amount of pressure can reverse.

Such a model of change can be prescriptive to academic health centers in their shift to change. Perhaps all orders of change must be journeyed; some settings will be limited by courage, will, and vision and will grow only haltingly. Others will, experience breakthroughs. Academia will be involved in reform; but mostly, it will tend to follow.

CONCLUSION

Academic health centers' response throughout the process of our country's health-care reform is and will continue to be a period of self-discovery. Just as we begin to respond to yet another "state-of-the-art" change for the better, we must prove our strength and stability by responding to an "improved" revision. When frustration abounds, however, it is time to seek the various opportunities presented to us. Our discovery of our purpose and our goals toward better health care for everyone is our strength; and our stability lies in our leadership.

REFERENCES

Association of Academic Health Centers. (1994). Critical data about academic centers: Survey report. Author.

Adams, J. D. (1984). *Transforming work.* Alexandria, VA: Miles River Press.

Drucker, P. (1994, November). The age of social transformation. *The Atlantic Monthly, 274* (5):53-80.

Genel, M. (1994, November). Presentation at National Science and Technology Council, National Academy of Sciences, Washington, DC.

Institute of Medicine Special Initiative (IOM). (1994). *America's health in transition, protecting and improving quality.* Washington, DC: National Academy Press.

Koerner, J., & McWhinney, W. (1994, November). *Transformation.* American Organization of Nurse Executives, Center for Nursing Leadership.

Land, G. T. L. (1973). *Grow or Die.* New York: Dell Press.

McWhinney, W. (1992). *Paths of change: strategic choices for organizations and societies.* Newbury Part, CA: Sage Publications.

Prigogine I., & Stengers I. (1984). *Order out of chaos: man's new dialogue with nature.* New York: Bantam Books.

Moore, G. T., Inui, T. S., Ludden, J. M., & Schoenbaum, S. C. (1994, August). The teaching HMO: a new academic partner. *Academic Medicine*, 8, 69.

O'Neil, E. H. (1993). Health professions education for the future: schools in service to the nation. San Francisco, CA: PEW Health Professions Commission.

Valberg, L. S., Gonyea, M. A., Sinclair, D. G., & Wade, J., (1994). Planning the future academic medical centre: conceptual framework and financial design. *Canadian Medical Association.*

Chapter 6

Key Elements of Nurse Case Management in Curricula

Mary H. Mundt, PhD, RN

OVERVIEW

Nurses lead educational reform for the health professions by applying concepts from nurse case management.

Successful reform of the health-care system must include reform of health professions education. As the largest group of health-care professionals, nurses are in a key leadership position to initiate the necessary educational changes. This chapter focuses on the values-oriented elements of case management, which include consumer orientation, coordination, outcome orientation, collaboration/cooperation, and resource efficiency. Attention to these elements can improve both the health care and the educational systems by improving the lack of continunity and coordination that has led to criticism of both systems. Restructuring curricula according to the principles of case management can lead to an educational program that teaches individualized client care that is more nurturing, more humanistic, and more holistic.•

HEALTH-CARE AND EDUCATIONAL SYSTEM REFORM

If restructuring of the health-care system is to occur, it must be done in tandem with a restructuring of health professions education. The need for educational reform goes deeper than simply revising the curriculum, offering new courses, and changing the titles of clinical experiences. A new orientation to the concepts of "health" and "caring" is required. The values underlying the current fragmented structure of health care must be examined and replaced with a value structure that supports coordinated and comprehensive client-centered care.

The need for significant reform of health professions education comes at a time when institutions of higher education, much like health-care institutions, have come under severe criticism. In fact, the criticism of the two types of institutions is strikingly similar. They are both accused of a lack of consumer orientation, ineffi-

cient use of resources, lack of coordination of services, and poor outcomes. Both systems are also faulted for overemphasizing specialty practice at the expense of more needed generalist services and orientations.

To truly reform health professions education, the issues facing reform of health care and higher education need to be addressed together. In many cases, students in higher education programs feel as disenfranchised as clients (patients) in the health-care system. Both suffer from institutional bureaucracies that operate as complex systems without appropriate attention to the coordination of care or instruction. Both systems allow clients to find their way through a maze of services and challenges, applauding the successful survivor as "self-reliant" and "self-directed." There is very little follow-up of "lost" clients in either system and a lack of responsibility for continuity and attention to outcomes.

While identifying these deficiencies in the health care and higher educational systems, it is only fair to acknowledge the fact that both systems have many strengths and successes. The point here, however, is that the social structure of these institutions works against many clients of the system. In addition, lack of attention to continuity and coordination leads to negative outcomes. True and significant change will require a renewed commitment to the realities of the human condition.

This chapter proposes that the key elements of case management constitute a value-oriented approach to improving both health care and educational systems. The key elements highlighted here are consumer orientation, coordination, outcome orientation, collaboration and cooperation, and resource efficiency. These elements form a cluster of concepts that are useful in reform of both systems. This can be accomplished by structuring the curriculum according to the principles of case management and using these same elements to guide patterns of interaction with students. In fact, students in educational programs who experience educational case management may learn the process of nursing case management more effectively.

NURSING LEADERSHIP IN REFORM OF EDUCATION AND PRACTICE

Because of the size and distribution of nursing education programs, there is tremendous potential for a key leadership role in health care and educational system reform. In addition, nursing has a long history of using case management approaches. Case management, as practiced in the historical tradition of nursing, is more than a technology for practice. It reflects an orientation to the care and nurturing of people in a humanistic and holistic framework. More contemporary models have shown that this kind of care is also cost effective and assures positive and measurable health outcomes (Miller, 1994). Nursing should invoke its history and expertise in exhibiting the kind of leadership that will enhance options for improved health care for all.

The kind of leadership required invites a renewed participation of all players in the health-care field and will be distinguished by the kind of consumer-client orientation missing in the current system. The structures and values needed in a reformed health-care system support client- and family-focused care that is of high quality, delivered in a comprehensive and coordinated way, at a reasonable cost, and with a high level of satisfaction for the client and the provider. The principles and practice of case management include this orientation to care. Current examples of nurse case management exemplify the kind of health care needed in a reformed health-care system (Del Togno-

Armanasco, Olivas, & Harter, 1989; Etheredge, 1989; Ethridge, 1991).

Nursing education should be a leader in contributing to and influencing health policy at all levels. It is essential to have demonstrations of comprehensive, coordinated care and nursing case management available as examples to show policy makers and consumers. These demonstrations are usually carried out in partnership with agencies and others in the community. They also develop a strong consumer group that can articulate the benefits of the care they receive. Nursing centers at many schools of nursing provide such examples of practice and serve as excellent laboratories for nursing and multidisciplinary educational experiences.

The primary reason that an educational institution should be involved in such demonstrations is to generate new knowledge and models to influence system change. Institutions of higher education should serve as "risk takers" in forwarding new models of care that can be used to promote system redesign.

KEY ELEMENTS OF CASE MANAGEMENT

The term "case management" as used here will refer to a system of care that is client centered, coordinated, outcome oriented, resource efficient, and collaborative with others in the care system. Bower (1992) describes case management:

> The fundamental focus of case management is to integrate, coordinate, and advocate for individuals, families, and groups requiring extensive services. The ultimate goal is to achieve planned care outcomes by brokering services across the health care continuum. Although case management may be directed toward other goals, and although the primary purpose for instituting a case management system may vary among programs . . . coordination of care is the basic component of all models and modalities of case management (p. 3).

The key elements of case management that are helpful to consider in the reform of health-care systems and health professions education are listed in Box 6-1 and discussed briefly here.

Client-Centered Approach

In case management, it is the needs of the client that are the focus of care rather than the needs of the institution or the professional.

Coordination of Care and Services Across Settings

In case management, the needs of the client may place them in a variety of settings or institutions. The role of the case manager is to coordinate, communicate, and manage the contacts across settings. In a sense, the

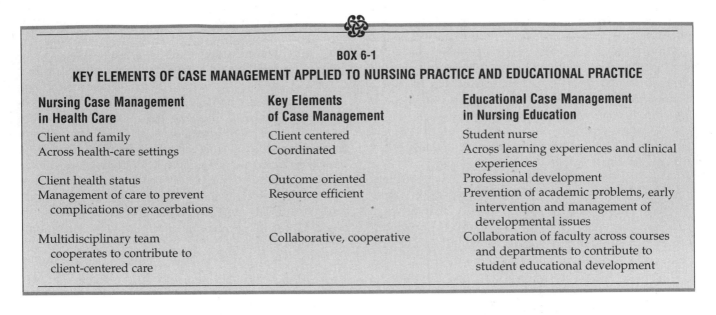

BOX 6-1
KEY ELEMENTS OF CASE MANAGEMENT APPLIED TO NURSING PRACTICE AND EDUCATIONAL PRACTICE

Nursing Case Management in Health Care	Key Elements of Case Management	Educational Case Management in Nursing Education
Client and family Across health-care settings	Client centered Coordinated	Student nurse Across learning experiences and clinical experiences
Client health status Management of care to prevent complications or exacerbations	Outcome oriented Resource efficient	Professional development Prevention of academic problems, early intervention and management of developmental issues
Multidisciplinary team cooperates to contribute to client-centered care	Collaborative, cooperative	Collaboration of faculty across courses and departments to contribute to student educational development

case manager holds a steady picture of the individual during movement from setting to setting.

Outcome Oriented

The focus of case management is to move the client toward successful meeting of planned outcomes. By constantly seeking outcomes, interventions are tied to a sense of movement, and constant evaluation occurs to measure progress. With an outcome orientation, there is a higher level of motivation to identify and remove barriers to success that occur during the course of care. The value of prevention and early detection is recognized because of the long-term effect on outcomes and the benefit to improving health status.

Resource Efficiency

Case management focuses on the client and seeks to move toward successful outcomes. Because of the high level of coordination and attention to reaching the outcome, there is a strong commitment to the prevention of useless setbacks and barriers that may interfere with progress. There is a strong commitment to achieve outcomes with the most efficient expenditure of resources.

Collaborative and Cooperative

Case management recognizes that collaboration with all parties involved in the client's care is essential and the key to successful outcomes. A case management model also recognizes the skills and abilities of a variety of providers. It seeks to match the client with the most appropriate provider at the most appropriate time. Although health professionals retain their identity and the clarity of their unique contribution to the care process, territorial barriers are reduced.

INTEGRATION OF CASE MANAGEMENT INTO CURRICULUM: HOPE FOR HEALTH-CARE SYSTEM REFORM

The health professionals of tomorrow must be educated in programs that are guided by values such as those identified as fundamental to systems of case management. If there is any hope of transforming our current confused and inefficient system, then it must be in the future professionals. They will carry out their practice in a yet-to-be-defined structure. In assuring that health professionals will be prepared to face the challenges of the future, those presently engaged in curriculum design carry a heavy burden but also share a wonderful opportunity.

Values and the Curriculum

It is important to remember that the work of designing a curriculum is essentially a value-based activity and that every curriculum is a value statement. In initiating any curriculum work, faculty must go through an exercise designed to explicate values important to the educational program and discuss them in some depth before determining the specifics of a curriculum design. This is an important step that all faculty should engage in as health-care reform movements are debated at the policy level. Health professions curricula should be reexamined in view of present policy debates.

An argument can be made that this values exploration should occur across disciplines. If this happened it would bring together varying perspectives and promote a better understanding of how the future health-care system could serve the needs of individuals, families, and communities. The current structure of health professions education does not readily allow for such joint exploration. It is, however, clearly a step that must happen along the way to true reform. If, in some fantasy, there were a collaborative retreat of medical, nursing, allied health, and business faculties to do fundamental values clarification and values building for the purpose of informing curriculum work, it would be a substantial step on the road to curriculum reform.

The key elements of case management clustered as a set of belief statements could be used as the template for discussion at such a session. Carefully exploring the meaning of "client centered" or "collaboration" would be an exercise for faculties who need to rethink the concepts of continuity of care and continuity of responsibility for care. To examine the concept of accountability from an interdisciplinary perspective leads to value exploration that will challenge all parties.

There are several methods that can be used in this values exploration. For example:

- A philosophy statement can be drafted for discussion.
- A set of value statements can be drafted and put forward for discussion and debate.
- A brainstorming technique can be used to identify values to guide the curriculum.
- A case review method can be used to present real situations and determine the value base for the care approaches chosen.
- Examples from nursing history or current practice can be shared as examples of value-based practice.
- Consumers can be brought into the discussion to clarify values from a nonprofessional perspective.

Whatever the method chosen to examine values as the foundation for curriculum, it is essential to prevent it from being only an "academic" discussion. The issue of values must be tied to the nature of the practice and the needs of clients.

Unfortunately, the distribution of power in the health-care system, and the embedded sense of ownership exhibited by different professional groups usually overshadows such discussions. For this type of interdisciplinary arrangement to work, it requires a restructuring of the reward system in both the health-care and educational systems, and "the development of a professional identity drawn from the needs of patients" (PEW, 1991, p. 23). The parties in the health-care system must see a value in working together to promote a common purpose. This is the real leadership challenge of interdisciplinary curriculum work in an era of health-care reform.

In addition to the development of values consensus for the curriculum, faculty must be given the opportunity to self-identify value conflicts that present barriers to their practice and teaching. Every effort must be made to seek resolution of these conflicts and develop plans to resolve them. In the event there are value incompatibilities with a reformed curriculum, the administration must significantly oversee these efforts to assure that these conflicts do not interfere with the curriculum implementation. Faculty freedoms must not be the rationale for failure in curriculum work. The ethical responsibility of health professions educators mandates an interpretation of academic freedom that has a strong accountability measure tied to it.

Curriculum Design

Following the essential examination of values, faculty proceed to develop the curriculum plan in concrete terms, identifying concepts, content, and process consistent with the philosophical underpinnings. This is a crucial transition point in curriculum work and one that needs constant clarification and validation to be true to the values work that preceded it. A recent national study (Valiga & Bruderle, 1994) surveyed nursing programs to determine the key concepts in the curriculum and asked faculty to identify those that were most critical. It was startling to note that all of the key elements associated with case management were missing from the list. Probably many case management concepts are assumed to be included in areas such as "community" and "advocacy"; however, it is disconcerting that such concepts as continuity of care, collaboration, and coordination are missing from the list of key concepts. These findings strengthen the argument for aggressive attention to philosophical orientation of case management and inclusion of the elements in the nursing curriculum.

If the key elements of case management provide the framework for curriculum, then attention must be given to both the content and process of the program and the type of clinical learning experiences best suited to the framework. The following discussion illustrates some suggested approaches to using case management to guide this process.

Development of Learning Experiences

Client centered. To design content and experiences that truly promote a client-centered approach, clients must be invited into the educational setting to tell their stories. For too long we have supposed how clients feel but have not clearly studied the client response to health care, and in fact, frequently ignored it. Student health professionals frequently apply rigid and simplistic frameworks to complex client situations and assume they are acting in the client's best interest. In the end, however, they often close a case or move on from a situation without adequate evaluation or outcome orientation. Students need continuous challenges to be comprehensive in their assessments, seeking validation from the client and family, involving other appropriate professionals, and clarifying expected outcomes.

For example, several things can be learned from the case of an 82-year-old man hospitalized for observation after a fall at home, followed by a 24-hour wait before a friend found him. A very short assessment was done by a social worker who, according to the client's perception, "asked me a few questions." No significant assessment was done by nurses related to his home situation or discharge plans and no family members were interviewed or consulted, although they were present and available.

Based on the short unvalidated assessment, and without consultation with the client or family, the social worker recommended assisted-living placement and determined that the individual was not safe to return to independent living in his home. This conclusion was challenged by family members who clarified the client's level of independence—he drove his own car, did his own shopping, volunteered at church, and essentially managed well in an independent capacity. In addition, because he had suffered only minor injuries, the family expected him to return to his independent living environment.

This example points out the dangers of imposing a professional model on situations defined without validation or clarification from the client and family. Clearly, this social worker, operating independently and from a "placement" perspective, made a recommendation that was contrary to the client's current state and experience. In fact, her recommendation was very disruptive to plans the client and family were discussing for potential changes in living arrangements.

This situation is an example of care that was not client centered, driven by the needs of the professional to make placement and handle cases in a short period of time, and based on unvalidated and incomplete assessment data. It also demonstrates the fragmented communication among professionals who share the care of a client. Turning this situation around for a curriculum learning experience is one way of clarifying the nature of client-centered care.

Outcome oriented. The curriculum design should include exposure to outcome-oriented practice across the life span. For example, students should be exposed to population parameters for health and wellness across the life span (USDHHS, 1992) and know health promotion and prevention interventions that support outcomes. In addition, the Agency for Health Care Policy and Research (AHCPR) clinical practice guidelines, critical pathways, and other outcome-oriented parameters should be included in the design of theory and practice courses.

Coordinated across settings. Clinical learning experiences should be designed to provide students with the flexibility to follow clients across settings and into the home, depending on the needs of the client and family and the skills of the student. As more and more agencies merge into integrated health-care systems it should become much easier to arrange such experiences for students. For example, as hospital systems adopt their own home care agencies and expand outpatient departments, referral, reporting and coordination of care across services should be enhanced.

In nursing education, this type of clinical experience will require a new kind of flexibility in staffing, scheduling, and organizing clinical learning experiences. The clinical instructor will need to adopt a client-centered focus and creative approaches to coordination of services. The learning goals in this type of experience should also be tied to outcomes with the student learning the linkage between coordination of services, improved outcomes, and the prevention of problems.

Collaborative. If collaboration is a valued goal of the curriculum, then it must be included in the design of learning experiences. This means providing opportunities for interdisciplinary learning experiences. The experiences may be anything from a joint discussion group around clinical issues to a planned clinical experience sharing clients in a complementary practice model. In this model, each profession provides the expertise best suited to the planned outcome for the client.

There is a great deal of discussion about nurses and physicians being educated together, especially in primary care. Mundinger (1994) states, "perhaps most important in the changes forecasted is the move toward coeducation of nurses and physicians" (p. 31). This type of collaborative practice is not easy to accomplish without a committed team of faculty on both sides who are willing to make it work from an educational standpoint. In reporting on a Kellogg-sponsored Community Partnership Initiative, Zungolo (1994) describes the challenges and barriers encountered in an interdisciplinary educational experience between medicine and nursing students:

This project has brought to the fore a number of barriers to a genuinely equitable collaboration. The medical dominance that is the hallmark of the American health care system is an integral component of the educational process for health professionals and influences the nature of any collaboration. This dominance underpins, and may even cause, some fundamental differences between medical and nursing education that threaten interdisciplinary efforts (p. 289).

The issues of interdisciplinary education are complex and must be addressed in order for an experience to be successful. It is important to note that the way in which students observe faculty in interdisciplinary collaboration is also an important modeling of the behaviors required for collaboration.

Resource efficient. The concept of cost-effective care is still foreign to most health professions programs. For so long, cost has been a invisible and seemingly uncontrollable part of the health-care equation. The design of learning experiences now requires a strong component detailing the issues of cost from multiple perspectives. It should include the consumer perspective, provider perspective, system perspective, and the national impact of health-care costs on the overall economy. A strong orientation to managing health-care resources in relation to the needs of clients and families is essential. Cost analysis of the care to clients who are case managed is an important component of the learning experience.

INTEGRATING THE KEY ELEMENTS OF CASE MANAGEMENT INTO INSTRUCTION

As mentioned earlier, the key elements of case management outlined in this chapter also have utility when applied to the instructional relationship between nursing students and faculty. There is a need to have a student-centered approach with attention to the coordination of learning experiences, and a focus on achieving expected learning outcomes. Box 6-1 displays the incorporation of case management elements into an instructional approach.

In this approach students will have the experience of "educational case management," feel the effects of educational coordination, and see approaches modeled by faculty. In addition, by assuming educational interventions that mirror a case management approach, faculty will be developing a response to the issues of instructional improvement that are challenging higher education.

The curriculum itself could become a vehicle for teaching case management. Instead of fragmenting courses and interactions with instructors (i.e., treating them as separate, independent experiences), the instruction could be designed around students and their educational development. In fact, case management might be learned more successfully by students if the curriculum and instruction of the program utilized the same principles in designing their education.

The process of professional development and clinical instruction that occurs in nursing education demands a comprehensive approach to coordinated learning experiences. Frequently, faculty believe that each clinical course should be viewed as a blank slate for both the student and the instructor to avoid prejudgment of the student's abilities or performance. Clearly, this is an antiquated concept and one that often disadvantages the student who must always start a clinical experience trying to "psych out" the instructor. In these situations, students rarely feel that their development is the focus

of concern and definitely do not feel that their clinical learning is coordinated and managed to promote the best possible learning outcome for them.

If the principles of case management were applied to clinical instruction, then the entire curriculum pathway would be viewed as a developmental process requiring attention to fit between the student and the learning experience to meet individual learning needs. Faculty would share information, observations, and evaluation of the students and their progress across courses, departments, and settings. Further, faculty would attempt to "manage" and coordinate the total experience of a particular student. This model assumes an integrated advising and instructional approach in which every student would be assigned a faculty "case manager" and faculty would carry a caseload of students that they follow throughout their educational program. Although this model may be used only with high-risk students, the philosophical orientation of case management is helpful with all students and consistent with educational reform.

In summary, case management is a system of care that supports a pattern of practice that is continuous, client centered, outcome oriented, resource efficient, and collaborative. In this chapter a model was presented (see Box 6-1) that identified key elements of case management and argued that the key elements were useful in informing both nursing practice and nursing education. The integration of a case management approach into curriculum and instruction will enhance the educational process for students and support a coordinated approach to meeting learning needs. It was proposed that learning nursing case management for application to professional practice is enhanced when the student is exposed to educational case management in the curriculum and instruction.

CONCLUSION

By structuring the health professions curriculum according to the principles of case management and using those elements to guide educational case management, we can achieve our goal of comprehensive client-centered care. It is this response to the ever-changing health-care reform agenda that will keep the health professions education orientation toward the care and nurturing of people in a humanistic and holistic framework a reality.

REFERENCES

Bower, K. A. (1992). *Case management by nurses.* Kansas City, MO: American Nurses Publishing.

Del Togno-Armanasco, V., Olivas, G. S., & Harter, S. (1989). Developing an integrated nursing case management model. *Nursing Management, 10,* 26-29.

Etheredge, M. L. (Ed.). (1989). *Collaborative care: nursing case management.* Chicago: American Hospital Publishing, Inc.

Ethridge, P. (1991). A nursing HMO: Carondelet St. Mary's experience. *Nursing Management, 22,* 22-27.

Miller, N. (1994). An interview with Phyllis Ethridge. *Nursing & Health Care, 12,* 65-70.

Mundinger, M. O. (1994). Health care reform: will nursing respond? *Nursing & Health Care, 15,* 28-33.

PEW Health Professions Commission. (1991). *Healthy America: Practitioners for 2005, an agenda for action for U.S. health professional schools.* Durham, NC: PEW Health Professions Commission.

United States Department of Health and Human Services (USDHHS). (1991). *Healthy people 2000: national health promotion and disease prevention objectives.* Boston: Jones & Bartlet Publishers.

Valiga, T. M., & Bruderle, E. (1994). Concepts included in and critical to nursing curricula: An analysis. *Journal of Nursing Education, 33,* 118-124.

Zungolo, E. (1994). Interdisciplinary education in primary care: the challenge. *Nursing & Health Care, 15,* 288-292.

Chapter 7

The Education of Nurses: Nurse Case Managers' View

Mary Sinnen, MSN, RN
Marita Schifalaqua, MSN, RN

OVERVIEW

Educating advanced practice nurses is crucial to the success of nurse case management.

Health care is changing at a rapid pace. The curriculum designed to prepare advanced practice nurses for future roles must be challenging and fluid. Core components of such a curriculum should include a mixture of theory, practice, and research. Nurse case management as a successful practice modality will become even more so given the shift toward complex, chronically ill patient populations. Within this chapter, core curriculum components that will prepare advanced practice nurses for future roles are discussed, and associated teaching strategies are identified.

Health care in America continues to change at a dramatic rate. Advanced practitioners must be prepared to meet the demands of a new climate and environment for the delivery of nursing care. The academic setting is likewise challenged to create a dynamic and fluid curriculum that is a stimulating mixture of theory, practice, and research. The ideal curriculum must assist in the formation of leaders who will know their theory well and be able to transfer the theory into practice.

Within the new health-care agenda, emphasis will change from an acute disease model to a chronic complex illness model. Causes of the diseases seen within society today have multiple contributing factors as opposed to single agents seen in the past acute disease model. The basis of illness for these chronic conditions is biopsychosocial as opposed to just an alteration in physiology. The aim of intervention changes to assisting toward optimal levels of wellness as opposed to curing illness. Temporal relationships become continuous versus a single isolated event, and the role of the patient is viewed as active rather than passive (Pawlson, 1994).

As the paradigm shifts or widens to include a concentrated effort on chronic diseases, changes will need to take place in financing, reimbursement, delivery, research, and the education of health-care professionals. For financing, this means universal and need-based coverage; for reimbursement, it means an illness-based, value-driven system; for the delivery of care, it means more ambulatory centers, a focus on prevention, and a network of linked providers who view the client as an active participant in care. Research and quality assurance must focus on longitudinal studies that concentrate on multiple risk factors and functional outcomes. The education of health professionals will need to broaden beyond social, behavioral, and biological sciences. This education should include a study of human systems, compassionate and technical knowledge of illness, finances, and longitudinal experiences (Pawlson, 1994).

Nurse case management is a prevalent theme within health care today and is defined as the *utilization of practicing professionals to focus on the complex needs of high-risk patients, families, and populations along the health-care continuum*. Nurse case management certainly has the capability to position advanced practice nurses (APN) to assist in the paradigm change from acute-centered to chronic-centered health care. Nurse case management is an exciting process that should be incorporated within the curriculum for APNs. Although individual professionals may have altered their specific focus within graduate school, there are identified core components that will prepare the APN for the future. These core components include:

1. The practice of nurse case management within integrated delivery systems
2. Climate creation
3. Systems theory
4. Change theory
5. Leadership
6. Ethics
7. Economics within health care including health-care reform
8. Continuous quality improvement
9. Research
10. Dissemination of knowledge

These curriculum components will prepare the APN to become positioned within an integrated delivery system. Advanced practice nurses will be qualified to collaborate toward goals of health promotion, maintenance, and restoration. As key players within the system, these nurses will be further qualified to assist in the improvement of outcomes related to satisfaction, access, and cost. The background in research and continuous quality improvement will prepare them for validation and evaluation of the achievement of both quality and cost outcomes in practice (Figure 7-1).

This chapter will further detail these core components. Also, included are suggested teaching and learning activities that correspond with the core components.

NURSE CASE MANAGEMENT WITHIN AN INTEGRATED DELIVERY SYSTEM

Integrated delivery systems will be the future of health care within this country. "Networks" will be formed that assume responsibility for the health care delivered to designated members of the population. Assigned populations will have varying degrees of health-care needs. The chronically ill and complex clients will require more intense interventions.

Hospitals will no longer function independently but will be linked with clinics, offices, long-term health-care facilities, public health departments, and wellness and prevention programs. Although the creation of integrated delivery systems remains at an infancy stage, there is no doubt that APNs will need to move with clients and families across the continuum of services by using case management interventions.

The goals of nursing case management are to:

- Provide quality health care along the continuum
- Decrease fragmentation of care
- Enhance quality of life
- Contain costs (ANA: Nursing Case Management, 1988)

These goals provide a solid foundation for the APN.

Committed to the philosophy of "care management," nurse case managers realize the need to "care" for the individual client and family while paying close attention to the "management" of resources and timely access to appropriate services. This approach links *one* APN with the client over time. The APN provides case management services, namely, health assessments, planning of care, procurement, delivery and coordination of services, and monitoring the multiple needs of the client and family. The nurse must be prepared to work collaboratively with the client, family, and other members of the health-care team. Attention is placed on health promotion, maintenance, and restoration while cooperating with the payors of the health-care services. The APN will need to experience caring for complex clients and families across various environments.

CLIMATE CREATION

It will be essential for APNs to have an understanding of human systems theory. Hanlon (1968, 1973, 1984) has done extensive work in this field and defines seven basic human operations that, when mastered, lead to self-actualization. These seven processes include learning, world-view construction, ideal pattern construction, conceptualization, climate creation, environment creation, and cybernetics.

The ability to create climate or the psychological environment will be an extremely important component of the role for the APN within the integrated delivery system. The role calls for a mastery of the art of communication and collaboration. In essence, APNs must have a pulse on the current climate within health care, be keenly aware of the process of climate creation, and help build healthy interpersonal relationships for the future.

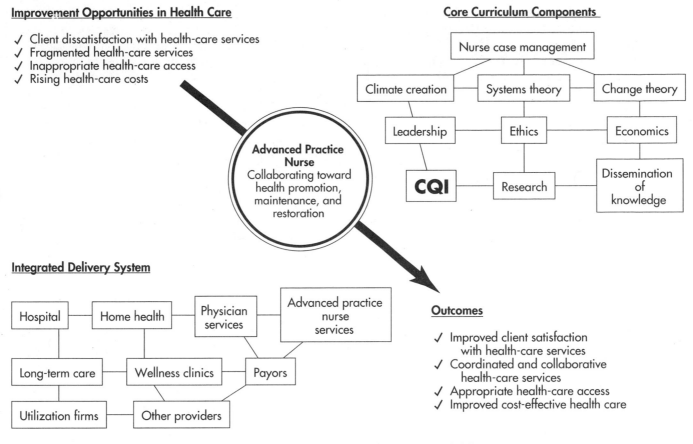

Improvement Opportunities in Health Care

✓ Client dissatisfaction with health-care services
✓ Fragmented health-care services
✓ Inappropriate health-care access
✓ Rising health-care costs

Core Curriculum Components

Nurse case management

Climate creation — Systems theory — Change theory

Leadership — Ethics — Economics

CQI — Research — Dissemination of knowledge

Advanced Practice Nurse
Collaborating toward health promotion, maintenance, and restoration

Integrated Delivery System

Hospital — Home health — Physician services — Advanced practice nurse services

Long-term care — Wellness clinics — Payors

Utilization firms — Other providers

Outcomes

✓ Improved client satisfaction with health-care services
✓ Coordinated and collaborative health-care services
✓ Appropriate health-care access
✓ Improved cost-effective health care

FIG. 7-1   Model of advanced practice nurse in an integrated delivery system

Within the client and family domain, the APN will need to promote a climate of responsible levels of wellness. Attention must be given to intrapersonal as well as interpersonal development. Likewise, within the integrated delivery system, healthy relationships among provider groups will be necessary to keep the system operating effectively. Intragroup and intergroup dynamics will be of importance. With an understanding of the process of climate creation, the APN will be able to assist clients, families, and coworkers toward healthier relationships.

According to Hanlon (1968), intrapersonal development must precede interpersonal development. Self-acceptance, self-support, and self-esteem need developing before a relationship involving mutual acceptance, mutual support, and mutual esteem can evolve. Each of these levels represents a hierarchy. One cannot support self without first developing acceptance nor esteem self without building in support. To the degree that one is able to relate to self, a person will be able to relate to others. In other words, that person cannot accept or support or esteem others if unable to accept, support, or esteem oneself. This principle has many implications for proceeding with climate creation and motivating others toward healthier lifestyles.

Beyond the realm of working with clients and families, the APN will be an essential link in the integrated delivery network. The study of climate creation can be translated to address groups within the network. The same principles apply to working with groups as those with clients and families, only the terminology changes to intragroup and intergroup. The dynamics remain the same. In other words, the group must develop from acceptance to support to esteem. As it is able to relate to itself as a group, it will be able to relate to other groups. To be truly integrated, the system must develop healthy segments that are able to relate to each other in the mission of delivering quality and cost-effective health care. No group can do it alone. No group can be less than or more than the others. The APN who practices nursing case management within such a network is in an optimal position to understand and stimulate the creation of a healthy climate.

SYSTEMS THEORY

The curriculum needs to be designed so the APN will gain an understanding of *basic systems theory*. The understanding of systems theory is necessary because health care is a complicated and dynamic system.

There are many key elements of general systems theory (Kast & Rosenzweig, 1981). The holism and synergism of systems theory view the system as a whole, not just the sum of its parts. This is true for all systems that are mechanical, biological, and social. Systems have boundaries which separate them from their environment; these relate to being an open or closed system. There are open systems that exchange information or energy. These systems are viewed as a transformational model. There is energy flowing between all systems and subsystems to transform inputs into outputs.

As integrated delivery systems are developed, the need to be open and dynamic will be necessary for the success of that system. There are closed systems in which the exchange of energy and information is relatively slow, but not completely closed.

Feedback is an important element in understanding how a system maintains a steady state. Feedback needs to occur so that effective change will be a priority. Open systems exchange information often in the form of feedback loops. That information is put into the loop and feedback is given. The APN will be an integral component of this feedback mechanism in this open system.

The APN will need an understanding that systems have a hierarchy of relationships with other subsystems, one part of the system will affect another part of the system (Kast & Rosenzweig, 1981; Senge, 1990).

CHANGE THEORY

The movement of change along a clearly defined continuum facilitates the evaluation of the circumstance and the process (Porter-O'Grady, 1992). Sullivan and Decker (1986) define leadership as an interpersonal process of influencing the activities of the individual or group toward a common goal. The transformational leader is one who can take the concepts of change and human relationships and has the ability to apply them to the changing environment.

The APN will be in an environment that will continue to be dynamic. The APN will have responsibilities for planned change and will need to understand this approach to achieve success. Lewin (1947) has described the planned-change approach to include unfreezing of the current approach, implementing the change, and then refreezing or creating an acceptance and consistent use of the new approach. Variation between these phases will often occur.

For each phase it will be necessary to identify the driving and restraining forces. The driving forces need to be identified to be able to use them in the attainment of the goal. It is also important to identify the barriers

or restraining forces so they can be eliminated or decrease their impact, so progress can be continued (Lewin, 1951). The APN will deal with factors both from within and outside the specific setting.

LEADERSHIP

Today the trend for leadership is to engage others, encourage teamwork, and empower others to feel capable and strong (McNeese-Smith, 1993). These attributes are essential components for the APN to be able to function effectively in the changing climate of health care.

Today the skills needed to direct people would include the domains of the human, technical, and the conceptual aspects (Smith, 1993). The human skill would include the nurse case manager's ability to harmonize demands and develop a personal view of human activity. The technical skills involve an understanding of methods and analytical ability of specialized management knowledge. The conceptual skills involve the ability of the nurse case manager to assess the driving and restraining forces of the area of responsibility.

ETHICS

There is no doubt that as the future of health care unfolds, many decisions will need to take place requiring ethical thinking and moral judgments. There will be controversy because of the forces inherent within society today. These forces include preferences for individual versus community or group norms, misuse of scientific advances, changes within political philosophy, and erosion of religious consensus (Harvey & Pellegrino, 1994). Abortion, euthanasia, assisted suicide, and the rationalization of health-care resources are examples of issues currently causing debate.

As professional health-care providers, APNs will need an understanding of ethics, morality, values, ideals, and cultural and societal norms. Hanlon (1968) refers to the operation of creating values as ideal pattern construction. It is one of the basic human operations within his human systems theory. As individuals, APNs will want to consider their own ideals, as well as to examine the process of ideal pattern construction so that they can assist others in clarification of values, which is a necessary step in the decision-making process.

The structure of the ideal pattern can be divided into three areas and diagrammed on a pyramid (Figure 7-2). The bottom rung represents chance ideals; these are adopted with little deliberation, such as language. The second plane represents opportunistic ideals;

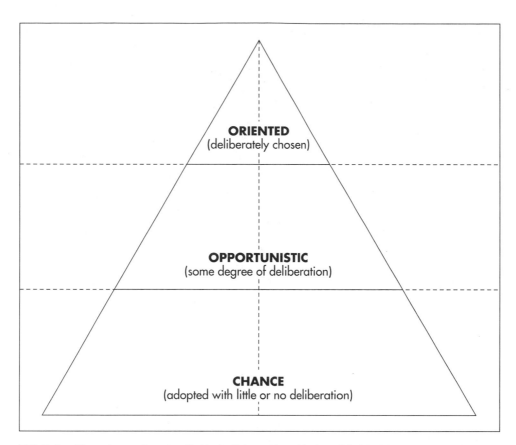

FIG. 7-2   Hierarchy used to classify ideals (Adapted from Hanlon, JM: Administration and education, Belmont, 1968, Wadsworth Publishing)

these are formed with some degree of deliberation. At the top of the pyramid are oriented ideals; these are deliberately chosen and represent the loyalties of adult life.

Values can and do change over the course of a lifetime. They move up and down on the pyramid. Situations happen that alter the world view and therefore the ideals in life. Ideals represent goals or intentions. They are carried out with a degree of aspiration. This degree of aspiration is the amount of energy or work devoted by the individual to that ideal. Oriented ideals should receive the greatest amount of aspiration.

Organizations have ideals, also. Just as it is important to examine the ideals of self and clients in making decisions, so it is vitally important for the APN to identify the values that coincide with the integrated delivery system. The practice in which the APN participates should uphold the ideals of the integrated delivery system in which it is positioned.

Difficult choices must be made within the health-care arena—it cannot be all things to all people. As these decisions are made, the good of ends as well as the good of means must be considered. Understanding the process of ideal pattern construction can assist the APN through these dilemmas.

ECONOMICS

For this nursing curriculum to come alive, many design influences need to be addressed. The bigger system that will have direct influence over this curriculum will be that of health-care reform and the managed care market. The APN must have a basic understanding of economics and politics that affect the health-care arena.

Some of the basic information needed is about health coverage plans. Currently, health-care coverage plans for managed care are separated into three areas. First, a health maintenance organization (HMO) is characterized as a prepaid service provided by a group to a group. The HMO places emphasis on prevention and efficiency. The second type of managed care coverage is an Independent Practice Association (IPA), which is a variation of an HMO. The services of the IPA are provided by private physicians to a group. The primary physician functions as the gatekeeper. The third variety of a managed care plan is the Preferred Provider Organization (PPO). A PPO has negotiated fees as a basis. The enrolled members of the PPO are required to use a PPO physician (Smith, 1993; Swanson & Albrecht, 1993). These managed care programs were developed as a cost-containment measure. The APN could be employed by any of the organizations.

Health-care networks would be developed as partnerships with the payor and provider. The role of the APN in the new networks is being developed at this time. Managed competition is being proposed to create an environment that would foster working with clients in a cost-effective manner. A paradigm shift would need to take place so the provider is rewarded for quality and economy (Curtin, 1993; Swanson & Albrecht, 1993).

Within this structure, it will benefit providers to promote prevention with a variety of innovative programs. The future of health care is in the community, to keep people well will be a priority (Westoff, 1992). The driving force for providers is all related to financial incentives, the better they do their job the more enrollees will be in their network. The education of APN and the priorities to promote prevention and maintenance are closely aligned.

The APN will need to effect both quality and cost outcomes. The essence of nurse case management is that of coordination and cost-effective care (Cohen, 1991). Coordination of care is often addressed to evaluate the client's needs and direct them to the correct access of care (Catholic Hospital Association, 1992; Swanson & Albrecht, 1993). The APN through the utilization of nurse case management principles can deliver individual, community-based, coordinated, quality, and cost-effective care. The managed-care influence will increase the market for nursing case management services.

CONTINUOUS QUALITY IMPROVEMENT

One of the theoretical models for the ANP curriculum is the Deming philosophy of quality improvement. The evolution of Deming's thinking includes statistical methods, system improvement, fourteen points, and the system of profound knowledge. The system of profound knowledge includes: knowledge of system, knowledge of variation, knowledge of psychology, and knowledge of a theory (Deming, 1993).

The *knowledge of system* consists of an organization in which customers, suppliers, and processes work interdependently toward a common goal (Deming, 1993). The sum of the components do not equal the functioning of the whole system. Thus, even if each component strives to perform its best individually, the system as a whole may not. The APN will be practicing in a variety of environments, and each setting will be a subsystem that will contribute to the whole. The professionals in these settings will need to collaborate within the integrated delivery network.

The *knowledge of variation* states that variation exists in all life processes. The APN must have an understanding of variation as it exists in different situations. This includes common cause versus common and special cause variation. The APN will play a key role in data evaluation related to variances in the integrated delivery system.

The *knowledge of psychology* is the interactions between people and systems. Motivation and learning take place on a very individual level. Change in people occurs through learning and understanding (Deming, 1993).

The *theory of knowledge* is gained through theory and experience. The focus-plan-do-study-act cycle is a method of acquiring knowledge, which is a cycle of learning (Deming, 1993). The definition of focus includes finding a process to improve, organizing an effort to work on improvement, clarifying current knowledge of the process, understanding process variation and capability, and selecting a strategy for continued improvement (Deming, 1993). The plan-do-study-act cycle includes plan, enact the plan and collect data, analyze the results of the data, and the action is to adapt or abandon the plan (Deming, 1993).

In today's environment, the most knowledgeable people are the ones who work with the product or are the closest to the delivered service. The APN is coordinating the care of clients, and thus has expert knowledge of the health-care consumer.

RESEARCH AND DISSEMINATION OF KNOWLEDGE

The role of the APN within the integrated delivery system is not well carved out at this point. It will take time and much energy to define the role as well as research to prove its worth. That is why it is essential for the graduate student to understand the core components of research and the dissemination of knowledge.

Theory, practice, and research form an interconnected link within professional studies. Research studies undertaken within the practice field verify theories and their relevance to the professional work. Both qualitative and quantitative methods are necessary and have the potential to assist in the development of models that will serve to position APNs within the integrated delivery system. Longitudinal studies in which complex, chronically ill clients and families are followed by APNs across the continuum of health-care services utilizing a variety of interventions are war-

BOX 7-1
SUGGESTED TEACHING AND LEARNING ACTIVITIES

1. Attain and maintain a case load of chronically ill clients.
2. Utilize case management process in providing care.
3. Evaluate the results of the case management process.
4. Map out the care for clients with similar diagnoses across the continuum; validate interventions and make recommendations for improving systems.
5. Analyze the climate of a client and family experiencing chronic or complex illness or trauma; include an examination of intrapersonal and interpersonal dimensions.
6. Analyze the climate created within an existing health-care group or department in a health-care setting; examine the intragroup and intergroup dimensions.
7. Discuss the interrelated parts of the health-care system as it relates to a client and flow chart the process.
8. Analyze the driving and restraining forces that relate to client care and to the integrated delivery system.
9. Define your leadership world view.
10. Identify your own ideals according to whether they are chance, opportunistic, or oriented.
11. Analyze the ideals of a health-care organization.
12. Analyze the interrelationships of public policy and the economics of health care as these relate to the health status of individuals, families, and communities.
13. Participate on a CQI team and analyze the process for improvement.
14. Design a research study involving the use of a NCM intervention with a specific client population.
15. Write a grant for funding of a certain project involving the use of APN within the community setting.
16. Participate in a grant writing process within the Nursing Department of the University or College.
17. Present knowledge gained through study within this curriculum at a professional gathering.
18. Submit one professional article for publication.

ranted. More importantly, these studies need to focus on the outcomes of care related to quality and cost.

The vast amount of knowledge gained through the work of nurse case management within this realm of practice requires dissemination to the public, politicians, colleagues, and other members of the health-care team. This sharing of information will require both written and oral communication skills. These technical skills should be interwoven with the curriculum. Mastery of these technical skills is necessary for the APN to carve out the pathway for the future of professional nursing (Box 7-1).

CONCLUSION

Leaders in both academic and practice settings must come together to create a shared vision for the future of professional nursing. This vision must concentrate on the preparation of advanced practice nurses. Curriculum development must include dynamic and stimulating courses. The associated teaching and learning activities as described should support the core curriculum. These activities are designed to integrate theory into practice. APNs will be challenged to demonstrate their own growth potential and their evolving role in client care. Future roles will demand practitioners who are knowledgeable in theory, practice modalities, and research.

REFERENCES

American Nurses' Association. (1988). *Nursing Case Management*. Kansas City, MO.: American Nurses' Association.

The Catholic Hospital Association. (1992). *Setting relationships right: a working proposal for systemic health care reform.* St Louis: CHA.

Cohen, E. (1991). Nursing case management, does it pay? *Journal of Nursing Administration, 21* (4), 20-24.

Curtin, L. (1993). Health reform: the shape of things to come. *Nursing Management, 24,* 28-30.

Deming, W. E. (1993). *The new economics for industry, government, education.* Cambridge: Massachusetts Institute of Technology.

Hanlon, J. M. (1968). *Hanlon: administration and education.* Belmont: Wadsworth.

Hanlon, J. M. (1973). *Theory, practice and education.* Fond du Lac: Marian College Press.

Hanlon, J. M. (1984). *Humanitas: a guide to the discovery and development of human potential.* Unpublished.

Harvey, J. C., & Pellegrino, E. D. (1994). A response to euthanasia initiatives. *Health Progress,* 36-53.

Kast, F. E., & Rosenzweig, J. E. (1972). General systems theory: Applications for organizations and management. In M. T. Matteson and J. M. Ivancevich (Eds.). *Management and organization behavior classics* (pp. 72-90. BurrRidge, IL: Irwin).

Lewin, K. (1947). Frontiers of group dynamic: concept, method, and reality in social science: social equilibria and social change. *Human Relations, 1,* 5-41.

Lewin, K. (1951). *Field theory in social science.* New York: Harper & Row.

McNeese-Smith, D. (1993). Leadership behavior and employee effectiveness. *Nursing Management, 24* (5), 38-39.

Pawlson, G. L. (1994). Chronic illness: implication of a new paradigm for health care. *Journal of Quality Improvement, 20* (1), 33-39.

Senge, P. M. (1990). *The fifth discipline: the art and practice of the learning organization.* New York: Doubleday.

Smith, T. C. (1993). Management skills for directors of nursing. *Journal of Nursing Administration, 23* (9), 38-49.

Swanson, J., & Albrecht, M. (1993). *Community health nursing.* Philadelphia: W. B. Saunders Company.

Westoff, L. (1992). Case management: quelling the confusion. *Nursing Management, 23* (12), 33-34.

Chapter 8

The Denver Nursing Education Project: Promoting the Health of Persons Living with HIV/AIDS

Carole Schroeder, PhD, RN
Gina Astorino, MS, RN

OVERVIEW

Partnering nurses with people who are living with HIV/AIDS is a successful strategy for promoting clients' self-care and personal autonomy.

Jean Watson's theory of nursing as the "art and science" of human caring is based on the belief that all persons possess inner resources and strengths that they can draw upon to meet health challenges. This theory is used to guide the Denver Nursing Project in Human Caring (DNPHC), a nurse-managed outpatient center for people living with HIV/AIDS. This chapter focuses on two innovative programs used by the DNPHC that both promote self-care and personal autonomy in people living with HIV/AIDS and provide the necessary education to help this diverse client population to make informed choices about health promotion, symptom management, and disease prevention. The in-depth discussion of the Nursing Care Partnership Program and the modular "Living with HIV" educational curriculum will enable other health-care professionals to implement similar programs to promote health in people living with HIV/AIDS.

The Denver Nursing Project in Human Caring is a theory-based, nurse-managed outpatient center for persons living with human immunodeficiency virus (HIV) and acquired immunodeficiency disease syndrome (AIDS). Designed to promote the health and well-being of people living with HIV/AIDS, the center is a practical example of Jean Watson's theory of human caring. Care is primary to cure at the center, and the mission statement emphasizes relationship and education to promote self-care and personal autonomy for persons living with HIV/AIDS. To that end, health promotion is a major emphasis of the center.

In this article, two programs will be outlined: the Nursing Care Partnership (NCP) model of nursing practice, and the Living with HIV program of modular education. We will describe initially the origins, theoretical foundations, and available outpatient services of the Center; next, the Nursing Care Partnership program; and finally, the Living with HIV program of education. The purpose of this discussion is to assist other health professionals to implement similar innovative programs that promote the health of persons with HIV/AIDS.

THE DENVER NURSING PROJECT IN HUMAN CARING

The idea for a nurse-managed outpatient center for persons with HIV/AIDS was originally conceived by hospital nurses concerned that the chronic health-care needs of persons with HIV/AIDS disease were not being met by the cure-oriented medical care system. In 1988, the center was originated through cooperative financial and practice agreements among three Denver hospitals and the University of Colorado School of Nursing, Center for Human Caring. In 1990, the Department of Health and Human Services, Division of Nursing (now called the National Institute of Nursing Research) awarded grant funding to the center to expand outpatient nursing services. Persons eligible to participate in services at the center are those who obtain their primary HIV/AIDS care through one of the three sponsoring hospitals. The center is used 400 to 500 times per month, primarily by men living with HIV/AIDS. Women comprise less than 5% of client visits, although numbers are increasing as more women are being diagnosed with HIV/AIDS.

The center employs baccalaureate, master's and doctorally prepared registered nurses, and levels of education differentiate levels of nursing practice at the center. The minimal level of preparation for nurses at the center is the baccalaureate degree. Newman's (1990) work on an integrated nursing practice model served as a model for the center. In this model, advanced practice nurses are professional nurses with a graduate degree based on a curriculum that is person-centered and focused on health, and who have direct responsibility for clients over time. At the center, doctorally prepared nurses serve as project director and researcher. Master's prepared clinical nurse specialists fulfill the three roles of education, research, and practice at the center and also serve as overall consultants to baccalaureate prepared nurses. Available nursing services include both independent and medically supportive nursing services. Independent nursing services offered at the center are therapies that promote health and healing, and assist people to negotiate the health-care system. In addition to the Nursing Care Partnership program, independent therapies include individual and family counseling and psychiatric support, education, various massage therapies, therapeutic touch sessions, Reiki, and so forth. Medically supportive nursing services include intravenous fluid administration, blood transfusions, Pentamidine treatments, medications, laboratory work, skin testing, and others.

Jean Watson's theory of nursing as the art and science of human caring (1970/1985, 1985, 1988, 1990) guides the practice of nursing at the center. Watson's work provides nurses with a theoretical focus for relationships of partnership with clients and their family, friends, and lovers. According to Watson, persons possess inner resources and strengths that can be drawn upon to meet health challenges. Health refers to unity and harmony within mind, body and soul, rather than the absence or cure of disease. The goal of nursing is to help persons gain inner harmony in order to generate self-knowledge, self-healing, and self-care processes (1985, p. 48). Care is primary to cure in Watson's work, and caring relationships are designed to enhance and preserve human dignity, rather than treat persons as objects. Watson's work presupposes reciprocal and nonhierarchical client-nurse relationships based on mutuality, as opposed to the more common approach based on unilateral professional expertise and authority. The Nursing Care Partnership program was designed to be an actualization of Watson's relational theory in nursing practice, and is discussed below.

Nursing Care Partnerships

During the conduct of client and staff focus group sessions early in 1990, it became apparent that the team nursing model then in effect at the center did not provide sufficient individualized, consistent client support. During these focus group sessions, clients and their significant others described how they needed more assistance to negotiate the complexities of the health-care system, including access to a nurse who knew their situation when a crisis arose. In response to these needs, the Nursing Care Partnership program was developed and put into practice at the center in 1991. Based on Jean Watson's theory of caring, Nursing Care Partnerships (NCPs) are defined as *a care-enabling method which establishes authentic caring relationships between clients and nurses based on partnership* (Schroeder & Maeve, 1992). Although the NCP idea evolved from notions of case management, traditional models of case management were deemed incongruent with the theoretical basis of the center for a variety of reasons. In traditional case management programs, professional-client relationships are usually acute in nature, professionally controlled, and require the person seeking care to meet the needs of the health-care system, rather than the reverse. Moreover, the case management relationship was initially designed to save health-care costs, rather than assist the individual and family to negotiate the complexities of the health-care system successfully.

Thorn (1990) describes the evolution of case management in terms of generations: traditional or first-generation case management was oriented toward cost containment, controlled by physicians, and the point of contact was limited to the episode of acute illness. Second-generation case management was similar to first, but involved some quality-of-care issues. Third-generation case management, most similar to the NCP model, is controlled by the person with the illness, and the entire course of a person's illness, rather than an acute event, is considered the point of contact. Cost containment, although one of the goals of third-generation case management, is not the overriding framework; rather, encouraging self-care, autonomy, and the ability to obtain quality care from the health-care system is emphasized.

The Nursing Care Partnership program is similar to third-generation case management. Role negotiation is important in the partnerships, and no prescription for relationship exists. Instead, nurses are guided by Watson's abstract theory of caring relationship in nursing. Participation in a care partnership relationship is voluntary, and not all clients actively participate. When planning the partnership model, clients and nurses alike expressed a desire to choose their care partners. Thus, both partners' wishes are equally considered when establishing and maintaining a care partnership relationship. The intensity of NCP relationships escalates as the needs of the client, family, and friends grow with progressing illness. NCPs consult during hospitalizations, for oftentimes, the nursing care partner is the most informed professional regarding the client's current level of health and emotional and familial needs. Through consultation, information can be quickly transferred to other professionals. Not only are hospital costs potentially reduced, but the client's wishes regarding such concerns as treatment plans, home care, and medical directives (living wills) are more quickly and easily carried out.

Evaluation research conducted at the center has determined that the NCP program is a well-utilized and popular program which is meeting its mission to promote the health of persons with HIV/AIDS. The center has recorded over 15,000 visits since it opened its doors in 1988, and client satisfaction is consistently high. Moreover, this research has also shown that the NCP program improves client access to cost-effective, quality health care. The 1991 and 1992 costs of HIV/AIDS were used to conservatively estimate that the center has saved over $700,000 in 1991 and over $1 million in 1992 in hospital charges for HIV/AIDS care. These savings resulted from prevention of hospital admissions and readmissions, reduction of prolonged length of stays, provision of less costly outpatient medical treatments, assistance to families to maintain home care during the dying process, and attraction of professional and nonprofessional volunteer services and donations. (For further information on the conduct, evaluation, and cost effectiveness of the NCP program, please see Schroeder & Maeve, 1992, Schroeder & Neil, 1992, and Schroeder, 1993.)

Education is an important component of the NCP relationships, and the center recently augmented its health promoting mission with a formal, self-paced modular HIV/AIDS curriculum. The following section outlines the development and content of this innovative program.

THE HIV/AIDS EDUCATION PROGRAM: LIVING WITH HIV

During the early years of the center's history, educational programs included group classes and individual teaching sessions with clients and others. When nurses or other resource specialists offered formal classes regarding specific problems, diseases, and issues related to living with HIV/AIDS, client participation in the scheduled classes was intermittent and often disappointing. It became evident that lack of participation was related to the pertinence of the topic to the individual client's perception of his or her health status, rather than because of variations of scheduling, content, presentation, or style. Information deemed relevant to potential participants included that information which concerned a current health problem, rather than specific or general information regarding manifestations and treatment of HIV/AIDS. It became clear that to provide consistent and relevant education to a diverse population, a self-paced, modular curriculum was needed.

In consultation with staff, clients, and their significant others, the HIV/AIDS educator/clinical nurse specialists developed the Living with HIV program. The goal was to provide a comprehensive HIV curriculum that not only met the needs of a diverse population, but assisted people to make informed choices regarding health promotion, symptom management, and disease prevention. The Living with HIV program ranges from content on asymptomatic HIV infection to manifestations and treatment of acute AIDS disease, and emphasizes how to obtain resources for self-care. For example, the first module of the system, "From HIV to AIDS," describes the progression of HIV disease and identifies human needs and issues that evolve from the various stages of disease. Other modules provide information about relief of symptoms, solutions to common problems, and positive coping strategies. "Living well" with HIV/AIDS is a common thread throughout the modules, and the content is continually revised as new information becomes available. With the Living with HIV program, NCPs assist clients to "take charge" of their own particular experience of health through knowledge; in this way, clients learn that positive choices do exist despite the reality of living with a chronic and terminal disease (see Table 8-1 for more information on the content of the Living with HIV program).

TABLE 8-1   Selected modules and content: Living with HIV/AIDS program

User's guide
 	
Subject index
	ALTERNATIVE AND COMPLEMENTARY TREATMENTS
	
	Accupressure
	Biofeedback
	Massage
	Meditation/
	  visualization
	Reiki
	Relaxation and guided
	  imagery
	Self-healing
	Therapeutic touch
		CHILDREN AND HIV/AIDS
		
		HIV epidemiology
		Health maintenance
		Immune system
		Parenting
		Resources
			CULTURAL AND SEXUAL ISSUES
			
			African American
			Gay
			Heterosexual
			Hispanic
				FROM HIV TO AIDS: SEQUENCE OF INFECTIOUS COURSE
				
				AIDS general
				  information
				AIDS CDC definition
				Asymptomatic HIV+
				Symptomatic HIV+
				HIV epidemiology,
				  immune system,
				  transmission

HEALTH MAINTENANCE
 	
Alcohol, drug use
Exercise
Nutrition
Oral hygiene
Risk reduction/
  staying healthy
Skin care
Spirituality
Stress reduction
Stretching
Symptom
  management
	MEDICAL MANAGEMENT
	
	AIDS Medical Guide
	Blood transfusions
	Central lines
	Clinical trials
	Drug information
	Experimental
	  drugs/treatments/
	  vaccines
	Opportunistic
	  infections
		NEGOTIATING THE HEALTH-CARE SYSTEM
		
		AIDS fraud
		Professional-patient
		  relationships
		See resources, health
		  maintenance,
		  nursing care
		  partnerships
			NEUROLOGICAL CHANGES
			
			Caregiving
			Dementia
			Living strategies
			Pathophysiology
			Peripheral neuropathy
				NURSING CARE PARTNERSHIPS
				
				Consultation
				Home Care
				Initiation
				Proactive approaches
				  to health care
				Services

NUTRITION
 	
AIDS and nutrition
Food groups and
  symptom
  management
Herbs
Holistic approaches
  and natural foods
Recipes
Supplements
Total parenteral
  nutrition (TPN)
Vitamins and minerals
	PSYCHOSOCIAL ISSUES
	
	Coping
	Depression
	Loss and grief
	Support groups
	When a friend has
	  AIDS
		PUBLIC SPEAKING & HIV/AIDS
		
		Audience: general,
		  teen/school age
		Becoming politically
		  active
		HIV in the workplace:
		  information for
		  workers
			RESOURCES
			
			Advance directives
			Colorado Aids Project
			Drug programs
			Funeral, burial
			  assistance
			Home care
			Hospice
			Legal assistance
			Medicare handbook
			Handicap resources
			Identifying personal
			  resources
			Mobilizing options
			Social services
				WOMEN & HIV/AIDS
				
				Children
				Health maintenance
				Relationships
				Symptom
				  management
				Transmission

Although the Living with HIV program was originally designed for clients, their family members and significant others, visiting or consulting health professionals and students also began to use the curriculum. Because of this unexpected usage, the program was revised and expanded to include a more technical and diverse content. The self-instruction modules are available in a variety of media, including written and audiovisual materials. Written materials include published articles, pamphlets, brochures, newsletters, information sheets, and reference books. Audiovisual materials include slide presentations, video and audio cassettes, and rotating bulletin board presentations on such topics as Medical Directives, Exercise and Nutrition, and Nursing Care Partnerships. In addition, a monthly newsletter is published by clients; staff persons regularly contribute educational articles to the newsletter.

The modules are color coded to improve ease of access, and all written materials except for books and periodicals are located in colored hanging file folders.

Video and audiocassettes are labeled with colored labels corresponding to the module to which they are indexed. At the end of each modular section a folder labeled "Additional Reference Materials" contains a list of video and audio cassettes, books, and periodicals that relate to the modular subject. Audiovisual presentations vary from short informational segments of 10 minutes to as long as 60 minutes and are located in the Center library for easy access.

Although the Living with HIV program is comprehensive and self-paced, it is designed to be used in conjunction with professional support as needed. Nurses at the center use the curriculum to reinforce individual teaching and learning sessions. Schedules of formal presentations and classes are posted, and individual meetings with nurses are scheduled to reinforce and individualize content and answer questions. Users may access the materials on their own or with guidance from a staff member. In practice, clients usually request information from their nursing care partner, who then directs them to the appropriate module. A *User's Guide* gives detailed instructions on use of the curriculum and a *Subject Index* is available for easy reference. Most of the program usage occurs at the center, although a lending library system is in effect for those who prefer to take materials home. Many of the program materials are available for people to keep, such as brochures, articles, and newsletters. Most importantly, the self-paced design enables each individual to complete a module on his or her own time, when the particular content becomes relevant to individual health status and needs.

EVALUATION

For evaluation purposes, records were kept regarding program usage over a two-year period. In that time, more than 325 clients and 260 family members, significant others, students, health professionals, and visitors have used the system. Individual nurses access the curriculum approximately three times per week, usually to augment individual client or family education with written materials, or in response to specific requests for information. The most frequently used modules during that time were Psychosocial Issues and Coping, Medical Management, Alternative and Complementary Healing Methods, Health Maintenance, Resources, and Negotiating the Health-Care System. Both staff and lay users agree that the Living with HIV curriculum contains comprehensive and current information that is easily accessible. An application has been made to a funding agency for the means to provide clients with access to computer-assisted instruction and an internet HIV/AIDS information network.

CONCLUSION

Two innovative programs currently in place at the Denver Nursing Project in Human Caring promote the health of persons with HIV/AIDS: the Nursing Care Partnership and the Living with HIV programs. Jean Watson's theory of human caring provides the theoretical basis for the programs, and client and staff response to the programs has been very positive. These programs were presented to assist other health professionals to develop similar programs that promote the health of persons living with HIV/AIDS.

REFERENCES

Newman, M. (1990). Toward an integrative model of professional practice. *Journal of Professional Nursing, 6* (3), 167-173.

Schroeder, C. (1993). Nursing's response to the crisis of costs and quality in health care. *Advances in Nursing Science, 16* (11), 1-20.

Schroeder, C., & Maeve, K. (1992). Nursing care partnerships at the Denver nursing project in human caring: an extension of caring theory in practice. *Advances in Nursing Science, 15* (2), 25-38.

Schroeder, C., & Neil, R. (1992). Focus groups: a humanistic means of evaluating an HIV/AIDS program based on caring theory. *Journal of Clinical Nursing, 1,* 265-274.

Thorn, K. (1990). *Applying medical case management: AIDS.* Canoga Park, CA: Thorn Publishing.

Watson, J. (1979/1985). *Nursing: the philosophy and science of human caring.* Boulder, CO: The Colorado Associated University Press.

Watson, J. (1985). *Nursing: human science and human care.* Norwalk, CT: Appleton-Century-Crofts.

Watson, J. (1988). New dimensions of human caring theory. *Nursing Science Quarterly, 4,* 175-181.

Watson, J. (1990). Transpersonal caring: a transcendent view of the person, health, and healing. In M. Parker, (Ed.). *Nursing theories in practice.* New York: The National League of Nursing.

Chapter 9

Academic Nursing Centers and Community-Based Nursing Information Systems

Sally Peck Lundeen, PhD, RN, FAAN
Barbara Friedbacher, MS, RN

OVERVIEW

Expert nurse case managers promote academic nursing centers' research and educational efforts by applying their skill, knowledge, and competence in informatics.

The complex nature of today's society and the fragmentation of the health-care delivery system in this country require that the coordination of services be an essential part of the care provided to consumers in community practice settings. Although nurses have also been key providers of case management services in many community settings, the need for expert nurse case managers has never been greater. Case management is a nursing intervention that requires a high degree of skill and knowledge. The improved outcomes of individuals who receive this intervention are known to all nurses who provide it; however, empirical evidence that documents both the nature and the impact of nurse case management in community settings is limited. This chapter presents a description of academic nursing centers and outlines their potential to provide a framework for the education and research of nurse case management in community settings. A community nursing center exemplar is provided to demonstrate the nature of nurse case management in community nursing center settings and to describe the computerized clinical documentation system developed to retrieve data related to case management interventions and outcomes. Implications for nursing education, practice, research, and health-care policy are presented.

Nearly all aspects of our society are becoming increasingly complicated. Health care is certainly no exception to this general rule. Many individuals and families with complex needs find that they are unable to successfully negotiate a fragmented and complicated health and human service delivery system to gain access to services. This situation has led, in turn, to more attention being directed toward case management as a strategy used by health service providers to improve the coordination of services. Concern about escalating health-care costs also has been a factor in the recognition of case management as a potential strategy to increase efficient resource allocation in many health-care organizations. It is not clear that these two philosophies are necessarily compatible; and it is not clear that case managers in different practice settings function in similar ways, but it is clear that there is a real interest in case management by providers, consumers, and payors of health care.

Case management has been accepted as an important aspect of the nursing role in a variety of practice settings. Acute and chronic care, wellness and primary prevention, institutional and community-based settings all acknowledge the important role of nurses as case managers. In fact, case management is considered by these authors to be the essence of professional nursing practice. Therefore, case management in some nursing center settings can be viewed "simply as a vehicle for practicing professional nursing" (Newman, et al., 1991). It is certain that nursing case management as a practice modality is here to stay.

NURSING CASE MANAGEMENT AS AN INTERVENTION STRATEGY

Nursing is not the only profession that lays claim to case management as a professional skill. Many reports of case management are cited in the social welfare literature (Weil, 1985). Although some suggest that case management is a fairly recent phenomena in health care, others note that public health nurses have been doing case management for over a century (Knollmueller, 1992). There also has been considerable confusion in the healthcare literature in recent years around the related but distinct concepts of managed care and case management (Zander, 1993). Although similarities and differences in various case management models have been analyzed by several authors (Austin, 1988; Cohen & Cesta, 1993; Del Togno-Armanasco, 1989), a review of the literature suggests that there is a lack of clarity and consensus about the actual nature and focus of case management as a nursing intervention strategy. Definitions from the current literature include:

- Case management varies in form and function according to the system within which it is developed but the central theme of case management is that responsibility for meeting the needs of the client is with an individual or team whose purpose is to link the client with services required for a successful outcome (Franklin, et al., 1987).
- Case management is a set of logical steps and a process of interaction with service networks which assures that a client receives needed services in a supportive, efficient, and cost-effective manner (Weil, 1985).
- Case management optimized the client's self-care capability, promotes efficient use of resources, and stimulates the creation of new services (ANA, 1988).

According to Karen Martin and associates, developers of the Omaha System used by many community health nurses to classify nursing diagnoses and interventions, case management includes:

> . . . the nursing activities of coordination, advocacy and referral. These activities involve facilitating service delivery on behalf of the client, communicating with health and human service providers, promoting assertive client communication, and guiding the client toward use of appropriate community resources (Martin & Scheets, 1992).

There is great need for additional research on both the nature and the impact of nursing case management intervention strategies. Case management strategies and skills, however, must become an integrated element in nursing school curricula immediately if nurse educators are to prepare professional nurses with the theoretical knowledge and clinical skills necessary to provide effective nursing practice in a variety of practice settings. Academic nursing centers provide the unique opportunity both to investigate the impact of effective nursing case management strategies and provide a nurse-controlled practice environment within which to teach these strategies.

This chapter will:

- Describe academic nursing centers as one innovative model that supports the further development of nursing case management strategies by linking elements of practice, education, clinical research, and public policy;
- Identify the potential role of academic nursing centers in the support of research and educational activities related to case management;
- Describe the computerized clinical documentation system that provides support for clinical research and education;
- Present a community nursing center's exemplar to illustrate these points; and
- Suggest future challenges for professional nursing related to nursing case management.

Nursing Centers

Nursing centers have been a growing phenomena in the United States since the late 1970s. Populations of service frequently include hard-to-reach or disenfranchised populations, including poor and homeless persons, isolated elders, young single-parent families, and hard-to-reach rural populations. Many agree that, although the nursing center concept has been heralded as a unique phenomena during the past two decades, the origins of these community nursing centers are over a century old and harken back to the very beginnings of public health nursing on Henry Street (Glass, 1989; Wald, 1915).

Nursing center models are not limited to disadvantaged populations, however. Other populations frequently served by nursing centers include college students, employed workers and their dependents, and retirement communities. Neither are nursing centers limited to community-based settings. Hospitals and other health-care institutions have developed nursing centers as means of expanding direct access to professional nursing care. Such centers may attribute their historical roots to the Loeb Center, among other early institutionally based nursing center models. In fact, since responsiveness to an identified population is a defining criterion of nursing centers, it is possible to suggest that there may be as many types of nursing centers as there are identifiable nursing centers. Several definitions, however, have been developed during the past decade which attempt to define the key characteristics of nursing centers.

A 1986 Task Force of the American Nurses Association defined nursing centers as follows:

Nursing centers—sometimes referred to as nursing organizations, nurse managed centers, nursing clinics, and community nursing centers—are organizations that give the client direct access to professional nursing services. Using nursing models of health, professional nurses in the centers diagnose and treat human responses to actual and potential health problems and promote health and optimal functioning among target populations and communities. The services provided in these centers are holistic and client centered and are reimbursable at a reasonable fee level. Accountability and responsibility for client care and professional practice remain with the professional nurse. Overall accountability and responsibility remain with the nurse executive.

Nursing centers are not limited to any particular organizational configuration. Nursing centers may be free standing businesses or may be affiliated with universities. The primary characteristic of the organization is responsiveness to the health needs of the population (ANA, 1987).

This definition implies that nursing centers must (1) provide consumers direct access to nursing services, (2) be based on holistic, client-centered, *nursing* models of care which include an emphasis on health promotion as well as illness care, (3) be under the administrative and clinical control of professional nurses, and (4) provide services that can be paid for either directly by clients, third-party reimbursement, or through contractual arrangement with an employer or other payor. In addition, collaborative, interdisciplinary team-based models of health-care delivery have been identified as nursing center models by these authors and others (Lundeen, 1990).

Nursing centers provide the opportunity for professional nurses to develop and test intervention strategies that promote and support enhanced levels of wellness in defined populations. Practitioners in nursing centers intervene to assist clients to cope with the many "human responses to actual and potential health problems" (ANA, 1980). Clinical practice in nursing centers requires nurses to teach and support individuals and families to negotiate the multiple and complex

segments of health and human service of delivery organizations. This is the essence of nursing case management. It is a key service offered to the clients of many nursing centers regardless of the specific practice setting.

Academic Nursing Centers

Dozens of academic nursing centers have been developed in this country during the past 15 years. Affiliated with university schools of nursing, these centers are organized as the service arm of schools of nursing. These centers seek to integrate the multiple research, teaching, and service missions of these institutions. A 1993 AACN survey of university schools of nursing identified 60 academic nursing centers during that program year. This was 19.4% of the responding schools of nursing. Many (59%) of these academic nursing centers are community-based and provide accessible primary health care and primary prevention services to various populations (AACN, 1993).

Academic nursing centers offer nursing faculty in higher education the opportunity to meet the sometimes conflicting demands of simultaneously offering a quality educational program, conducting scholarly research, engaging in clinical practice, and providing community service. Some have also identified an important health policy role for academic nursing centers by providing innovative models of health-care delivery that can also generate the outcomes data necessary to inform policy makers about important issues related to access, quality, and cost of health-care delivery (Lundeen, 1994). The further development of academic nursing centers as models that facilitate the integration of the various aspects of professional nursing seems certain in coming decades. The expansion of the number of these centers and their positive impact on professional nursing and health-care delivery is anticipated with great interest by many. There is a potential for a significant impact on nursing practice, education and research, and public policies related to nursing case management through the contributions of community nursing centers.

The quality of the educational preparation of future generations of professional nurses will depend in large measure on the degree to which their teachers and mentors understand and respond to the ever-changing practice arena. To educate nurse clinicians who are prepared to meet the case management challenges of the health-care delivery environment and to participate as effective change agents within the practice environment, a critical mass of nurse educators must increase their own competence to practice in that environment. In short, academic nursing centers provide an important means for nurse educators to become and remain expert case management clinicians.

Case management intervention strategies also must be devised that are sensitive to the constantly changing needs of health-care organization environments as well as those of individual clients. Academic nursing centers are by definition under the control of nurses who recognize the necessity of developing strong collaborative partnerships with consumers and other providers. These settings allow experimentation with innovative practice models and intervention strategies. The eventual clarification of effective nursing case management philosophies and techniques will most likely result from the ability of nurse clinicians to implement and evaluate innovative strategies in practice settings controlled by nurses. Academic nursing centers provide the opportunity to develop just such environments that support both the research and educational agenda.

Research issues. Academic nursing centers offer rare opportunities to conduct clinical research in the area of case management by melding the resources of academe with those of specific clinical practice settings. The opportunity for expert clinicians to assume the researcher role is also greatly enhanced in these centers. This close affiliation between the practitioner and the researcher roles is particularly important to the further investigation of nursing case management intervention strategies for several reasons. First, the most accurate assessment of population needs and strengths are frequently obtained through the interactions of community residents and expert nurse clinicians over time. Case management activities must be designed that are responsive to the complex needs of a variety of consumer populations or communities while acknowledging the strengths of these same populations. Practicing nurse clinicians are perhaps the best qualified of all nurses to pose the most crucial research questions which most need to be addressed in these areas in relation to nursing case management.

Academic nursing centers provide the opportunity to translate research expediently into clinical practice settings where new knowledge and nursing/interdisciplinary intervention techniques can be further tested and refined. Nurse clinicians are in a position to implement research findings best and convey the impact of new techniques to policy makers in an expedient way. It is through the development of these research/service/policy links in centers developed by institutions of higher learning that practice-based research will be efficiently looped back into the education of tomorrow's practitioners. Expert clinicians working in academic nursing centers have a very important role to play on any research team investigation of case management.

Academic nursing centers also provide an excellent environment for the development and testing of clinical information systems for nurse case management research. There is a great need to implement clinical documentation systems that specifically record data related to the provisions of case management activities. Case management is a core nursing intervention and may, in fact, be one of the most unique aspects of clinical intervention that distinguish nursing practice roles from those of other health-care providers. To teach this skill to others, educators must be able to describe the nature of the techniques used and facilitate a transfer of knowledge to students. Likewise, to study the impact of nurse case management intervention on various populations, there is a need to collect and analyze reliable and valid data about this intervention strategy.

Many clinical documentation systems only capture data on those activities related to the hands-on clinical interventions of assessment and management of acute and chronic illnesses. These systems, even when used by nurses, are based on medical model traditions and fail to capture the essence of good nursing practice. Without the development of clinical documentation systems that record important aspects of nursing practice, such as nurse case management, the nature of professional nursing's contribution to positive client outcomes will never be fully recognized.

There is also a great need to develop computerized clinical documentation systems that specifically record data related to the provision of case management activities. In most practice settings, nurses are extremely conscientious about documenting the nature and substance of their clinical interventions in extensive narrative notes. Unfortunately, however, the actual utility of this form of clinical documentation must be questioned for most practice settings for several reasons. First, the use of nursing data recorded in this way by other health-care providers is frequently limited. In some institutions, nurses notes are still kept in a separate part of the chart and may never even be reviewed by other members of the team. From a practice standpoint, this is unfortunate because important data that could contribute to positive client outcomes are consistently lost on a case-by-case basis. From a research standpoint, there are even more serious repercussions if clinical data related to core nursing interventions are not retrievable for systematic analysis.

Currently, there is great interest in outcomes research within the professional nursing community as well as within other health-care disciplines. There is too little empirical evidence of the impact of specific intervention strategies on client outcomes. This is perhaps most particularly true of interventions that are not considered to be traditional medical interventions, such as case management. There will continue to be limited information in this area until we revise the clinical data that we collect and the ways in which we record and retrieve clinical data. It is imperative that we carefully identify the common data elements that nurse clinicians must collect and then we must collect these data in systematic ways in a variety of clinical settings.

It is not enough, however, simply to collect the appropriate data systematically. We also must develop management information systems that will allow us to store and retrieve these data in databases that are structured to facilitate analysis. The ability to provide reasonably accessible clinical data for analysis usually demands computerized systems. Computerization, per se, does not offer any guarantee of accessible and useful data, however. In fact, there are many examples of large computerized clinical databases that are structured in ways that have little relationship to the research questions of interest to practitioners or policy makers. Many health-care organizations have computerized a wealth of clinical data that can be used efficiently to meet important but limited objectives such as case documentation, audit of reimbursement procedures, or for analysis of organizational utilization from a marketing standpoint. Key data elements related to nursing practice are frequently omitted entirely from these management information systems and, even when nursing data are collected, the relational linkages between these data and other key data elements are not in place. Without these data linkages, the information of interest cannot be "teased out" of the system.

Before adopting or developing an information system, it is important to identify the type of information that is being sought. What are the questions of interest related to nurse management interventions? Secondly, it is critical that nurses who are knowledgeable about and interested in the documentation and study of nurse case management become involved in the development of clinical documentation systems. Nurses must specifically (1) identify the information that they need related to this and other areas of nursing practice and (2) identify the actual data elements to be included in an information system and work with informatics experts to develop the relationships between the data elements that will result in retrievable, useful data. Academic nursing centers facilitate the collaboration of colleagues with expertise in a broad array of subjects and allow the creation and testing of clinically relevant management information systems within an academic research environment.

Educational issues. It is important to develop learning laboratories that truly reflect the nature of the practice environment in society today where students learn nurse case management techniques. The nature of nurse case management is such that the skills required to become an effective practitioner must be developed in settings that serve clients with complex needs. Nursing educators cannot effectively teach sophisticated case management skills solely in the classroom or through simulated learning methods. Nursing case management is a complex and highly interactive strategy. When effectively practiced by skilled nursing professionals, nursing case management is a sophisticated form of the nursing process which requires the integration of assessment, communication, knowledge of community resources, advocacy, and other clinical skills. It, therefore, must be taught in a clinical laboratory that provides the opportunity for students to observe the case management process as implemented by skilled clinicians as well as to become innovative and creative in developing and testing their practice skills.

Nurse case management skills also are best taught in practice settings that offer opportunities for students to develop these skills without undue pressure from other professionals or organizational structure which might inhibit the broadest practice of professional nursing. Nontraditional community-based settings frequently provide excellent opportunities to teach these skills because the practice of nurse case management may be most challenging and have the greatest payoffs in settings where innovative solutions to client problems can be mutually developed in a collaborative process between provider and client. Academic nursing centers can provide this type of excellent learning environment.

Another type of education open to nurse educators and other professional nurses lies in the public policy arena. The challenges to nursing in both practice and education are changing rapidly, and professional nurses must look beyond nursing itself to a broader health-care context. In a recent article outlining practice realities, Barnum (1994) suggests that "nursing has become a full-fledged partner [with administration and medicine] in the organization. We got what we wanted at the worst possible time, becoming a powerful player when it might have been easier to fade into the woodwork." Academic nursing centers provide an important means for representatives from the country's leading schools of nursing to be legitimately present "at the table" with other service providers and policy makers as decisions are being made that affect the nature and delivery of health-care services to all residents in this country. This participation with other nurses representing practice, as well as other providers, administrators, and policy makers can provide the necessary forum for nurse educators to establish credibility both within and beyond the nursing profession on health-care policy issues. Professional nurses must be actively involved with other disciplines in the important policy issues affecting health-care delivery at this time.

Health-care practice strategies are frequently driven by reimbursement or other fiscal concerns. The current lack of funding for case management interventions by most private and public funders is an example of the type of policy issues that must be addressed in the immediate future if nurse case management is to survive in an increasingly competitive marketplace. Nurses who advocate for nursing practice models, including case management, must become active in public policy debates. Academic nursing centers can provide the means to develop and test innovative strategies that can affect public policy development; they serve as showcase centers to highlight the potential of effective models of care; and they facilitate the recognition of nurses as key players in the public policy arena.

THE SILVER SPRING COMMUNITY NURSING CENTER: A CASE MANAGEMENT MODEL EXEMPLAR

In 1979, the University of Wisconsin-Milwaukee (UWM) School of Nursing (SON) established one of the earliest academic nursing centers in the country as a strategy for integrating the multiple university missions of teaching, research, and community service. For more than a decade, innovative health promotion and primary prevention programs were provided to the greater Milwaukee community by SON faculty, nursing students, and academic staff at the original campus-based nursing center site. The center was developed as a clinical laboratory for undergraduate and graduate nursing students providing them ample opportunities for learning through observation and participation in the design, delivery, and evaluation of health promotion, education, and screening activities. Research activities conducted by faculty and graduate students through the nursing center during the first decade of operation included community health assessments, program evaluations, and intervention studies on issues such as family interaction, impact of various teaching interventions with young families, coping patterns of blended families, coping styles of families in transition, lifestyle modification, imagery, and self-efficacy. Although much of the emphasis of the UWM Nursing Center during the past few years has been focused on community-based practice sites, the campus-based Cunningham site continues to provide leadership in the development of community assessment techniques and the development of innovative health promotion and wellness programs that target a variety of consumer groups in the Milwaukee Metropolitan community.

The Silver Spring Community Nursing Center (SS CNC) was developed in 1986 as the school's first community-based nursing center in response to UWM urban mission and a School of Nursing commitment to the development and testing of community-based nursing intervention models. SS CNC is located in (and developed in partnership with) the Silver Spring Neighborhood Center (SS NC) a large multiprogram family service agency that serves residents of the largest low-income subsidized housing development in Wisconsin and the surrounding community area. The UWM shift from a campus nursing center site into the community was precipitated by the recognition of the need for viable primary care and primary prevention demonstration projects based on nursing models of practice. Such demonstration projects were seen as necessary to provide a firm foundation for a successful move by professional nurses into the health policy arena.

Through the collaborative efforts of UWM School of Nursing and the Silver Spring Neighborhood Center and other partner agencies, this demonstration project has become a nationally recognized model of comprehensive, coordinated service delivery that addressed the interrelated health, social service, educational, employment, and recreational needs of economically disadvantaged urban families in one accessible location (Ludeen, 1993). The success and stability of this Community Nursing Center (CNC) model has facilitated the increasing involvement of UWM nursing faculty and staff in health policy work at the local, state, and national level in recent years.

The SS CNC is currently staffed by a team of five master's prepared nurse clinicians (including a family nurse practitioner, three clinical nurse specialists, and a mental health nurse), a bachelor's prepared community health nurse, a full-time master's prepared nurse associate director, a half-time clinic assistant, and a half-time administrative assistant. A UWM School of Nursing faculty member directs the project. Undergraduate and graduate nursing students also participate as team members in the course of their clinical placements each semester. Six of the ten team members are African American and four are Caucasian. This arrangement mirrors the racial composition of the community. Individual team members were recruited for their unique skills and qualifications, their demonstrated cultural competence, and their strong desire to be part of an innovative community health initiative. Prerequisites for hiring of all of the Community Nursing Center nurse clinicians included extensive experience in community health and case management in impoverished, ethnically diverse, urban neighborhoods. Through a collaboration with the UW Madison Medical School-Milwaukee clinical campus and Sinai Samaritan Medical Center, two physician faculty members and two fourth-year medical students are on-site team members one day each week. In keeping with the philosophy of integration of the multiple missions of the university, all staff team members play an important role in the provision of services to community residents, the education of undergraduate and graduate students, and the research activities of the initiative.

The services currently provided through the SS CNC include comprehensive health assessments for persons of all ages, health education and health promotion programs, screening, counseling, community outreach, care coordination, and surveillance activities. A family-oriented case management philosophy guides all nursing practice. This is an autonomous nursing practice, with referrals to onsite and offsite physicians, other offsite health-care providers, and other onsite and offsite resources made as necessary for the delivery of comprehensive, holistic, primary health care. Nursing services are provided in various ways including daily walk-in clinics, scheduled appointments, telephone consultations, home visits, group screenings and health education programs, and informal contacts throughout the neighborhood center and in community locations such as stores, parking lots, street corners, and fast food restaurants.

The most innovative feature of the service delivery model is the integration of health promotion into virtually all programs for all age groups throughout Silver Spring Neighborhood Center. These SS NC programs include day-care classes and alternative middle school, youth, and adult recreation and support programs for elementary and school children, a family resource center, meals for elders, a food pantry, community development activities, and adult education courses. By integrating nursing care into all aspects of center programming, health and social services are provided in a more continuous, coordinated way to the 1000 or so persons who are served by the neighborhood center each day. In short, the entire delivery model has embraced a case management philosophy.

Service Population

The population served by the SS CNC includes the residents of the largest federally subsidized housing development in Wisconsin and the surrounding four census tracts. This area is relatively devoid of other health and social service providers. Indicators related to health and family stability in this community are common to many in urban care. Of the residents, 95% are persons of color with over 90% being of African-American descent. The total number of households receiving public assistance is 89%. Of the residents, 50% are minors, and over 85% of these households are headed by single female parents. The surrounding neighborhood has undergone a dramatic transition in the past 20 years. A strength of the community is that it is currently one of the few integrated neighborhoods in Milwaukee. Three of the four census tracts, however, have a higher percentage of families living below poverty and a higher percentage of families headed by single females than the city average. The 1990 census and other data indicate that this is an area of expanding poverty, decreasing home ownership, and increasing crime.

The needs of families in the housing development and the surrounding area are complex and require coordinated, interdisciplinary programs and services that address multiple issues and needs. At the same time, and perhaps more importantly, the partner agencies recognize and respect the inherent strengths of individuals and families within the community, their resiliency and ability to survive in the face of unending hardship and stress. They demonstrate an amazing capacity for survival and personal growth. It is the understanding of those factors, not just the assessment of problems and needs, that drives the philosophy of all service delivery by the partner agencies. SS NC and SS CNC represent a community-based effort to provide a coordinated program of individual and family support services through multiple agencies committed to collaboration *with community residents* in planning, provision and evaluation of those services. This comprehensive range of prevention- and strength-focused programs and services provided at one location is geared toward capacity building for individuals and families, the reduction of the interaction effects of multiple risk factors, and the elimination of barriers to growth and goal attainment. Working *with* the individuals who live in the community rather than simply working *in* the community sets this case management model apart from many others.

Case Management Strategies in a Community Nursing Center

In the SS CNC primary health-care delivery model, family-oriented case management is used by the nurse clinicians as a foundation nursing intervention strategy. The goal of all case management activities is to support and empower individuals and families to use their personal and community resources to achieve an optimal level of health and well-being for all family members. Decisions about the nature, intensity, and duration of services are made by the nurse case manager in partnership with the individual, the family, and other collaborating health and human service providers. This plan of care is based on an ongoing assessment of developing strengths of individuals and family, their changing needs and their progress toward goals related to health and well-being.

The Silver Spring case management model is based on three fundamental assumptions:

1. All individuals and families have the capacity to maximize resources to increase well-being

and achieve progress toward health related goals.

2. Many individuals and families who fail to maximize the resources on behalf of their health and well-being are unable to do so largely because of the failure of the health-care and social service delivery system to provide services that appropriately support the clients' inherent capacities.

3. The overwhelming majority of individuals and families who receive services which recognize and support their inherent capacities will use resources effectively to achieve long-term positive outcomes.

The case management philosophy that characterizes the Silver Spring model is, therefore, responsive, reciprocal, interactive, and participatory in nature. SS CNC nurse clinicians have the opportunities to gain an in-depth understanding of (and sensitivity to) the wide range of interrelated environmental, psychosocial, physiological and health behavioral factors affecting the health and well-being of individuals families and whole communities. Throughout the case management process, this holistic viewpoint allows the nurse clinicians to respond to and address those factors that constitute the "real world" for the individuals and families receiving the services. Throughout the process the emphasis is on a client-provider relationship that will support and empower the capacity of the client, rather than the tasks of doing things "for and to" the client.

The service delivery model focuses on "continuous versus episodic care" and "neighborhood-based versus community-wide services." This allows clinicians to build relationships with consumers, communities, and other providers which are characterized by mutual trust, respect, and understanding. These positive relationships lead to partnerships in which there is a sharing of information, resources, and responsibility in the case management process. It is the mutual trust that develops between the nurse clinicians and the community residents which serves as the basis for the "art of effective nursing case management" as practiced in this community setting. This, perhaps more than any other factor, sets such models as this apart from case management models that focus primarily on information and referral, brokerage of service, gatekeeping of resources, and monitoring of service patterns and outcomes on an episodic basis. A common SS CNC client scenario is presented here to explicate the type of case management services provided in this setting. This example is based on a compilation of several clients seen at SS CNC to protect client anonymity; however, the scenario is consistent with many clients seen at the center.

CASE STUDY

Lakretia, a 20-year-old single mother of two preschool children, came to the Silver Spring Community Nursing Center in January of 1990. Her initial concerns focused on parenting issues and concerns over the health-care needs of her young children. Although the nurse clinician in the SS CNC Walk-in Clinic found Lakretia to have very limited knowledge about her children's needs, one obvious strength was her genuine concern for the well-being of her children. Although there were no specific actual problems with parenting identified in the initial evaluation, a number of risk factors were clearly present.

Lakretia's violent interpersonal relationship with her boyfriend (the biological father of one of the children) compromised her emotional stability and safety. In spite of her efforts to provide good parenting, the periodic crises involving her victimization in the abusive relationship seriously threatened her children's safety and emotional well-being. The nurse clinicians made intensive efforts to assist her in resolving the situation and in coping with and managing her stress.

For the next three years, Lakretia visited and telephoned the CNC periodically. Case management and health teaching and counseling interventions were the predominant focus of the services provided to her at the center. Her major concerns included managing a violent interpersonal relationship, learning effective parenting skills, surviving on a very limited income, and dealing with frequent problems related to housing and transportation. She also came to seek assistance when she and her children were acutely ill. In addition to Lakretia's clinic visits, a nurse clinician also visited her in the home, and she was referred to the Silver Spring Family Resource Center (FRC), where she received services from a Community Parent Advocate and a Parent Educator.

The frequency of her visits varied from crisis periods, during which she was seen as often as twice a week, to periods when she dropped by the CNC periodically to report that "things are going pretty good right now." Follow-up calls were made to her when she had not been in for longer periods. Visits were characterized by supportive counseling and patient and persistent referrals and linkages to the appropriate community resources. The nurse case manager provided a consistent source of guidance. Lakretia was encouraged to participate in an ongoing parenting support group and to see the mental health nurse clinician to explore healthier ways to cope with stress and develop a more positive self-image. She was assisted to find appropriate child care and return to a G.E.D. program to complete her high school education. Healthy life options and alternatives were constantly presented to her.

During this three-year period, Lakretia made many changes in her life. She left her abusive boyfriend, completed her G.E.D., was hired for her first job, and grew significantly as a parent. Her children are healthy and doing well in a subsidized day-care program. She still comes to the center for routine visits and attends the parenting group as her work schedule allows. She "touches base" with the nurse case manager at least once every three months. Her next goal is to establish a loving relationship.

Opportunities for Student Learning

Nursing case management is undoubtedly one of the most sophisticated and complex of all nursing intervention skills. When practiced effectively, it requires the nursing professional to simultaneously draw upon a broad scope of knowledge and a diverse set of distinctly separate, but interrelated skills. Those who have witnessed both the power and the gentleness of a nursing case management process which gradually supports a client or family in taking their own bold steps toward a higher level of health and wellness can attest to the fact that case management can exemplify the nursing process in action at its highest level. The knowledge and skills required for the effective delivery of nursing case management at this level can only be learned in clinical laboratories where nursing professionals consistently model the integration and application of clinical knowledge and case management skills in their daily practice. Furthermore, the best learning environment will be a setting in which the nursing professionals who practice case management are simultaneously committed to and integrally involved in the education of students. Based upon this philosophy, SON faculty and graduate and undergraduate nursing students who come to the site as part of their course work for various clinical courses are viewed as integral members of the service research team.

Academic nursing center models, such as the one developed at UWM, integrate the university's missions of education, research, and service and provide ideal settings for nursing case management to be taught to students at both the undergraduate and graduate levels. Members of the SS CNC clinical team play a critical role in teaching of various aspects of community health nursing and community-based primary care at the center. Since the establishment of the SS CNC in 1986, hundreds of undergraduate and graduate nursing students have had community health learning experiences at the site. Educational experiences for master's level nursing students have included community health assessments and the design, implementation, and evaluation of aggregate-focused nursing interventions; multi-semester clinical practice as integral members of the nursing team to learn the advanced practice nurse clinician role; and a wide range of nursing research activities. Several doctoral students also have been extensively involved throughout their program of study as integral members of the SS CNC research team.

Nursing Center Research Related to Case Management Issues

There is an active research program in place at the UWM SS CNC, much of which relates to investiga-

tions of nurse case management interventions. A doctoral dissertation was completed in 1993 entitled, "Case Management at a Community Nursing Center" (Coenen, 1993). Analysis of five years of nursing intervention data is currently under way to determine the intensity of case management activity at the center as compared with all nursing intervention activities. Another project, "Project APPLAUD: An Intensive Case Management Intervention Model for Pregnant and Parenting Teens" is currently in the third of a five-year grant funded by the Wisconsin Department of Community Services. To conduct these research projects, a computerized database has been developed based directly on the clinical documentation of nursing practice in this setting.

A Computerized Clinical Documentation System for Nursing Practice and Research

The Automated Community Health Information System (ACHIS) was developed for the purpose of recording clinical data related to the users of nursing services (client descriptors), the actual or potential problems that affect them (nursing diagnosis), the nursing interventions implemented with these clients, and the outcomes related to nursing interventions. This management information system has been developed and tested as part of a comprehensive program of community-based clinical research implemented at the University of Wisconsin-Milwaukee in 1987. The ACHIS was developed after a search for a computerized clinical documentation system that was (1) based on a nursing taxonomy, (2) sensitive to primary health care and community health practice, and (3) capable of relating important data elements proved fruitless.

ACHIS was designed to serve as a computerized clinical database that would support the practice aspects of the community nursing center while simultaneously fulfilling the administrative requirements of reporting to multiple revenue sources. In addition, ACHIS was designed to provide a longitudinal research database that could be used to develop new knowledge about the impact of community-based nursing interventions, including nurse case management, on various populations. Such research is critical to provide the basis for changes in clinical practice and in the policies that affect the delivery of community-based health services. The ACHIS was designed with several criteria in mind, including (1) a sound conceptual fit with community nursing practice, (2) affordability for community agencies, and (3) efficiency of data recording and retrieval by clinicians (Lundeen & Friedbacher, 1994).

Specific data needs for every clinical site vary based on the nature of the organization and the nature of the practice. The ACHIS was structured to allow the SS

CNC administration to report to multiple funders each of whom were interested in specific data on different populations. It was also designed to facilitate reporting on both clinical and administrative data related to these populations on a complex reporting schedule. All nursing organizations will need to customize data elements for various reasons; however, some common themes have been identified when adapting the ACHIS for use in other nursing center sites.

A list of the actual data categories included in the ACHIS is presented in Table 9-1. The data elements included the 16 items recommended by the Nursing Minimum Data Set. The nursing elements of diagnosis, interventions, and outcomes are coded in the ACHIS according to the Omaha System taxonomy. The Omaha System, developed and tested at the Omaha VNA during a 15-year period, consists of a broad, community health-focused, client-problem classification scheme and a two-level system for coding nursing interventions (Martin & Scheets, 1992). The system includes a five-point rating scale for client outcomes specific to each nursing diagnosis in three categories: knowledge, behavior, and health status. The Omaha System also allows the provider to code whether the identified nursing diagnosis is an actual problem (AP), a potential health problem (PP), or is a concern related to health behaviors of the client (HP). Further specificity is provided through a coding of the diagnosis as a "family" or "individual" problem.

It is important that a clinical documentation system be responsive to the need for individualized client data reports. The ACHIS was developed predominantly for the collection and study of aggregate data; however, it is also able to produce individual status reports that can serve as client record documentation and case study material for analysis. A sample of an individual client encounter record is presented in Table 9-2. This example has been developed to correspond to the compiled client scenario presented earlier. This record demonstrates the frequency with which case management is used as a primary prevention strategy as well as an acute care intervention.

The ACHIS provides data for the study of many other issues related to case management. For instance, although cost control (particularly short-term or episodic cost control) is not the driving force that determines the characteristics of services provided in the SS CNC model, it has served as an important element in the development of the intervention strategies. The model is based on a philosophy that projects that over the long term, improved resource utilization and improved health outcomes for individuals and

---

TABLE 9-1   Selected data categories recorded in ACHIS

Patient descriptor categories	Nursing practice categories	Other data categories
Client I.D. number	Nursing diagnosis 44 Omaha problem categories	Unique clinic code
Social security number	Signs and symptoms Omaha codes	Type of visit
Date of birth	Nursing interventions 4 Omaha scheme categories	Site of visit
Race/ethnicity	Intervention target areas 63 Omaha categories	Visit status
Marital status	Knowledge outcome rating Omaha 5-point scale	Type of problem Actual, potential, health-related behavior
Gender	Behavior outcome rating Omaha 5-point scale	Problem modifier Individual, family, both
Years completed in school	Status outcome rating Omaha 5-point scale	Point of encounter
Current education status	Length of encounter	Encounter contact person
Employment status	Disposition	
Number in household	Unique provider code	
Number of children		

TABLE 9-2 Individual client report (selected visits) Silver Spring Community Nursing Center

Visit	Nursing diagnosis (domain/focus)	HP, PP, AP* (modifier)	K, B, S** (outcome)	Intervention & target area
#1	Psychosocial: Communication with community resources	Potential problem	2, 3, 3***	Case Management re: Other community resources
				Health teaching, guidance & counseling re: Parenting; medical/dental care (of child); physical symptoms (of child); support systems
			2, 3, 3	
	Psychosocial: Caretaking, parenting	Potential problem	3, 3, 3	Case Management re: Parenting; other community resources
#4	Psychosocial: Caretaking, parenting	Potential problem	3, 2, 2	Surveillance re: Parenting; safety (of child)
	Psychosocial: Interpersonal relationships—inappropriate suspicion/manipulation; compulsion/aggression	Actual problem		Health teaching, guidance & counseling re: Communication; interaction; other community resources; safety; support systems
				Case Management re: Other community resources; support group
	Psychosocial: Abused adult—attacked verbally; violent environment	Actual problem	2, 2, 2	Health teaching, guidance & counseling re: Interaction; legal system; other community resources; safety; social work/counseling; support group; support systems
				Case Management re: Legal system; other community resources; social work/counseling; support group
	Psychosocial: Emotional stability—apprehension; difficulty managing stress	Actual problem	2, 2, 2	Health teaching, guidance & counseling re: Coping skills; relaxation/breathing techniques; stress management; support systems; emotional symptoms
#8	Psychosocial: Abused adult	Potential problem	4, 3, 3	Surveillance re: Interaction; safety; support systems
	Psychosocial: Interpersonal relationships—prolonged unrelieved tension	Actual problem	3, 3, 2	Health teaching, guidance & counseling re: Communication; coping skills; interaction; support systems
	Psychosocial: Caretaking, parenting	Potential problem	3, 3, 3	Health teaching, guidance & counseling re: Parenting; safety (of child); stimulation/nurturing; emotional systems (of child)
				Case Management re: Other community resources health teaching, guidance & counseling re: Nutrition; physical symptoms; sickness/injury care
	Physiological: Digestion—nausea & vomiting	Actual problem	3, 3, 2	Case Management re: Medical care
				Health teaching, guidance & counseling re: Finances; other community resources; transportation
	Environmental: Income—low/no income	Actual problem	2, 2, 2	Case Management re: Finances; other community resources; social work/counseling

*HP, Health Promotion; PP, Potential Problems; AP, Actual Problems.
**K, Knowledge; B, Behavior; S, Status.
***Five point Likert Scale.

families can be expected to result in significant cost savings to society. When these capacity-building services are made imminently accessible in community settings to large numbers of families who typically use resources ineffectively and are at risk of costly negative health outcomes, the potential cost savings over time are significant. In the comprehensive Silver Spring case management model, long-term cost savings are projected in (1) potential reduction of emergency room visits, (2) more appropriated utilization of secondary and tertiary medical services, (3) improvements in self-sufficiency indicators including delayed childbearing, (4) increased job readiness, (5) levels of completed education, (6) improved self-esteem, and (7) the improved capacity to parent effectively. Case management is one very important nursing intervention being tested as one variable likely to increase effective and efficient use of health-care resources and also to increase health outcomes for nursing center clients. The ACHIS has provided the opportunity to examine this issue and various others through a longitudinal program of research.

Nursing Interventions

6-month period in 1994 (N = 8,567)

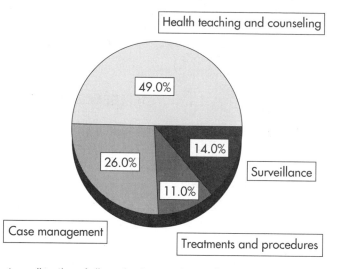

FIG. 9-1   Percentage allocation of all nursing interventions at Silver Spring Community Nursing Center

One of the questions being analyzed at this time involves the degree to which case management as a nursing intervention is utilized by nurse clinicians at the SS CNC. Preliminary analysis indicates that the use of case management as an intervention varies based on certain client descriptor variables and provider type. Nevertheless, Figure 9-1 shows the percentage of nurse case management interventions compared with all other nursing intervention categories (as defined by the Omaha System Intervention Classification Scheme) for a six-month period. The ability to differentiate case management interventions from other nursing interventions categories through the use of a standardized clinical documentation format facilitates the investigation of many clinical- and policy-related questions about this important strategy. In short, academic nursing centers provide outstanding opportunities for research on nurse case management and other issues related to nursing practice in community settings. If we are to better describe and evaluate nursing case management as a fundamental health-care intervention, there may be no better site than academic nursing centers where clinical excellence and research expertise can be integrated in challenging community-based practice settings.

CHALLENGES FOR THE FUTURE

Poor access to health care is an issue at the heart of health-care policy, particularly for vulnerable populations such as ethnic minorities, children, the unin-sured, and the underinsured. The economic and human costs of poor access are enormous. The frequent use of emergency rooms for primary care and the high rates of serious preventable diseases among Medicaid recipients across the country is evidence that more and different strategies are needed to reach the most vulnerable with primary prevention and health promotion services. The majority of families served by SS CNC are Medicaid recipients; however, simply having insurance, public or private, does not guarantee access. Because access to health care is complex and multidimensional in nature, evolving from the interplay between political, social, health, economic, and demographic factors, none of the factors can be effectively addressed in isolation. The comprehensive case management model developed by SS NC and the UWM SS CNC addresses the interplay of these factors for the high-risk population of a public housing development and the surrounding community.

Implications for changes in policy related to the organization and funding of health-care services have been highlighted by SS CNC studies and program evaluations again and again over the years. The CNC serves as a living demonstration of a program that works and has been host to a variety of important dignitaries, including U.S. Secretary of the Department of Health and Human Services, Dr. Donna Shalala, representatives of several major foundations, and Wisconsin's governor. The center also has been visited by nearly a dozen state and federal legislators, city and county officials, and other health-care administrators and providers. Staff provide leadership on more than a dozen city, state, and national task force or policy development groups. Testimony is developed and submitted at key legislative hearings and staff have been asked to serve as consultants on many demonstration initiatives locally and nationally. The strength of having a viable, successful, innovative project to showcase cannot be overstated in the discussions of public policy involvement. The ability to invite policy makers to "see for yourselves" an effective case management primary care model has made it possible for SS CNC staff to be actively involved with the shaping of health-care policy at many different levels.

For academic nursing centers to continue to provide an environment in which practice, research, and education related to case management can thrive, several important challenges must be met. First, nursing centers must survive. The current policies on the reimbursement of nursing services through these centers are frequently limited to those services basically medical in nature. Professional nursing services including primary prevention, health education, and counseling and case management must be designated as reimbursable under both public and private insurance plans if these centers are to become fiscally viable health-care delivery organizations. The challenge will be to describe and document these services and their positive impact on both client outcomes and the cost of providing health care.

A second related challenge is the development and consistent use of documentation systems that are built on *nursing* models of practice. Current clinical documentation systems are almost exclusively based on medical models of care. These symptoms, for the most part, do not include data elements that make it possible to collect and analyze nursing practice, including nurse case management. Nurses must accept the challenge to become active members of the interdisciplinary teams developing these systems and advocate for the inclusion of nursing practice elements in data management systems across all types of practice settings.

CONCLUSION

Colleges of nursing must acknowledge and support the development of affiliated clinical settings, such as academic nursing centers, to integrate the elements of practice, education, research, and policy development related to nursing practice. The ability of professional nursing to effect real change in practice and education rests, in part, on the ability of nurse educators, researchers, and practitioners to develop coordinated strategies for change and present them effectively to a wide variety of policy makers. Academic nursing centers provide an excellent mechanism for the imple-

mentation of significant changes in the delivery of coordinated, comprehensive care. We must accept the challenge by developing, testing, and teaching effective case management strategies. Finally, we must disseminate information about these strategies to a broad audience of providers, consumers, and policy makers. It is perhaps the greatest contribution that nursing will make to health-care reform efforts in this generation.

REFERENCES

American Academy of Colleges of Nursing. (1993). *Special report on institutional resources and budgets in baccalaureate and graduate programs in nursing.* Washington, DC: Author.

American Nurses Association. (1980). *Nursing: A social policy statement.* Kansas City, MO: Author.

American Nurses Association. (1987). *The nursing center: concept and design.* Kansas City, MO: Author.

American Nurses Association. (1988). *Nursing case management.* Kansas City, MO: Author.

Austin, C. D. (1988, Fall). History & politics of case management. *Generations.* 7-10.

Barnum, B. S. (1994). Realities in nursing practice: a strategic view. *Nursing and Health Care, 15* (8), 400-405.

Coenen, A. (1993). *Case management at a community nursing center.* Unpublished doctoral dissertation. Milwaukee, WI: University of Wisconsin-Milwaukee.

Cohen, E. L., & Cesta, T. (1993). *Nursing case management: from concept to evaluation.* St Louis: Mosby.

Del Togno-Armanasco, V., Olivas, G. S., & Harter, S. (1989). Developing and integrated nursing case management models. *Nursing Management, 20* (1), 26-29.

Franklin, J. L., Solovitz, B., Mason, M., Clemons, J. R., & Miller, G. E. (1987). An evaluation of case management. *American Journal of Public Health, 77* (6), 674-678.

Glass, L. K. (1989). The historical origins of nursing centers. In A. Arvonio (Ed.). *Nursing centers: meeting the demand for quality health care.* New York: National League for Nursing.

Knollmueller, R. N. (1989). Case management: what's in a name? *Nursing Management, 20* (10), 38-41.

Lundeen, S. P. (1990). Nursing centers: models for autonomous nursing practice. In McCloskey, J. and Grace, H. K. (Eds.). *Current issues in nursing.* (3rd ed., pp. 304-309). St Louis: Mosby.

Lundeen, S. P. (1993). Comprehensive, collaborative, coordinated, community-based care: a community nursing center model. *Journal of Family and Community Health, 16* (2), 59-67.

Lundeen, S. P. (1994). Community nursing centers: implications for health care reform. In McCloskey, J. and Grace, H. K. (Eds.). *Current issues in nursing,* (4th ed., pp. 382-386). St Louis: Mosby.

Lundeen, S. P., & Friedbacher, B. K. (1994). The automated community health information system (ACHIS): a relational database application of the Omaha System in a community nursing center. In S. J. Grobe, & E. S. P. Pluyter-Wenting (Eds.). *Nursing informatics: an international overview for nursing in a technological era.* Amsterdam: Elsevier, 393-397.

Martin K. S., & Scheets, N. J. (1992). *The Omaha System: applications for community health nursing.* Philadelphia: Saunders.

Newman, M., Lamb, G. S., & Michaels, C. (1991). Nurse case management: the coming together of theory and practice. *Nursing & Health Care, 12* (8), 404-408.

Wald, L. D. (1915). *The house on Henry Street.* New York: Holt.

Weil, M., & Karls, J. M. (Eds.)(1985). *Case management in human services practice.* San Francisco: Jossey-Bass.

Zander, K. (1990). Differentiating managed care and case management. *Definition, 5* (2), 3-4.

Chapter 10

Case Management in Community Nursing Centers

Gerri S. Lamb, PhD, RN, FAAN

OVERVIEW

Nurses revitalize community nursing centers, offering nurse case management and other health-care services to enhance integrated delivery and managed care.

Community nursing centers are a vital and uniquely nursing component of community-based care delivery systems. For these centers to continue to develop and thrive, their mission and goals must be linked to the evolving themes and needs of health care today. Case managers, with their focus on the needs of vulnerable and high-risk populations, fill a critical gap in the services offered at nursing centers. This chapter examines the contributions of nurse case managers to the survival and ongoing evolution of community nursing centers.

The popularity of community-based practice and the use of community health services have grown in direct response to dramatic shifts in health-care delivery and reimbursement. Managed care and capitated (per person) financing, in particular, have created strong incentives for offering preventive and health promotion services in the community to avoid or reduce the use of costly technologies and hospital days. Current models of health-care delivery emphasize the need to provide services in the most appropriate setting and at the lowest cost.

Today, nurses have an important opportunity to revitalize a unique nursing model of care delivery, the community nursing center, and to demonstrate that these centers are integral to the goals of integrated delivery systems and managed care models. The viability of community nursing centers will rely on our ability to frame

their function and worth in the context of dominant health-care concerns. The purpose of this chapter is to (1) explore issues related to incorporating community nursing centers into the mainstream of health care and health-care contracts, and (2) propose that nurse case managers are essential to the work of community nursing centers in a new health-care environment.

COMMUNITY NURSING CENTERS

Community nursing centers have served as innovative nurse-managed sites of care in the community for several decades. Based on early models of public health nursing practice, community nursing centers have sought to bring health promotion and primary, secondary, and tertiary prevention services directly to people where they live, work, go to the school, or seek recreation.

According to Riesch (1992a), there are three basic types of community nursing center models: (1) community health or outreach models, (2) health promotion models, and (3) independent practice models. Each of these models offers direct access to professional nursing services and emphasizes nursing control over nursing practice and the delivery of holistic, family-focused care (Riesch, 1992a).

Community health and outreach models include hospital- and university-affiliated clinics (Lundeen, 1993) as well as parish nurse (McDermott & Burke, 1993) and block nursing programs (Jamieson, 1990). The wellness and health promotion types of community nursing centers emerged during the late 1970s and early 1980s in response to a national focus on healthy lifestyles and healthy communities. Riesch (1992a) noted that most of these centers were developed by academic faculty seeking student experiences in working with well populations. She emphasized that the health promotion-oriented centers were not integrated with the formal health-care system yet substituted for available services. Independent practice models included faculty practice sites, as well as centers run by nurse entrepreneurs.

PAST OUTCOMES AND PAYMENT SOURCES

In the past, the growth of community nursing centers has been severely limited by lack of research to demonstrate their cost effectiveness and the limited sources of reimbursement for their work. In her recent review of research on various nursing centers models, Riesch (1992b) concluded that although there is considerable support for client satisfaction with these models, there is very little information about clinical outcomes or costs of care, particularly in the nonacademic community nursing centers. This lack of outcome and cost data will continue to plague contracting efforts and must be remedied.

Reimbursement for community nursing centers has relied primarily on self-pay by consumers and funding through government initiatives and foundation grants. Riesch (1992a) provides an excellent history of funding for community centers, including initiatives by the Division of Nursing, federal and state mandates, as well as private grants provided by such well-known foundations as Robert Wood Johnson and W.K. Kellogg.

Until recently, there have been few opportunities or incentives for nursing centers to become a part of integrated care networks of managed care contracts. Few centers have had experience with fixed or capitated reimbursement.

Several decades ago, the Frontier Nursing Service began financing their community health centers by charging each household in the community—an important predecessor to current capitated reimbursement. More recently, Carondelet Health Care in Arizona began to incorporate community nursing centers in capitated managed care contracts (Ethridge, 1991). Since 1985, nurse practitioners at Carondelet, with extensive support of community volunteers, have provided health promotion, prevention, and early disease detection and treatment services in neighborhood-based centers. Located in such convenient sites as mobile-home parks or churches, these centers have attracted managed care members who might otherwise wait until their health problems become acute before seeking care.

PARTNERING WITH MANAGED CARE

In 1991, Carondelet moved to formalize the relationship between the centers and its managed care contracts. Members of HMOs contracting with Carondelet were encouraged to use the preventive and health promotion services available in the community nursing centers.

In 1992, the community nursing centers at Carondelet became the hub of a new nurse-managed capitated delivery system that includes home health, outpatient therapies, durable medical equipment, and other community-based services. As one of four national sites selected to participate in the Community Nursing Organization (CNO) demonstration, Carondelet began a three-year project to design, implement, and evaluate a capitated model of community and ambulatory care for Medicare beneficiaries. Within the evolving CNO delivery model at Carondelet, community nurses, nurse practitioners, and nurse case managers work side by side in the centers developing programs that will meet the needs of the population of people enrolling in the Carondelet CNO.

Community nursing centers share distinctive features that make them ideal participants in current managed care contracts and integrated delivery systems. Most importantly, the centers are located in the heart of local neighborhoods and communities and are an integral part of daily life. Often they meet a variety of needs for local residents—a source of health care for adults and children, a home base for basic social programs (meals or transportation), and a comfortable place for meetings and socializing with friends and neighbors.

Translated into the goals and incentives of managed care contracts, community nursing centers are an ideal setting from which to promote a grass-roots approach to primary care, prevention, and low-cost management of potentially high-risk populations. Research has shown that nursing centers are viewed by their users as accessible and acceptable (Riesch, 1992b). Local residents often will come to the centers when they will not go to more institutionalized settings, such as primary-care clinics or hospital outpatient departments (Ethridge, 1991). They will tell their nurses about family members and neighbors experiencing health and social problems who may be reluctant to seek timely care.

In contracting discussions, nurses need to assist administrators and payors to visualize the benefits of using community health centers as the point of entry into integrated delivery systems. Key words are *accessible*, *acceptable*, and *cost effective*. The focus of these centers has been and needs to continue to be the provision of primary care and prevention services; however, primary care and prevention services need to be delivered in the context of population-based care. Particular attention needs to be paid to identifying at-risk individuals and groups served by the center and implementing and evaluating programs designed to reduce personal and social risk factors and improve the cost effectiveness of the care delivery model.

In the next sections, the concept of population-based care is described and the role of nurse case managers as "high-risk specialists" in community nursing centers is advanced. Nurse case management is viewed as an integral feature of the population-based work of nursing centers and a major benefit in selling community centers to integrated delivery systems and managed care organizations.

POPULATION-BASED FINANCING AND CARE

Much of the current emphasis on community and community-based care delivery systems is being driven by changes in reimbursement. Prospective payment, particularly capitation, offers clear financial incentives to provide services in the least costly setting, which in the majority of situations, is in the home or local community settings. All participants in capitated risk contracts benefit when the use of the most expensive health services, hospitals and emergency rooms, is reduced. Thus, health care administrators, physicians, third-party payors and others increasingly see the benefits of providing preventive and supportive services in the community. The opportunities for expansion of community-based programs and for linking them financially to integrated health networks are unprecedented.

Increasingly, the financing of health care is concerned with managing the health needs of populations, rather than individuals or families. Under fixed methods of reimbursement, like capitation, there is a preset amount of funds to cover all agreed-upon services for a designated population. The challenge of population-based financing is to develop strategies and programs that create incentives to use preventive services, reduce use of expensive services, and at the same time, assure access to all covered services.

According to Greenlick (1992) and Hegyvary (1993), a population-based approach to care relies on systematic attention to the common needs of a large group of individuals as well as the unique needs of defined subgroups. Population-based care requires that administrators, professionals, and payors work together to:

- Develop systems and structures that encourage widespread use of primary care and preventive services.
- Implement case-finding techniques to identify high-risk, vulnerable individuals and groups before they enter a downward health trajectory and a cycle of using expensive acute-care services.
- Design cost-effective strategies to maintain contact with nonusers of services and anticipate patterns of increased service use.
- Recognize and track marker events and conditions that signify gaps or failures in coordination and preventive efforts (e.g., the incidence of hospital readmissions).
- Use public health and epidemiological models to anticipate commonly occurring and potentially expensive health problems.
- Interact with the broader community in which members live and work to understand the factors that influence the health and lifestyles of members.

None of the precepts of population-based care are new to nursing or to nurses who have been leaders in community health. We have not, however, always systematically linked our understanding of these principles to the incentives that drive health-care contracting today. The survival of community nursing centers may rely on our ability (1) to articulate clearly the link between population-based care and successful managed-care contracts, and (2) to demonstrate that the goals of population-based care are best achieved in neighborhood-based community centers managed by nurses who are skilled in primary care and case management.

THE ROLE OF CASE MANAGERS IN COMMUNITY NURSING CENTERS

Until recently, few of the community nursing center models included nurse case managers. The vast majority of nurses providing case management have been located in hospitals, HMOs, and insurance companies. Their work has focused on identifying individuals at risk of expensive service use, long hospital stays or readmissions, and coordinating services to prevent these complications. In a few isolated examples, case managers have worked on an "as-needed" basis as consultants for coordinating care for high-risk clients in community centers and primary care clinics and as a referral source when more intensive nursing intervention and coordination of services were indicated (Ethridge, 1991; Shelton, et al., 1994).

In the past, common case management functions, including case finding, risk appraisal, and coordination of care, have been carried out in community nursing centers by public health nurses, home health nurses, nurse practitioners, and other professionals. Why add case managers to current nursing center practice models? Will case managers bring anything unique to these models? Can they be expected to make significant contributions to the achievement of cost-effective care in these settings?

In light of the dearth of research on the quality and cost outcomes of community nursing centers and nurse case management, key arguments in favor of incorporating case managers in these centers must rely more on theoretical than empirical support (Lamb, in press). Once the functions and benefits of case managers are better specified, it should be possible to design studies that compare and contrast outcomes of models with and without identified case managers. The following discussion is intended to lay beginning groundwork for describing key case management interventions in various community nursing center models.

Nurse case management, as it is currently evolving, is concerned with the health of high-risk populations. Nurse case managers work with individuals with multifaceted and complex health needs to enhance their ability to care for themselves and to access the services they need in a timely and cost-effective manner. More recently, case managers, using their insights and knowledge about characteristics and situations that place people at risk, have become proactive in developing programs aimed at prevention. Thus, there are growing numbers of descriptions of programs implemented by case managers to reduce the number of high-risk pregnancies or reduce repeated heart attacks (Erkel, 1993; Ounce of Prevention, 1994).

As noted earlier, the development of systematic approaches to the care of high-risk populations is core to population-based care models and to cost-effective management of capitated contracts. In the Medicare population, for example, it is well known that a small percentage of Medicare beneficiaries consume the vast majority of resources and spend the bulk of the Medicare dollar (ProPAC, 1994). Without effective management of the needs of this relatively small high-cost, high-risk group, there are limited resources to address the health and wellness needs of the larger group.

Care that acknowledges the special needs and costs of high-risk groups within the population at large must attend to a series of key case-management functions including:

1. Case finding and risk appraisal
2. Interventions matched in type and frequency to the characteristics and needs of the risk group
3. Coordination of services
4. Evaluation of individual and group outcomes (Bower, 1992; Mullahy, 1995)

To address whether case managers are needed in community nursing centers, it is necessary to look at the effectiveness with which the total set of these functions is currently being carried out. My observation has been that although there is usually common recognition of a set of individuals who appear to have greater needs and exert more demands on the health-care system, there are few systematic attempts to organize care and services for these individuals. Care tends to be organized individual by individual rather than by subgroup or population. Reliable and valid risk appraisal instruments are in short supply and those that are used are inconsistently applied and evaluated. Nonusers of services are overlooked until they become members of the high-cost, high-service group (Greenlick, 1992).

NURSE CASE MANAGERS AS HIGH-RISK SPECIALISTS

The presence of case managers can focus attention on the special and complex needs of high-risk populations and the potential to avert costly health crises and complications through carefully orchestrated programs. Through their work, case managers can assist community nursing centers to analyze service delivery and use patterns that significantly affect quality outcomes and budgetary concerns. In effect, the role of the case managers is to translate the principles of population-based care into the daily work of the centers. Programs and services are designed and evaluated in response to the following questions:

- What are the characteristics of the population currently being served by the centers?
- Are there groups of individuals served by the centers who require more time and resources than other groups?
- Are there groups of individuals who could use the centers, but do not, and often seek expensive crisis-oriented care in local emergency services and hospitals?
- Are there local health and social problems that affect the effectiveness of care provided at the centers?
- How is care currently being provided to identified high-risk groups?

- What are the costs of care for high-risk groups in the centers? What proportion of overall expenses is accounted for by services provided to high-risk groups?
- What treatment modalities are used with high-risk populations? How are individual, group, and community interventions used?
- What are the potential benefits of better managing the needs of high-risk populations? To the clients, to the professionals and organization? To the local community?
- What changes are needed to realize these benefits?

In effect, the case manager is the "high-risk specialist" for the community nursing centers assisting the organization and professionals to evaluate and improve their service delivery patterns and costs for targeted high-risk populations. By better organizing care for high-risk populations, case managers enable professionals to focus their time and energies more effectively and efficiently and to use budgets to meet the needs of whole populations better.

NURSE CASE MANAGERS, COMMUNITY CENTERS, AND INTEGRATED CARE NETWORKS

Management of the needs and service-use patterns of high-risk populations is pivotal to the success of integrated care networks. Systems in which programs and services are closely linked through capitated financing have powerful incentives to maximize the likelihood that their clients use the most appropriate and least expensive services (Shortell et al., 1993).

In this context, the availability of skilled case managers is an effective marketing tool for community nursing centers. Their presence suggests that the centers and their staff understand quality and cost issues related to managing the needs of high-risk populations and that they are prepared to achieve desirable quality and cost goals.

Obviously, case managers must be more than a means to obtain managed care contracts. The case managers must be prepared to implement and evaluate programs for high-risk populations. This requires knowledge and skill in areas that may not be possessed by all case managers, including family and community assessment, risk appraisal and modification, group dynamics and leadership, and program evaluation. Today, most of these competencies are addressed in graduate-level nursing education programs. In contrast, the majority of nurses practicing as case managers seem to be graduates of associate-degree and baccalaureate-degree nursing programs. The lack of adequately prepared nurses may present a serious obstacle to realizing the benefits of nurse case management in community nursing centers.

We have just begun to address the role of case managers in prevention and health promotion programs. Although it makes good sense to anticipate health risks and avert potential complications, in many areas of clinical practice, there is insufficient research to assist case managers to predict individuals and groups who (1) have a high probability of experiencing adverse events, and (2) have a high probability of responding to nursing interventions in ways that will significantly reduce their risk (Erkel, 1993). Assisting individuals to make substantial lifestyle changes is a complex iterative process that often defies direct cause-and-effect explanations. Recent research, however, in the area of fall prevention in the elderly, for example, suggests that it is possible to develop and test clinical models that successfully predict risk for significant adverse events and guide effective interventions (Tinetti et al., 1994).

In our recent experience expanding a community-based nursing model to include health promotion and prevention services, it has been evident that many nurses feel ill-prepared to offer basic instruction and support in such core areas as exercise and nutrition (Lamb, 1995). Hospital-based professionals in other disciplines are used to working with acutely ill people using one-to-one treatment modalities and have needed extensive reeducation and support to shift their thinking about the focus of care and possible treatment alternatives.

To maximize the effective use of nurse case managers in community nursing centers models, we need to align educational requirements with the demands of the role. This requires that we take a serious look at the knowledge and skill required to serve as a high-risk specialist and hire only those nurses able to deliver the quality and cost outcomes to which we have made a commitment. In addition, it is imperative that we design and implement information systems to evaluate the cost-effectiveness of nurse case management services.

CONCLUSION

To remain viable in a rapidly changing health-care environment, all programs and professionals must examine their contribution to the quality and costs of health care and their role in an increasingly integrated care delivery system. For several decades, community nursing centers have symbolized the importance of providing care in the community and the benefits of direct access to professional nursing. Today, changes in the structure and financing of health care have set the stage for the "rediscovery" of community health centers. The challenge for nurses is to capitalize on the incentives for community-centered care and to develop the language and outcomes data to support successful contract negotiations.

Ten years ago, Sara Barger (1985) suggested that the future of community nursing centers depended on aligning the goals of the centers with the needs of the broader health-care environment. In a message that sounds strikingly similar to more recent critiques of nursing centers, Barger emphasized the importance of using the language of the health-care marketplace to sell the nursing center concept and the critical need to develop a body of research to document outcomes of care in the centers. Unfortunately, we appear to have made little movement on these fronts. In her 1992 review of the state of the community nursing centers, Riesch recommends the same priorities as Barger and observes that our approach to the development of nursing centers has continued to be "fragmented" (p. 22), and we have done little to integrate centers within the mainstream of health care.

Changes in health-care delivery and financing have once again opened a window of opportunity for nursing centers. The future of community nursing centers will be determined by our actions. We must articulate how these centers contribute to current goals in the health-care environment in language and outcomes that can be heard by the people writing the contracts. We must define the nursing skills and expertise required for management and delivery of primary care and case management services in the centers and then consistently adhere to these requirements. Further, we must document quality and cost outcomes by using measures that capture nursing's contribution to health care and convince people in key administrative and financial positions that we offer integral and irreplaceable services to individuals and populations.

REFERENCES

Barger, S. E. (1985). Nursing centers: here today gone tomorrow? In J. C. McCloskey & H. C. Grace (Eds.). *Current Issues in Nursing* (2nd ed., pp. 752-760). Boston: Blackwell Scientific.

Bower, K. (1992). *Case management by nurses.* Washington, DC: American Nurses Publishing.

Erkel, E. A. (1993). The impact of case management in preventive services. *Journal of Nursing Administration, 23* (1), 17-32.

Ethridge, P. E. (1991). A nursing HMO: Carondelet St. Mary's experience. *Nursing Management, 22* (7), 22-29.

Greenlick, M. (1992). Educating physicians for population-based clinical practice. *Journal of the American Medical Association, 267,* 1645-1648.

Hegyvary, S. (1993). The shift in focus from provider processes to population outcomes. *Nursing Administration Quarterly, 17* (3), viii-ix.

Jamieson, M. (1990). Block nursing: practicing autonomous professional nursing in the community. *Nursing and Health Care, 11,* 250-253.

Lamb, G. S. (1995). Early lessons from a capitated community-based nursing model. *Nursing Administration Quarterly, 19* (3), 18-26.

Lamb, G. S. (in press). Case management. *Annual Review of Nursing Research.*

Lundeen, S. P. (1993). Comprehensive, collaborative, community-based care: a community nursing center model. *Family and Community Health, 16,* 57-62.

McDermott, M. A., & Burke, J. (1993). When the population is a congregation: the emerging role of the parish nurse. *Journal of Community Health Nursing, 10* (3), 179-190.

Mullahy, C. M. (1995). *The Case Manager's Handbook.* Gaithersburg, MD: Aspen Publishers.

An ounce of prevention. (1994, September). *Case Management Advisor,* pp. 127-131.

Prospective Payment Assessment Commission (ProPAC). *Medicare and the American Health Care System, Report to the Congress,* June 1994 (Washington, DC: ProPAC, 1994).

Riesch, S. K. (1992a). Nursing centers: an analysis of the anecdotal literature. *Journal of Professional Nursing, 8,* 16-25.

Riesch, S. (1992b). Nursing centers. *Annual Review of Nursing Research, 10,* 145-162.

Shelton, P., Schraeder, C., Britt, T., & Kirby, R. (1994). A generalist physician-based model for a rural geriatric collaborative practice. *Journal of Case Management, 3* (3), 98-104.

Shortell, S. M., Gillies, R. R., Anderson, D. A., Mitchell, J. B., & Morgan, K. L. (1993). Creating organized delivery systems: the barriers and facilitators. *Hospital and Health Services Administration, 38,* 447-466.

Tinetti, M. E., Baker, D. I., McAvay, G., Claus, E. B., Garrett, P., Gottschalk, M., Koch, M. L., Trainor, K., & Horwitz, R. I. (1994). A multifactorial intervention to reduce the risk of falling among elderly people living in the community. *New England Journal of Medicine, 331* (13), 821-827.

Chapter 11

Integrating Services across the Continuum: The Challenge of Chronic Care

Becky Trella, MSN, RN

OVERVIEW

Nurse case managers develop a process to integrate acute and long-term care for chronically ill clients across the continuum.

As a large segment of our population continues to age and technology increases the life span of people with chronic conditions, our health-care system needs to refocus from an acute care orientation to a chronic care perspective. Individuals with chronic conditions require multiple services which currently operate within distinct organizations with their own set of policies, procedures, finance and billing structures, rules and regulations, and methods of care delivery. Efforts need to focus on integrating primary prevention, acute, transitional, and long-term care services into one comprehensive continuum of health-care services with easy access, simplified financing, and providers who collaborate to manage care throughout an individual's entire condition. This chapter will discuss the three key ingredients necessary to integrate health care and present one health-care system's approach to developing an integrated continuum of care.

As the number of individuals who suffer from chronic conditions continues to rise in our country, health care needs to be reshaped to offer a continuum of care. As defined by Evashwick (1987), a *continuum of care* is *an integrated, client-orientated system of care composed of both services and integrating mechanisms that guides and tracks clients over time through a comprehensive array of health, mental health, and social services spanning all levels of intensity of care.* This chapter will overview the primary mechanisms necessary to integrate care across settings for individuals with chronic conditions and describe

one health-care system's attempt to operationalize this concept.

Although many large health-care organizations offer the complete array of services expected in a continuum, these services are not usually integrated into a system of care. (Box 11-1; Evashwick, 1987). The following case study illustrates this lack of integration.

As illustrated in this case study, each service or site of care operates as a distinct organization with its own set of policies, procedures, finance and billing structure, rules and regulation, and methods of care delivery.

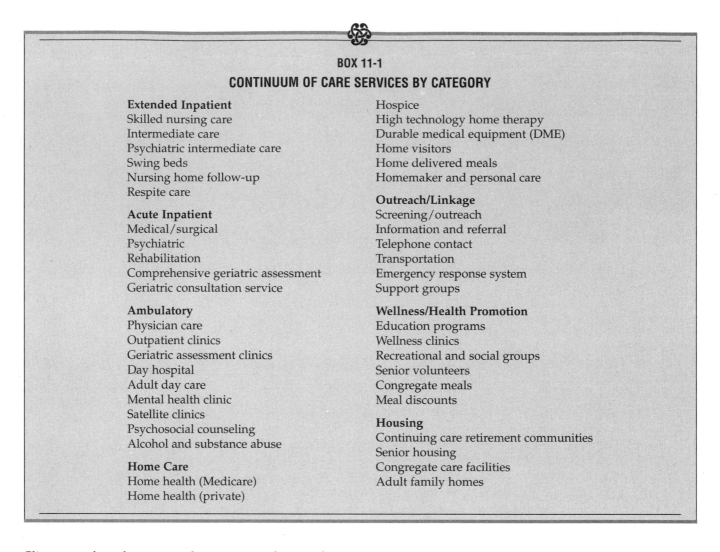

BOX 11-1
CONTINUUM OF CARE SERVICES BY CATEGORY

Extended Inpatient
Skilled nursing care
Intermediate care
Psychiatric intermediate care
Swing beds
Nursing home follow-up
Respite care

Acute Inpatient
Medical/surgical
Psychiatric
Rehabilitation
Comprehensive geriatric assessment
Geriatric consultation service

Ambulatory
Physician care
Outpatient clinics
Geriatric assessment clinics
Day hospital
Adult day care
Mental health clinic
Satellite clinics
Psychosocial counseling
Alcohol and substance abuse

Home Care
Home health (Medicare)
Home health (private)

Hospice
High technology home therapy
Durable medical equipment (DME)
Home visitors
Home delivered meals
Homemaker and personal care

Outreach/Linkage
Screening/outreach
Information and referral
Telephone contact
Transportation
Emergency response system
Support groups

Wellness/Health Promotion
Education programs
Wellness clinics
Recreational and social groups
Senior volunteers
Congregate meals
Meal discounts

Housing
Continuing care retirement communities
Senior housing
Congregate care facilities
Adult family homes

Clients are forced to access the system each time they use a new site or services, providing the same information repeatedly. Health providers in the different sites duplicate their efforts by not sharing the client's clinical information or developing a plan of care beyond their site or service. Each of the individual's illnesses is treated as a distinct episode while the individual receives care at that site instead of as an ongoing condition that needs continual monitoring and management. Quality and cost outcomes are monitored and collected by site or service, instead of over an entire condition and for outcomes that are meaningful for the individual. Clients are billed separately by each site and financial coverage is provided through multiple sources.

Mr. J is one of the three million people in our country who suffers from a chronic illness and whose health-care needs are inadequately met by our current system. Individuals with chronic illnesses require multiple medical, nursing, rehabilitation and social services. Figure 11-1 illustrates the annual movement of persons 75 years and older through the health-care system. These services are currently fragmented into two

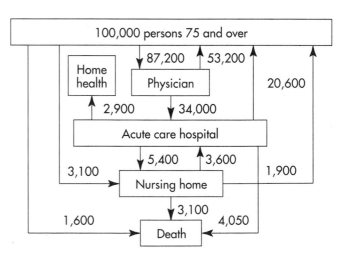

FIG. 11-1 Movement of persons 75 years and older through the health-care system (Source: NCCC; adapted from Denson, Paul M, AHCPR Monograph, Tracing the elderly through the health-care system, January, 1991, p. 7)

CASE STUDY

Mr. J was an 80-year-old male who lived independently in his own apartment in a senior housing building. He had minimal health problems including mild emphysema and high blood pressure. Mr. J rarely saw his physician and tended not to take his blood pressure medication because he felt fine and the cost strained his budget. His physician was concerned about his living alone and knew he did not take his medication, but felt there was little that could be done to change this situation. His only relatives were a niece and grandniece who lived about 30 minutes from him. Although they only visited about once a month, they frequently contacted him by phone to check on him.

One day, after no one had seen him for a few days, Mr. J was found unconscious in his apartment by the building manager. He was rushed to the nearest hospital where he was diagnosed with a stroke. The emergency room had no access to his medical history, information about his physician, or advance directives. It took hours and many phone calls to obtain this information. This information was used to complete an assessment and plan in the emergency room. A more detailed assessment and care plan was redone on the medical floor.

Mr. J stabilized and did well in the hospital and after seven days was transferred to a nearby rehabilitation facility. A short summary of his hospital stay and status was sent to the rehabilitation facility. The rehabilitation staff conducted another detailed assessment and care plan for this site. A key piece of information was unknown and not included. While in the hospital, Mr. J had difficulty voiding and was catheterized longer than expected. His output was closely monitored in the hospital after being decatheterized. Although Mr. J progressed well in the rehabilitation facility, on the tenth day he became lethargic and spiked a temperature.

Mr. J was sent back to the hospital and diagnosed with sepsis, UTI, and urinary retention. A short summary was sent to the hospital with no details of his rehabilitation plan or current functional status. A new detailed assessment and care plan was developed in the hospital. It was three days before Mr. J's physical and occupational therapies were restarted in the hospital and at five days he was ready for discharge. Unfortunately, he was unable to return to the rehabilitation facility because his function had declined so rapidly in the hospital. The niece, unwilling to accept the advice of nursing home placement, insisted on taking him home. A visiting nurse and home therapy were arranged upon discharge. The visiting nurse was provided with limited information except for a brief excerpt of Mr. J's last hospitalization. She conducted another detailed assessment and developed another care plan. Her perception was that Mr. J had limited potential for rehabilitation considering that it was now 23 days after his stroke and he had regained little function. She felt the niece was unrealistic about her ability to care for him and tried to encourage the niece to reconsider nursing home placement. Much to the niece's dismay, a very nonaggressive approach was taken with Mr. J's therapy at home and after two weeks therapy was discontinued because of lack of progress. Shortly after this, Mr. J's niece placed him in a nursing home.

During these episodes, Mr. J had six separate assessments and nursing care plans completed and received 18 different bills.

---

different areas: acute care medical services and long-term care services. The lack of integration between acute and long-term services leads to poor quality and increased expense. As a large segment of our population continues to age and technology increases the life span of people with chronic illness, our health-care system needs to refocus from an acute care orientation to a chronic care perspective. If a new health-care system is unable to meet this challenge, it will not effectively reduce the spiraling cost or widespread dissatisfaction in the current system.

To provide an integrated *continuum of care,* sites and services need to operate as a system of interdependent components that work together to accomplish a common aim, that is, improve the health status of people we serve. A continuum needs to be "customer oriented" and find out what the clients expect and put their needs and expectations first. A continuum needs to be seamless for clients so they do not have to reregister and repeat information each time. Planning needs to be done across sites and disciplines for all of an individual's conditions.

In the past, many attempts have been made to integrate the care of individuals who need multiple services (Cohen & Cesta, 1993). Most of these attempts have used case managers to coordinate the individual's care through the fragmented health-care system. Case managers have served an important function as client advocates, assisting clients to obtain necessary services and maximize the financial reimbursement. Although using case management has helped clients maneuver the complicated health-care system, it has not forced the health-care community to cure the ills of the system. Future efforts need to focus on integrating the acute, medical, and long-term care systems into one comprehensive continuum of health-care services with easy access, simplified financing, and providers who collaborate to manage care throughout an individual's entire condition. Case management should be reserved for the highest risk individuals who cannot manage their own care in a seamless integrated continuum of care.

KEY INGREDIENTS TO INTEGRATION

There are a few key movements in the nation which have focused their efforts on the integration of acute and long-term care. The most well-recognized efforts are the social health maintenance organizations and the Pace demonstration programs (Abrahams, 1990; Zawadski, 1988). Both of these efforts have integrated the finance mechanisms for acute, medical, and long-term services and have provided case management to frail elderly to coordinate the management of their health-care needs. Using a team approach, the Pace Models have been most successful at integrating all the clients' care into one comprehensive long-term plan. These models, however, serve a small and distinct population in a separate, special program. Neither of these models has changed how health care is delivered overall, so that care of individuals with chronic conditions is integrated and appropriately managed and financed.

The National Chronic Care Consortium (NCCC) is an organization of 25 leading-edge health-care systems who are committed to developing integrated chronic care networks (CCN) (NCCC, 1993). Each CCN will include an integrated continuum of primary prevention, acute, transitional, and long-term care services. A CCN provides a customer-centered, system-oriented approach to integrating chronic care across time, place, and profession. Three key ingredients are necessary to integrate a health-care system into a chronic care network:

- Integrated financing mechanism
- Integrated information systems
- Integrated care management

Integrated Finance Management

As illustrated by Figure 11-2, the financing of chronic care is very complex. Individuals are often forced to seek more expensive forms of care which are covered by insurance rather than low-cost services that are not covered by insurance. For example, the client may use skilled home care instead of homemaking services.

Clinicians frequently provide unnecessary care so that other services may be covered. For example, pain medication may be given by injections instead of orally so that the nursing home costs are covered. Clients, families, and clinicians waste much of their time trying to understand the finance system and completing forms to obtain reimbursement. A key aspect of caring for individuals with chronic illness is community-based supportive services. These services, however, have been greatly underfinanced in the current system although acute care and medical services have received most of the resources.

The separate finance structure for acute and long-term care has led to the fragmentation in how we deliver care. As providers, we have alliances to the system that pays our salaries and tend to focus only on the individual's needs while at our institution. Even case managers have had a tendency to focus primarily on coordinating the client's needs that are covered under the system that employs the case managers. For example, case managers employed by the Department on Aging may deal with the client's psychosocial and supportive needs in the community while overlooking their medical needs. Medical case managers employed by the insurance companies focus on meeting the client's short-term medical and skilled needs and may overlook their psychosocial and supportive needs.

Because of these issues, integrated financing to link reimbursement methods with positive outcomes over a condition's duration and across settings is necessary to deliver integrated care (Bringewatt, 1992). Integrated financing mechanisms will allow flexibility to provide the right care at the right time to maintain individuals at their highest level of functioning. For example, if reimbursing a grab bar will prevent a fall and a hip fracture it will be covered. Integrated financing will

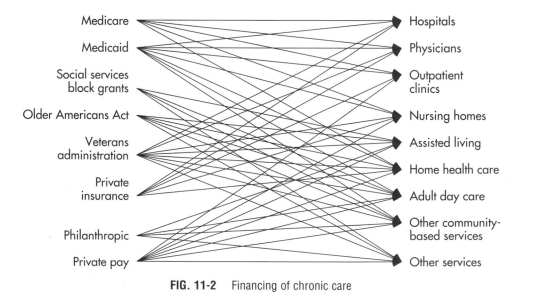

FIG. 11-2   Financing of chronic care

provide incentives for clinicians to provide care that will optimize the client's long-range outcomes and the overall cost even if it appears their bottom line is not optimized. For example, a client may spend one additional day in acute care if the client is able to return directly home instead of going to a nursing facility for three days.

Developing integrated finance mechanisms will mean creating capitated finance programs that pool funding for both acute care and long-term services (Figure 11-3). Unfortunately, health-care reform, while advocating funding through capitated finance mechanisms for medical and acute care services, is not ready to make the leap to include long-term services. Many proposed bills have included Medicare and long-term care reform but these now seem to be losing momentum. The nation needs to offer comprehensive health-care coverage for individuals requiring more than medical or acute care services. Until we are able to accept this challenge, an opportunity to truly impact cost and quality will be missed. As discussed in Part One, nursing as an organized group must respond to the issue of integrating health care.

Integrated Information System

The technology for user-friendly, multipurpose, multisite computer systems exists and has been implemented in industries other than health care. Currently, in health care each site has its own information system or systems and often the systems are not integrated, such as billing, cost accounting, registration, clinical data, and order entry. To manage care efficiently and effectively for individuals with chronic conditions, appropriate information needs to be shared across all sites and services (Box 11-2). Clients should not have

to repeat the same information as they access the health-care system each time.

The paper trail is an inefficient and inaccurate method of transferring information. Because of human error, key pieces of information are not shared from site to site. In an era when clinical decisions should be based on efficiency and effectiveness, information should be put on line for access by the clinician. For example, it would be helpful for a clinician to know that a particular antibiotic is just as effective but costs half as much as another antibiotic. Many new information systems for health-care systems are being marketed to integrate their information needs. Unfortunately, most of these companies are catering to the acute care and medical sites. Although it will be advantageous for a physician to access the daily lab reports of hospitalized clients from the office, the information needs of a social worker in a community-based program are very different. The social worker needs to have access to a client's living situation, functional abilities, and how the person copes over time. This is not information that medical or acute care systems are likely to offer in the near future.

To manage care across sites and services efficiently in an integrated capitated continuum, an information system will require the capacity to input and access clinical information across multiple sites, track and monitor clinical and cost data by client and diagnoses, integrate clinical and financial data, have the ability to monitor research outcomes and quality indicators (variance analysis), and assist with clinical decision making for diagnosis and treatment (Barrett, 1993). Many information systems have been developed that have some of these capabilities. A few systems have extended their capabilities across multiple sites. No one information system will provide all data across all

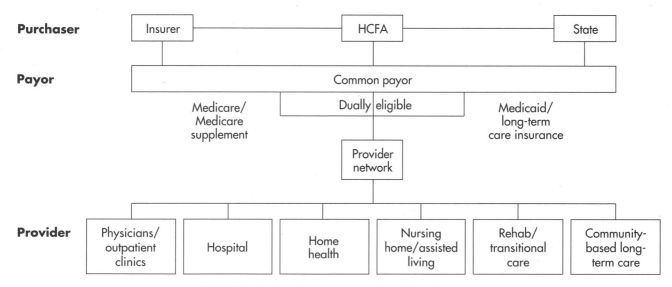

FIG. 11-3 Pooling financing for acute and long-term care

BOX 11-2
FEATURES OF A CONTINUUM'S INFORMATION SYSTEM

Core data set:
- A common client identifier
- Social security number
- Date of birth
- Sex
- Family indicators
- Household indicators
- Mother and baby indicators
- Leading and trailing digits
- Population and classification indicators

An electronic medical record, which includes the following information:
- Complete demographic
- Encounter history
- Social history

- Transition summaries
- Medication profile
- Test results
- Current plan of care
- Client problem list
- Financial history

A single billing account and format:
- Consistent format and appearance
- Single account for all services under the continuum
- Single current balance for client responsibility
- Ability to encompass all providers

A common client registration system:
- Common registration process
- Standardized information collection and verification process

---

sites. Therefore, an integrated information system will need to be composed of smaller systems that can be integrated into one large system through open system architecture as illustrated in Figure 11-4. This will require smaller systems that have compatible data structures that can be fed into the larger system.

Health-care systems will need to plan and centralize carefully all information system needs to fit together the pieces of the puzzle. Unfortunately, this type of strategic planning has not occurred, causing many organizations to abandon costly, incompatible systems. Before choosing information systems, organizations need to have representatives from all sites agree on the common data requirements (what information all sites need to access), individual site needs, and system requirements (i.e., ability to interface with cost accounting) (Box 11-3). An information systems specialist who can translate computer language into everyday language and understands the clinical needs is an important member of the committee. Clinicians who specialize in computer technology will be highly sought after in the future. Information specialists will understand whether the chosen computer systems can eventually be integrated and accessed across sites.

At vendor demonstrations, one must be suspicious of a company that states it can integrate all information across your continuum. Many times you will find the company's definition of a continuum of care is from unit to unit in the hospital. Rather than allowing acute care clinicians and physicians to choose a system for everyone, all the sites, both those owned and those not owned but contracted with, should be represented at the demonstration. During the demonstration, the vendor should be asked to show specific examples of how the system integrates information. For example, the vendor could be asked to demonstrate the system's ability to list Mr. J's medication from the physician's office, the hospital, the rehabilitation unit, and home care. Vendors tend to answer, "We are working on developing this capacity and will have this on line soon." Although it can be helpful to be part of a company's product development, choosing a company that can actually meet your future goals is a challenge. The company's solvency should be investigated. Other health-care systems that have worked with this company must be contacted, and if possible, visited. The company's security and confidentiality policies and how they deal with client identification numbers must be discussed. Because most sites establish different identification numbers for the same client, having one common client identifier may seem minor but is a large hurdle to overcome.

A totally integrated information system across the entire continuum of care does not yet exist; thus, organizations will find this a time-consuming, expensive developmental process. Hopefully, a few health systems who decide to take the lead in this development will find many solutions that can be applied to other health-care systems.

Integrated Care Management

Individuals with chronic conditions receive care from multiple providers and from multiple sites and services. Unfortunately, the planning and management of a client's care tends to be limited within that discipline

Future Network

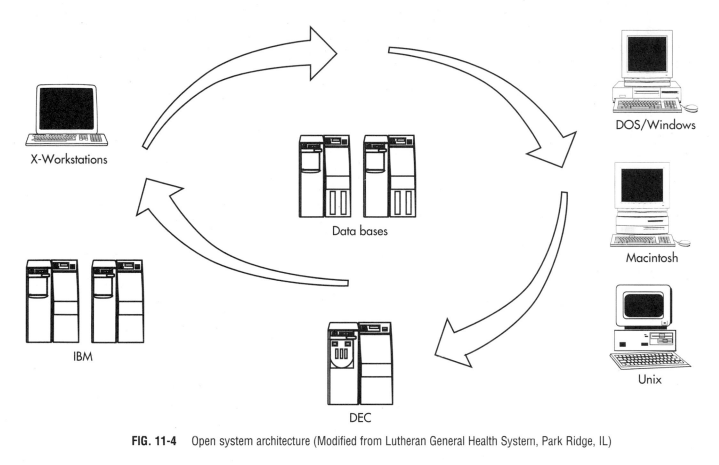

FIG. 11-4   Open system architecture (Modified from Lutheran General Health System, Park Ridge, IL)

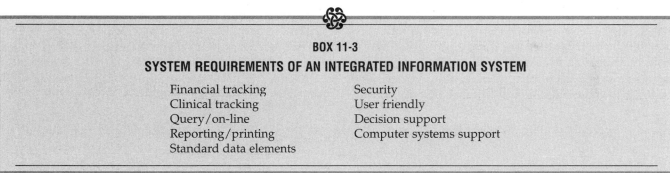

BOX 11-3

SYSTEM REQUIREMENTS OF AN INTEGRATED INFORMATION SYSTEM

Financial tracking	Security
Clinical tracking	User friendly
Query/on-line	Decision support
Reporting/printing	Computer systems support
Standard data elements	

or site. Some organizations have developed an interdisciplinary team approach to planning and managing care (Trella, 1993). Few organizations have developed methods of cross-site interdisciplinary planning and management. Normally, each site and discipline does its own assessment and plan of care by using very different tools. Providers from two different sites who are serving the same client at the same time, such as home care and a physician's office, typically communicate only at a time of crisis. Communication is often incomplete and provides no formal method for collaborative planning and follow-through.

Most health-care continuums have focused on integrated financing and information as the key to integrating care. Although capitated financing provides the incentives for clinicians to better manage care across a client's conditions, it does not automatically lead to mechanisms that will integrate care. Despite the fact that an integrated information system should support the clinician's ability to manage care by providing appropriate information, it cannot provide the actual planning and management. Thus, many programs have found it necessary to use case managers to plan and manage client care across settings.

What if tools and mechanisms are put in place to allow the actual providers to plan and manage care together across sites and disciplines? The challenge is not only the physical distance between providers but the differences in the way we deliver care. As illustrated in Figure 11-5, acute care and long-term providers have had a very different orientation toward care. Acute care is high tech and short term, but long-term care is high touch and continuous. The language we use is different and our goals are very diverse. For example, the goal may be to cure the clients in acute care but to support the clients to maximize their functional abilities in long-term care. In addition, rules and regulations have developed within each area and are inconsistent across sites and services. In today's uncertain economic climate, each site is focused on its own existence and not what is necessarily better care for the client.

Despite the barriers, clinicians from various sites need to develop methods of collaborative planning and management. This cannot be accomplished unless they are willing to meet at the same table and agree on the same goals. In essence, they must define the most appropriate care based on the client's needs instead of the needs of the site. Clinicians from all sites and services who provide the daily care need to be involved in the planning. Because it is not practical to meet and plan one individual's care at a time, designing a mechanism to provide integrated planning for large populations of clients across the continuum should be the focus of cross-site initiatives. For example, clinicians in the system may develop a tool that can be used to guide and monitor care for all stroke clients throughout the entire condition and across all sites. The tool needs to be individualized to adapt to a client's specific needs, and there needs to be a mechanism to communicate a client's progress and deviations from the expected plan from site to site.

Most importantly, clinicians who are accountable for using the tools must coordinate the client's care and provide smooth hand offs to the accountable clinicians at the next site.

Methods for monitoring the system's ability to meet the client's needs and then improving the system to exceed the client's expectations must also be in place. This philosophy is consistent with the goals of Continuous Quality Improvement (CQI), which many health systems have begun to adapt over the last few years (Berwick, 1989). The challenge for a continuum will be to monitor the ability to meet the client's goals over time and across sites, instead of focusing improvement efforts on each individual site. Before a process can be improved, however, it needs to be standardized (Figure 11-6) (Carey, 1995). Most continuums will find they do not have a standard process to manage care of clients across their sites and services. This needs to be the starting point—designing a mechanism to standardize care management across the continuum. Using the philosophies of CQI, such as including the people who know the process, can also assist them on this quest.

LUTHERAN GENERAL HEALTH SYSTEM CONTINUING CARE PATHWAY: A CASE STUDY

Lutheran General Health System (LGHS), a network of health and human service organizations, offers a full array of services that include a 712-bed teaching hospital, outpatient services that register approximately 158,000 visits annually, a comprehensive psychiatric-behavioral health program, a geriatric fellowship program, a parish nurse program, an 18-bed inpatient geriatric medical unit, a 12-bed geropsychiatric unit, a senior community services program with four adult day-care centers that provide 156,337 units of service

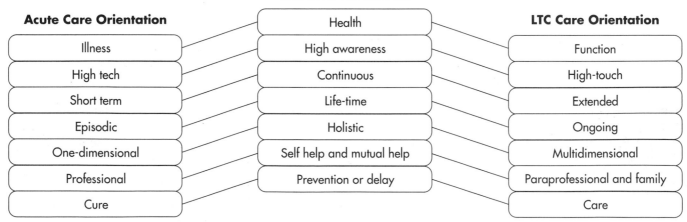

FIG. 11-5   A trinocular view of care

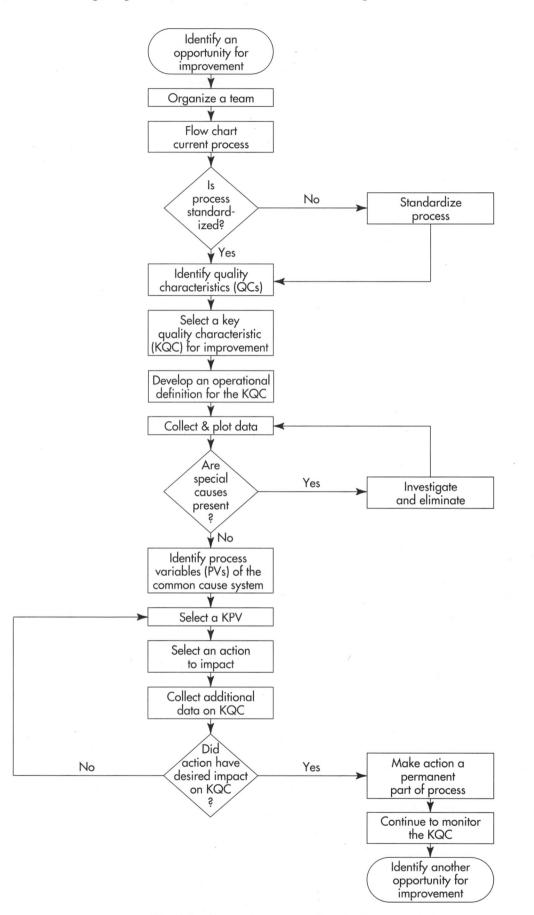

FIG. 11-6   Process improvement flow chart

annually, an Information and Referral-Central Intake office that handles 3,546 calls per year as well as other programs to support the chronically ill elderly and their families.

The primary deficiency within existing LGHS services, and one which exacerbates any other weaknesses, was the lack of integration. Until recently, services geared toward the elderly were located in several subsidiary corporations of the system. They have evolved as very separate, and sometimes competitive, entities with their own culture, priorities, and goals. Clients suffered because they could not locate services they required, and service providers within LGHS lost potential referrals and duplicated the efforts of one another.

Clinicians managed care in their own sites and then passed the client to the next site with minimal information and communication. Although ideally the primary-care physician provides the overall care management, this was rarely the case. Many times a different physician followed the client in the nursing home. When the physicians did stay involved, they found it difficult to manage care of the client in different sites with limited information and inadequate communication with other key providers such as home care nurses. The providers in the sites felt the physicians did not adequately communicate with them; they sent the physicians long summary reports but the reports did not address key physician concerns about the clients. Each site used its own assessment and care plan tools. None of these tools were passed on to the next site, so each site conducted a new assessment and gathered much of the same data to develop a new plan of care.

In 1990, Lutheran General Health System joined the National Chronic Care Consortium. The goal of the NCCC, to integrate acute and long-term care, was consistent with the goals of Lutheran General Health System. The NCCC defined the key ingredients to integrate a continuum of care and developed resource groups to design in detail the components of the integrated mechanisms. The care management resource group defined the key component of integrated care management as "common protocols" that enable network providers collectively to prevent, delay, or reduce the ongoing effects of disability throughout a condition's natural progression (NCCC, 1992).

In September 1991, LGHS convened a committee to examine the development of common protocols as a tool to manage geriatric clients across a continuum. Committee leaders invited the clinicians who provide care management from all the different sites considered part of the geriatric network to join the committee. The clinicians included nurses, social workers, physicians, and therapists. The committee included clinicians from acute care, ambulatory care, skilled nursing facilities, home care, and community-based services.

The committee began by agreeing that there was not a standardized formal process in place to manage clients continuously across multiple sites. Lutheran General Hospital had developed critical pathways to standardized care within the acute care setting. The committee agreed that care pathways could be used to manage and standardize care not only in acute care but also across multiple sites. The goal of the committee was to "develop and implement care pathways that apply to all levels of care and professional domains in responding to the needs of the individuals with chronic disabilities."

Because LGHS invited the community-based provider into the process from the beginning, their end product, Continuing Care Pathways (CCP), is very different from the typical critical pathway. The CCPs are longer than critical pathways and have more detail especially in the areas which cover function, therapies, discharge planning, and psychosocial needs. The CCPs are also not as specific and directive as critical pathways since the chronically ill elderly do not fall easily into treatment categories. See Table 11-1 for an example of a CCP. Involving clinicians at the next site of care also improved the care pathway's ability to address readiness for transition and how to prepare clients for transitions. Because of these findings, the committee found it necessary to rewrite previously developed critical pathways. Working on the committee together also improved the communication between clinicians at the different sites.

Over an 18-month period, LGHS protocol committee developed five sets of pathways that crossed all major sites of the continuum, for the diagnoses of dementia, depression, stroke, hip fracture, hip and knee replacement. Table 11-2 lists the pathways developed by sites. Flow charts were also developed to assist clinicians in the appropriate diagnosis of dementia and depression. Separate guidelines and client educational material for managing specific geriatric issues were chosen and referred to in the pathways when appropriate. Many of these guidelines and educational material were being used in certain areas in the system. The creation of CCPs encouraged their use throughout the continuum, again creating consistency.

There was little detail on the best strategies for implementing care pathways in the literature and the latest research findings indicated compliance tended to be very poor over time (Health Care Advisory Board, 1993). The literature on practice guidelines warned that much more focus should be placed on the implementation process (Mittman, 1992). To obtain adequate resources for implementation, a grant for

TABLE 11-1	Continuing care pathway (dementia—physician office)	

Components	First 3 visits	Follow-up visits every 4 months and as needed
Assessment (monitoring)	▪ H&P focus on recent neuro changes: new lacunar infarct, EPSE from neuroleptic, parkinsonian features, cognitive changes ▪ Care coordinator to complete assessment forms	——————————————>
Consults	▪ SW ▪ Consider PT, OT, rehab, psych, neuro geriatric assessment	▪ If client status changes, reconsider need for consults ▪ Periodic communication w/other MD involved in care re: status & tx plan
Tests	▪ Dementia W/U if not already done (see protocol W/U of memory loss/confusion) ▪ Repeat bld work as needed	——————————————>
Functional rehab	▪ Assess for changes in function, cognition, behavior, gait, sleep, falls, wandering (helpful tools Folstein MM, Katz ADL) ▪ Assess ability to continue driving ▪ Assess for sensory loss-referral for evaluation/prn (audiology, etc.) ▪ Exercise program to maintain conditioning	▪ Assess each visit for changes in function, cognitive & behavior
Nutrition	▪ Baseline wt ▪ Compare __ intake last 4 mos-1 yr ▪ Assess nutritional status & ability to chew, swallow & feed ▪ Swallow eval prn ▪ Assess need for changes in consistency of diet-finger food mech. diet, thick liquids etc. (see nutrition guidelines) ▪ Explore goals of long-term nutritional support (i.e., comfort vs. life prolonging methods) ▪ Referral to outpt nutrition prn (696-7770)	▪ Assess each visit for changes in wt, nutritional status appetite & ability to feed, chew & swallow ▪ Reconsider need for nutritional consult prn
Meds	▪ Review current & past meds including OTC ▪ Assess for compliance to med regimen ▪ Assess teaching needs re: meds, indication, dose, time, SE ▪ Check for SE especially psychotropics-orthostatic __, anticholinergic, sedation, urinary retention, ↑ confusion, falls, EPSE, tardive dyskeness	▪ Evaluation effectiveness & ongoing use of meds ——————————————> ——————————————> ▪ Ongoing instruction re: meds, indication, dose, time, S. E.
Treatment teaching	▪ Review course of dementia including common problems: behavior, falls, incont., sleep disturbances, wandering, etc. (see teaching material) ▪ Provide education material on disease and community resources ▪ Provide instruction for fall & safety precaution, B&B program, good skin care ▪ Review advance directives & client's goals of tx	▪ Re-evaluate ongoing teaching needs re: disease ▪ Behavior management ▪ Safety issues ▪ Incontinence & toileting ▪ Communication
Psychosocial	▪ Determine client's ability to make decisions & need for surrogate decision maker ▪ Assess for S & S of depression (helpful tool-depression scale) ▪ Assess caregiver burden & social support-refer to support group and to Alzheimer's Association (708-933-2413) ▪ Family mtg prn to address issues & goals ▪ Refer client/caregiver for counseling prn	▪ Ongoing assessment of impact of condition on client/caregiver ——————————————> ——————————————>
Continuing care needs	▪ Assess current living situation & ability of caregiver to provide care ▪ Assess client safety at home especially for client living alone ▪ Consider referral for adult day care (696-7770), VNS (824-7720), for skilled needs or other in home support services, or NHP ▪ Transition plan & paperwork provided to other sites of care ▪ S.W. evaluation to assist with decision & referrals (696-7770 Senior I & R) ▪ If no service in place periodic f/u phone calls by care coordinator	▪ Reassess need for supportive services especially if client status changes or support network changes ▪ Periodic communication with other health professions providing care (VNA, day care) especially when client, meds or tx plan changes

Signature: _____   Signature: _____
Date: _____   Date: _____

TABLE 11-2 Pathways

	Acute care	Inpatient rehab	Nursing facility	Home health	Adult day care	Physician's office	Outpatient rehab	Flowchart for work up
Stroke	X	X	X	X	X	X	X	N/A
Dementia	X	N/A	X	X	X	X	N/A	X
Depression	X	N/A	X	X	X	X	N/A	X
Hip and knee replacement	X	X	X	X	N/A	X	X	X
Hip fracture	X	X	X	X	N/A	X	X	N/A

$177,000 from the Retirement Research Foundation was obtained. The grant provided two and a half FTEs for two project managers and a half-time project director to provide the education and data collection, and to oversee the process. The grant would allow the project to be piloted in seven sites: five units in the hospital, two nursing homes, the home care agency, two physician offices, and elderly services.

Each site agreed to appoint a care coordinator who was accountable for using the continuing care pathways to coordinate care and who would serve as the key contact person for the project managers. The care coordinator was typically a clinician who was familiar with the client's needs and was currently responsible for coordinating care.

Clients could not be managed appropriately with the pathways if clinicians did not obtain correct information from site to site. An assessment tool was developed that could be updated and accompany the client from site to site. The assessment tool was meant to deter clinicians from duplicating their assessments as the client moved from site to site. It would also provide a better means of tracking the client's progress over time and place. Although some sites would have to continue to use their current tool such as the Minimum Data Set regulated in the nursing homes, the goal was to replace the old tools with the common assessment tool.

A communication tool was developed to be sent to the physician office on the day of the client's visit (Figure 11-7). The purpose of this tool was to provide brief notes to the physician about the key area of concern upon which to focus during an office visit. It has space for the physician to write recommendations and orders and then send back to the originating site, such as home care. The communication tool was designed to improve communication between physicians and the care coordinators.

Sites agreed to use the CCP as the care plan knowing that otherwise the pathways would not be used consistently. To meet the requirements that the care plan be individualized for each client, the back of the pathway has an area to list individual needs, interventions, and necessary adjustments in the pathway (Figure 11-8). Similar to a variance record originally developed as a part of the critical pathway process, most hospitals have started to use this as a method to individualize the care pathway and chart by exception. The sites agreed to pilot this system as part of their care plan with the hope that it would eventually replace their old tools. Most agreed it was a far superior tool; however, they were not ready to relinquish their old care plan because they feared that the new system would not meet Medicare, JCAHO, and other regulations.

As clients transition to the next site, a copy of the assessment tool and previous pathways is sent with them so the receiving site knows everything that had previously occurred, how the client's deviated from the plan, what interventions worked, and any individual needs. These tools provided a model of care management that used coordinated transition, standardized interdisciplinary management plans, and providers who were accountable care coordinators.

It was agreed that the focus during the first year of implementation should be documenting and evaluating the implementation process. This coincided with the current literature that indicated the need to document and evaluate the implementation of practice guidelines and critical pathways. Three tools were developed to measure clinicians' perception of this new model of care management: a pre- and post-survey to measure clinicians' perception about care management and coordination across sites, a quarterly survey that measured clinicians' perception about what it was like to use the new tools and system, and a weekly log to document whether each pathway was reviewed, if not why, and whether the interventions listed on the pathways were done and if not why (Figure 11-9).

The implementation phase of the pathway project is near completion. Every day is a new learning experience leading to a small readjustment in the process. The biggest challenges have been targeting the right clients and coordinating care in the physician office. The project managers, who were providing care coordination in the physician office, have found this difficult to do part

CLIENT'S NAME: _____

Completed by:	Date:
Sending agency:	Receiver agency:
Fax number:	Fax number:

Summarize any problems/concerns or recommendations in these areas, focusing on unmet needs.

Assessment/monitoring of physical health

_____

Consults

_____

Tests

_____

Functional/rehab

_____

Nutrition

_____

Medication

_____

Treatments/teaching

_____

Psychosocial

_____

Continuing care needs

PHYSICIAN USE

Comments/change in treatment plan

Signature: _____

FIG. 11-7   NCCC project assessment summary and communication tool

Date	Individualization or Variance	Cause	Intervention	Outcome

FIG. 11-8   Interdisciplinary care plan or variance record

LOG

Continuing care pathway project

Name of client: _____

Discipline completing log: R.N.   A.C.S.W.   Therapist   Other: _____

Setting: 6E   8W   6W   11W   8E   Abington   Ballard   Health connections   Nesset   Touchy   OAS

Type of pathway: Stroke   Dementia   Depression   Orthopedic

DATE	ABLE TO REVIEW PATHWAY? (Y/N)	IF NO, WHY NOT? Enter letter from key below and/or write own description	ABLE TO USE INTERVENTIONS? (Y/N)	IF NO, WHY NOT? Enter letter from key below and/or write own description	MINUTES SPENT REVIEWING THE PATHWAYS q weeks/q days	NAME OF CARE COORDINATORS

a = not enough time
b = not enough staff
c = interventions were not appropriate for my client
d = interventions were not realistic for my setting

e = I did not understand the interventions
f = other clinicians involved in care refused to cooperate
g = not enough information was provided about the client to follow the pathway

i = other involved clinicians do not understand the purpose of the pathways
j = the communication between myself and other involved clinicians is inadequate

FIG. 11-9   Weekly log for evaluation of interventions listed on pathways

time. The pathway process was not integrated into the normal office routine and was not embraced by the staff. In one office, a staff member agreed to become the care coordinator and was then able to integrate the process. Learning that the providers at the sites should be the managers of the process was an important lesson. The project has also discovered that paraprofessionals such as LPNs and therapy assistants can use the pathways and coordinate care. Because the pathways already establish a plan, it is appropriate for non-professional staff to use the tool to guide their care. When a client deviates from the pathway, the paraprofessionals work with the project managers to plan alternative interventions.

Another challenge is keeping the lines of communication open. It is easy for the care coordinators to go back to blaming each other for what was not done at the previous site now that the project has established certain expectations. To control this problem, the project has monthly care coordinator meetings to problem solve and work on issues together. The monthly care coordinator meeting is also used as a process improvement forum to address variances on the pathways. For example, the first trend noticed on the variance forms was physician's orders not being received in a timely manner for home care and nursing homes. To address this problem, pretyped orders which have the usual orders needed for these sites have been developed.

The orders can be individualized and then sent with the other tools to the next site. Other trends have documented specific problems in certain sites, for example, a site which was not able to accept a new client in a timely manner. These quality issues are given back to the individual sites to resolve.

The project is documenting in what site the pathways and process are working well and where they are less effective. Although project staff have some ideas about why this is occurring, it is too soon for conclusions. The results of the surveys and logs will be carefully analyzed at the end of the year. Six-month data indicated that clinician compliance was at 87%, and that communication and coordination have improved across the sites. This may be in part to the project managers doing weekly site visits to encourage compliance and communication. Some sites consistently have problems completing the expectations without close monitoring. Staff turnover and limited staffing have been problems in other sites. Having at least one committed staff who understands the project benefits can lead to successful implementation in a site.

Although the care coordinator has the ultimate responsibility for the process, the interdisciplinary team should be part of the process. This too has worked better in some sites than others. In sites where there has always been a strong team focus, such as rehabilitation, the review of the pathway fits well into their team meetings. In other sites, such as home care, the pathways have encouraged the need for team planning for the first time.

It is difficult for clinicians when the change is only a pilot project and is being done for only part of the population. When a change is integrated into the usual process of care delivery, it is easier to manage. The Retirement Research Foundation has funded two more years of the grant with the goal to expand and integrate the process into the sites. Until this time, the pathway project will continue to need project managers who oversee the process and fill in the gaps. The project managers have also been more involved with the very complex clients who tend not to follow the standardized plan, thus serving as case managers for highest-risk clients.

Unfortunately, some clinicians continue to have difficulty understanding the need to plan and manage care beyond their site or even their shift. Incentives and expectations need to be aligned to encourage clinicians to manage accordingly. LGHS has ventured into its first Medicare managed care program in September 1994. Physicians and system administrators are more concerned than ever regarding the efficient management of older adults. Plans to integrate the pathway model into the managed care program are under way and physicians and administrators are taking a much more active approach in its progress. Contracted sites have an added incentive to follow the pathways and address issues that affect quality.

Generic pathways that will guide care of any frail older adults despite their diagnosis, as well as guidelines for wellness and health promotion are being developed. Use of the pathway model will facilitate the management of this population as they move throughout multiple sites with much less manpower than case managing each individual client. LGHS now has freedom to manage these clients according to the best practice in the pathway, instead of following Medicare reimbursement requirements.

Key to continued growth and expansion of the project is an integrated information system. The current courier system for the pathway client record is inefficient and cannot keep up with the flow of the clients. LGHS has purchased an information system (Senior Information System, SIS), which will connect the sites with personal computers and modems (Mack & Associates). This system is relatively inexpensive and will be connected to the open system architecture the LGHS is in the process of implementing. Unlike hospital systems, the SIS has already developed software that links multiple types of community-based providers. Although data on line are currently limited to demographic and basic assessment data, project staff hope to acquire more grant dollars to develop the system further.

Although the Continuing Care Pathway project at LGHS is in the early stages of implementation, it has been well received. Five new sites (one nursing home, three physician offices, and the preadmission testing area) have been added at their request and others are being evaluated. A committee addressing pediatric chronic care is examining the pathway project as a method to coordinate care for pediatric clients. Clinicians agree that the process is going smoothly and have rated a high satisfaction with the project. Although evaluating effectiveness was not the focus of the first year, preliminary data have demonstrated that stroke patients in the project have a two-day shortened length of stay in acute care and on the rehabilitation unit. Plans for next year include a more detailed evaluation of clients' outcomes in the project including cost of care and satisfaction.

Key to the success of this project has been the sponsorship from the system. In January of 1993, LGHS committed itself to developing an integrated continuum of care for all its populations. A 15-member design team developed a plan that is being implemented by 11 continuum teams (Box 11-4). The pathway project has been successful because of the support and understanding that have been gained through the continuum effort. At the same time, the pathway project has been embraced as a project that has operationalized the continuum concepts (see Case Study).

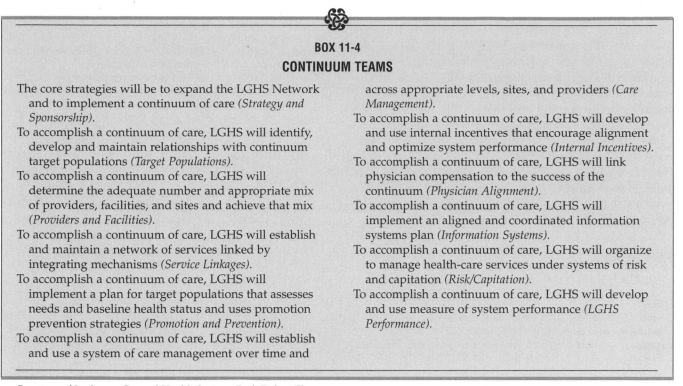

BOX 11-4
CONTINUUM TEAMS

The core strategies will be to expand the LGHS Network and to implement a continuum of care *(Strategy and Sponsorship)*.

To accomplish a continuum of care, LGHS will identify, develop and maintain relationships with continuum target populations *(Target Populations)*.

To accomplish a continuum of care, LGHS will determine the adequate number and appropriate mix of providers, facilities, and sites and achieve that mix *(Providers and Facilities)*.

To accomplish a continuum of care, LGHS will establish and maintain a network of services linked by integrating mechanisms *(Service Linkages)*.

To accomplish a continuum of care, LGHS will implement a plan for target populations that assesses needs and baseline health status and uses promotion prevention strategies *(Promotion and Prevention)*.

To accomplish a continuum of care, LGHS will establish and use a system of care management over time and across appropriate levels, sites, and providers *(Care Management)*.

To accomplish a continuum of care, LGHS will develop and use internal incentives that encourage alignment and optimize system performance *(Internal Incentives)*.

To accomplish a continuum of care, LGHS will link physician compensation to the success of the continuum *(Physician Alignment)*.

To accomplish a continuum of care, LGHS will implement an aligned and coordinated information systems plan *(Information Systems)*.

To accomplish a continuum of care, LGHS will organize to manage health-care services under systems of risk and capitation *(Risk/Capitation)*.

To accomplish a continuum of care, LGHS will develop and use measure of system performance *(LGHS Performance)*.

Courtesy of Lutheran General Health System, Park Ridge, Ill.

CASE STUDY

Mr. J's Story in an Integrated Continuum of Care

When Mr. J was diagnosed with hypertension, a guideline focused the office staff to provide extensive education on the importance of medication compliance. Mr. J was a member of a Medicare HMO that provided the physicians and office staff with incentives to keep Mr. J well. Mr. J's medication was part of the benefit package so cost was not a concern. Mr. J's history and functional status, goals of treatment, and advance directives were entered into the integrated information system. This system also reminded the office staff when to send a card reminding Mr. J of his next office visit. The HMO provided Mr. J with access to a low-cost exercise and wellness program for seniors, accessible by public transportation. At this program, Mr. J was encouraged to purchase a low-cost emergency call system because he lived alone and was at risk for a stroke.

If Mr. J had had a stroke, he would be quickly found and when he arrived at the emergency room his clinical information would be accessed on the integrated information system. His current status and findings would be entered into this system, and a flow chart would guide the emergency staff in efficiently diagnosing and treating his stroke. On the medical floor, his past independent functional status would encourage staff to take an aggressive approach by using the stroke pathway to start his rehabilitation. His urinary retention would quickly be assessed and

documented as a variance, and appropriate interventions would be instituted to resolve this problem. Staff would enter his current status into the information system that would provide a chronological picture of his progress and his plan as outlined on the pathway. When Mr. J was transferred to the rehabilitation facility on the fifth day, this information would again be accessed and updated from the new site.

The pathway for the rehabilitation facility would outline extensive family education and discharge planning to prepare Mr. J for transition into home care after 10 days. The home care clinicians would be able to access his current status and progress in the plan from the information system. The HMO would cover extensive home care to provide Mr. J with the opportunity to remain in the community if possible. Throughout Mr. J's care, there would always be at least one accountable clinician who was aware of every detail of Mr. J's progress and plans. When Mr. J reached his maximal functional potential and skilled care was no longer necessary, Mr. J's care would be coordinated through the physician's office by using the maintenance stroke pathway. At this point, the focus would be to keep Mr. J at his maximal function. If Mr. J exhausted his finances for any necessary custodial care, these benefits would then be provided and managed by his HMO.

CONCLUSION

Although no completely integrated continuum of care yet exists, the dream has become a focus of many health-care initiatives. Nurses have long been a driving force in integrating an individual's care and overcoming fragmentation. As we learn the benefit of focusing on improving and integrating care for populations instead of each individual, we will become part of the movement to integrate health care. Even though individual nurses may not have the opportunity to be involved with a specific initiative, they can still support these efforts by promoting health-care reform policies that encourage the integration of health care for people with chronic conditions.

REFERENCES

Abrahams, R. (1990, August). The social/HMO: case management in an integrated acute and long-term care system. *Caring Magazine,* 30-40.

Barrett, M. (1993, May 26). Case Management a must to survive managed care. *Computers in Health Care,* 22-25.

Berwick, D. (1989). Continuous improvement as an ideal in health care. *New England Journal of Medicine 320* (1), 53-56.

Bringewatt, J. (1992, June). Provider-based managed care—A health network imperative. Bloomington, MN: The National Chronic Care Consortium.

Cohen, E., & Cesta, T. (1993). *Nursing Case Management: from concept to evaluation.* (pp. 22-35). St Louis, MO: Mosby.

Evashwick, J. (1987). Definition of the continuum of care. In Evashwick, J. & Weiss, L. (Eds.). *Managing the Continuum of Care* (pp. 23-36). Rockville, MD: Aspen Publication.

Health Care Advisory Board. (1993). Special research: Second generation lessons on critical care path. Washington, D.C.

Mack, Charles H., & Associates. Senior information system. Cincinnati, Ohio.

Mittman, B., Tonesk, X., & Jacobson, P. (1992, December). Implementing clinical practice guidelines: social influence strategies and practitioner behavior change. *Quality Review Bulletin,* 413-421.

National Chronic Care Consortium (1993, September). An overview of the consortium's purpose, structure, accomplishments and future, Bloomington, MN.

National Chronic Care Consortium (1992). Extended care pathway component project.

Trella, R. (1993). A multidisciplinary approach to case management of frail, hospitalized older adults. *Journal of Nursing Administration, 23* (2), 20-26.

Zawadski, R., & Eng, C. (1988). Case management in capitated long-term care. *Health Care Financing Review,* Annual Supplement: 75-81.

Chapter 12

Innovative Delivery Systems: Freedom, Trust, Caring

Annette McBeth, MS, RN
Alice Weydt, MS, RN

OVERVIEW

Nurse leaders are well positioned to facilitate the transformation of health-care services in the community by coordinating services along a continuum of care from birth to death.

Innovative strategies based on the concepts of freedom, trust, and caring will be key to empowering communities, clients, and families to take responsibility for their health and health care. The life health continuum must address all levels of health and health-care services in order to develop a delivery system that is seamless and without duplication and fragmentation. Nurse case management provides the framework to build a quality, cost-effective delivery system across the entire life-to-death health continuum. Nurse case management is a collaborative process that develops options and services to meet an individual's health needs through communication and resource allocation (Case Management Society of America, 1994). Florence Nightingale's vision more than a century ago will remain in the twenty-first century: to minister to whole beings with tender loving care and to create an environment in which the patient (client) can find healing (Nightingale, F. [1860]). Ultimately, our communities and nation will be better served when we build a delivery system that focuses on holistic prevention, health promotion, and early intervention instead of episodic illness care.

We are at the crossroads of transitioning from an illness system to a health system. Historically, the illness or disease model has been the driving force in formulating health-care policy and reimbursement. The nation's current health-care system was designed and developed around 10% of our population who are "sick" or "super-sick." The other 90% of our population is where we need to focus as we move forward (Westberg, 1990).

The clinical discipline of nursing is ideally positioned to facilitate the transition from an illness model to a "health" model. Nurses, by the very nature of their practice, intimately touch people's lives in ways other disciplines do not. Nurses, therefore, have the opportunity to provide the proactive leadership in facilitating coordination of services on a continuum of care from birth to death. Our communities and nation will be better served if we begin to focus on prevention, health promotion and early intervention instead of episodic illness care.

Innovation addresses old problems in new ways. As providers, we believe innovation is linked to three key concepts that will be discussed in this chapter:

- The concept of freedom
- The concept of trust
- The concept of caring

THE ART OF NURSING
Freedom

Nurses need to have freedom to learn and then understand the physiological, spiritual, mental, and emotional problems of clients and families. Nursing's scientific knowledge-base in biological, social, and behavioral science provides the foundation for understanding what it is to be human. Nurses study disease and know that there are some things that are very predictable. When nurses address human behavior or thought, however, the variables become enormous. There is no protocol or set methodology about what is needed when different kinds of human experiences are encountered. Nurses need to have the first concept—freedom—to explore what options are available for each client and family.

Trust

Trust cannot occur unless there is freedom to learn about the potential. Through trust, nurses build a relationship wherein they can elicit responses from clients and families to learn more about what clients and families believe, feel, think, and know. As a result, nurses can develop a strategy that will maximize client and family health potential. It does not necessarily mean that they will get well, or be cured. It does mean, however, that nurses will assist them to adapt, adjust, or to hold out hope that life can still be good. Nurses need to have the freedom to explore what it is that people believe and value. Nurses then assess the value system of others, internalize it within nursing practice, and then educate people about the kinds of options available to them, thus allowing clients to make an *informed* choice about their health and wellness. It is at this point that nurses build and maintain the concept of trust. The client and family have to trust what it is that nurses know, and nurses have to trust that the client and family know what can be accomplished. Erickson, Tomlin, and Swain (1983) have said that people know intrinsically what has made them sick, and they also know what will make them well. Nursing's role is to facilitate that discovery and then work with people to develop health options so that they achieve improved health.

Caring

Caring communicates to clients and families that they are valued and understood. Nursing is inherently grounded in caring. Definitions of nursing discuss caring for people as it relates to human responses to whatever it is that crosses their paths. The invitation to care is expressed through nursing practice. Using Erickson, Tomlin, and Swain's (1983) nursing theory and Lamb and Stempel's (1994) work on the insider-expert, the caring relationship can be explored and applied to meet health and wellness needs.

Erickson, Tomlin, and Swain's (1983) nursing theory continues to state that just as people know what has made them sick together with what will make them well, they also know what will optimize their effectiveness, fullfillment, and what will promote their growth. If people do not know this consciously, a skillful nurse case manager (NCM) can help them to learn and to know themselves. This knowledge leads clients to take more control and responsibility over their health. People will take control when they are permitted, invited, and patiently encouraged to do so. According to Erickson, Tomlin, and Swain (1983), modeling is the development of a mirror image of the situation from the client's perspective. Modeling is a scientific process of aggregation and data analysis to synthesize and integrate essential elements into a holistic unit. Having thus modeled the client's world, in subsequent interactions, the NCM thoughtfully and purposefully role models that world with the client so that the client can grow healthier. This promotes self-worth and a hopeful future. Role modeling is more than setting a good example. It facilitates the client's perception of being in a new role without experiencing the loss of the old (Redford, 1992).

Lamb and Stempel (1994) describe a bonding process that occurs between the NCM and the client. The bonding facilitates an understanding of the client's world which allows the NCM to know and understand the client for the purpose of better meeting the client's needs. The NCM is viewed as an "outsider" expert. When the clients can manage their own health issues, they become the "insider" expert. Lamb and Stempel's description of the bonding process is similar to Erickson, Tomlin, and Swain's modeling process. This process addresses everyone's perspective in developing an effective individualized plan of care. Additionally, modeling implies that empowerment is central to successfully meeting the client's health and wellness needs.

People need the freedom to explore health options. They need to trust their health-care providers; however, it is through the concept of caring that nurses gain insight into what people think and feel. Nurses can then nonjudgmentally internalize the family experience into nursing practice. Nurses may not agree with the clients' interpretation of the experience but can understand it and then role model different ways in which their health needs can be addressed.

Essential to promoting health and wellness is understanding what clients and their families think, believe, and feel as well as how their thoughts, beliefs, and feelings affect their perceptions about quality of life and health experiences. When nurses see the world through the eyes of those who are receiving or need the care, they facilitate client-centered decisions. Historically, perceptions of the client and family are seldom considered when changes in the health-care system have occurred; however, the Medicare Hospice Election is an exception. Hospice is an excellent model to replicate as we make the transition from a fee-for-service system to a capitated system. In the Hospice Election, clients and families can make health-care decisions consistent with their thoughts, beliefs, and feelings.

THROUGH THE CLIENT'S EYES

Many changes have been made in the health-care system in the last 10 years. Making the transition from a fee-for-service to a capitated system requires system changes in the ways in which today's health-care system is organized. We believe the Hospice Medicare Election provides an excellent model for replication in the other areas of health-care delivery.

To qualify for the Hospice Medicare Election, people have to be diagnosed with a terminal illness with a life expectancy of six months or less. To access Hospice capitated funds, people opt out of the traditional Medicare reimbursement and then become eligible for Hospice funding to meet their needs. Clients, families, and health-care providers are aware of the available funds. These funds become the checkbook to finance the decisions. The parameters are known in advance and mutual decisions are made at the time based on what the client and family need and what can be financially supported.

The three concepts of freedom, trust, and caring become evident in listening to the stories of Hospice clients, families, and staff. The outcomes of these stories have general themes whereby family members are given the freedom to render care to their loved one. Through the support and teaching from the Hospice staff, families experience the freedom to learn and then to trust what they know. This freedom thus empowers them to share in the care of their loved one and gives them a sense of having some control in an otherwise uncontrollable situation. For instance, it has been learned that someone with huge knarled hands can tenderly deliver care to a dying loved one. Scientific knowledge is not a prerequisite to caring.

In chronic or terminal conditions, the permission to care for a loved one or one's self is facilitated by the NCM. People who are free to determine their own destination can better control it. In this freedom to control

their destiny, even if their destiny is death, clients and their families have a wellness focus rather than an illness or disease focus. Clients and families can then make choices that maximize available time. Health-care providers must trust that people know what is best for them and collaboratively develop the plan of care that fits within the value systems of clients and families.

In addition to knowing financial parameters, Hospice also provides a model for a collaborative delivery system. Needs become so complex in Hospice that a single discipline cannot possibly address all of them. Providers share their expertise with one another and respect the complementary expertise that each brings to the situation. Our Hospice experience has shown that through collaboration, instead of competition, effective quality outcomes can be obtained. Collaborative alternatives based on client and family goals, not the providers' goals, must be offered within the context of known parameters.

We believe the Hospice model offers a framework to manage other chronic diseases such as COPD and cardiovascular diseases. Clients and families need the freedom for themselves to explore options with members of the health-care team. The relationship between the NCM and the client and family is based upon trust. When there is trust in the humanistic and scientific knowledge that is collectively possessed, the clients and families will be better able to manage their disease effectively.

The concepts of freedom, trust, and caring will be key to empowering clients and families to take responsibility for their health care. When clients and families accept this responsibility, rather than looking to health-care providers, significant and lasting changes in lifestyle behaviors occur which ultimately affect the quality of people's lives and the costs incurred to maintain that desired quality.

The Hospice experience and journey becomes a template for transitioning into a capitated delivery system and environment. Hospice prescribes a nurse case management model. Nurse case management offers significant opportunities to address the issues of cost, quality, and satisfaction. The nursing literature is rich with case management testimonies supporting the notion that nurse case management has an important role to play as health-care reform reshapes the health-care delivery system.

Nurse case management provides the framework to build a delivery system across the care continuum. The following case study demonstrates collaboration among five separate fragmented systems to build an individualized continuum of care. The catalyst to make it happen is the nurse case manager.

Because health-care facilities and agencies cannot be all things to all people, the health-care continuum must

CASE STUDY

A 56-year-old white male was admitted seven times to our hospital for life-threatening hypertension and gastrointestinal episodes. In addition, there were multiple emergency room visits within a year. It was decided that a clinical nurse specialists would case manage the man to address his needs better and to monitor the cost of his care. The NCM found that the man had a history of chronic alcoholism that was contributing to his medical instability. Also, she discovered that he was living alone in an apartment that posed fire and health risks. The man had slipped through the gaps in the health-care system and was only being seen in crisis situations. He had no one to advocate for his needs, and no one seemed to know what options were available to him. Although he was known to the county human services system, the county felt powerless to address his needs within the county system. The physician, an internist, did not trust the chemical dependency model to address the man's needs because he had been in treatment multiple times. The NCM realized that her expertise in mental illness and chemical dependency was inadequate.

The NCM made several home visits over a two-month period and collaborated with another clinical nurse specialist who had expertise in chemical dependency and mental illness. The NCM collaboratively developed strategies with the client, physician, county C.D. counselor, and a community rehabilitation social worker to meet the man's needs better. The client was not able to keep his commitment to his contract to abstain from alcohol. This commitment was a condition for him to be in partnership with the NCM. The client also knew that commitment to a state regional treatment center would be pursued if he broke his contract by resuming alcohol intake. The health-care team assessed that it was only a matter of time before a medical emergency would occur. When the client was readmitted to the hospital, the team enacted their plan to pursue commitment because of his incompetence to manage his medical needs. Within two days of hospitalization, the transfer from the hospital to a state facility was made. The physician stated that he did not believe that what had transpired could really happen and felt relieved from feeling solely responsible for providing the client's care. Although it was not a voluntary commitment, the client's well-being was foremost in every team member's mind. To discharge him back into the community would have ensured another crisis that could have ended his life. This case exemplifies the freedom this NCM had to collaborate with key stakeholders involved in this man's care. They developed a trusting relationship which facilitated the care that was rendered in order to provide a safe and caring environment for this vulnerable individual to manage on a daily basis.

address all levels of service and develop systems to meet needs without duplication and fragmentation. Again, capitation will enhance the collaborative efforts and decrease competition. The following is a case study of one of our cardiovascular clients who exemplifies

the problems encountered when clients and families try to negotiate a fragmented delivery system.

Unfortunately, this scenario is not an isolated incident. It was, however, the impetus to begin examination of how care is delivered in a fragmented regional environment. As a result, our hospital nurses in three communities in South Central Minnesota collaborated with a tertiary care center in Minneapolis and developed a nurse case management model to address care across the care continuum. A nurse group practice of case managers has evolved among the three rural settings together with the urban tertiary center. Outcome measurements at this time include the client's and family's perceptive quality, provider satisfaction, as well as clinical and financial outcomes. The following case study is an example of the collaborative outcomes achieved by the group practice of these NCMs.

Nursing's challenge in the present world of competition is to mentor others to develop insight into clinical issues, thereby enhancing collaboration. When nurses are supported by those who understand cost and quality outcomes, nursing's work becomes quantified. Nursing cannot and should not do this alone or in isolation. The people who work in health care do care about humanity; they want to be of service.

When nurses involve other stakeholders in the process by saying, "You can make a difference in peoples' lives even though you are behind the scenes," these individuals become further motivated to help nurses find better ways to address people's needs. These wonderful minds have all the expertise at their fingertips. With their help, nurses can quantify what is intuitively known. By including others in the process, these individuals become stakeholders with vested interests in the outcomes.

A case management executive committee has been formed in our organization to develop a case management model and process. Members selected have expertise in medicine, nursing, information systems, finance, continuous quality improvement, client care evaluation, and utilization review. Nursing has the opportunity to mentor nonclinical members of the case management executive committee to bring them into the client's world by mutually developing a common language. Just as nurses are being mentored, nonclinical team members are mentored by nurses. This process parallels the modeling and role modeling that is done with clients. The role of the committee is to facilitate the development of a case management or managed care system that enhances the quality and decreases cost of client care across the continuum. This is done in collaboration with NCMs who are currently delivering the care. The committee serves as a resource to the NCMs by allocating necessary resources and by providing outcome and cost information. Monthly meetings are held

---

CASE STUDY

One morning, a well-educated and productive man in his mid-sixties arrived at our hospital's Education Department with a gallon jug filled with urine. He had been instructed by tertiary care physicians who were some 90 miles from our hospital to take a urine sample to his local hospital. No one at the Education Department knew about his history. Upon further investigation, it was learned that he had been admitted to our local hospital with a myocardial infarction and transferred to the tertiary hospital for a coronary artery bypass procedure. He had been discharged from the tertiary facility with instructions to collect a 24-hour urine for analysis one week after his discharge. The man could not clearly remember his discharge instructions and was obviously confused about the follow-up care. In addition, he expressed his frustration about feeling abandoned because he was not sure about whom he needed to contact should an emergency arise and also voiced his fear about his inability to meet his own needs.

CASE STUDY

A 73-year-old white male who had no previous history of coronary artery disease was admitted to our local hospital with chest pain. The client had been widowed for 30 years and had raised eight children by himself. Angiography was done, and as a result of the tests, he was transferred to the tertiary care center for a six-vessel coronary artery bypass surgery. The NCM at our local hospital contacted a NCM at the tertiary care facility to relay necessary information to facilitate a smooth transfer. This process was repeated when the client was discharged from the tertiary care facility. The NCM at our local hospital learned that the client had been followed by a Public Health Nurse (PHN) and wanted to continue with that service. Honoring the client's request, the NCM from our local hospital contacted the PHN rather than the hospital home care service. When the client no longer meets criteria for home care services, the NCM will become more involved in helping the client manage his care over the next 12 months. In the meantime, the NCM is a collaborative resource to the PHN.

---

to share information and to problem solve. NCMs periodically update the committee on their activities. It is the client and family stories that tie this committee to client care. A family story related in a recent letter to coauthor Annette McBeth by a family member eloquently describes the essence of case management:

Dear Annette,

I would like to take a moment of your time to express my sincere thoughts and feelings about K.V., Dr. N's colleague.

I would have preferred to have this on letterhead, typed and formalized, however, I'm on a flight back home to Denver, Colorado, have two- and four-year-old boys waiting for me, in addition to working as a Medical Center Nursing Supervisor for two very busy surgical subspecialties. Felt it was far better to send the letter in handwritten form than not at all.

My father was diagnosed with brain cancer in August, 1993. After being able to almost fly home without the help of the plane (a few hours later), K.V. was the first person I spoke with on arriving at the hospital, as my family and I held hands and could barely accept the situation. She spoke calmly, professionally, and with a tremendous knowledge base. She also had a sincerity about her that has been unmatched by anyone else I've ever had the pleasure to meet within the nursing arena.

This past year has been an emotional roller coaster for our family, it truly has been the biggest tragedy we've faced as a family. The thing that has held us together, has helped us make medical decisions, and simply make it through the day is K.V. We children all live out of state, K.V. is like the sister in Mankato we all wished we had. She has been an unbelievable emotional and physical support to all of us, especially my parents.

It doesn't matter what time of day or night it is, K.V. is there for my parents, or whether it's Monday or Sunday, she still calls, gives us her pager and home phone numbers.

She has literally for one year, talked to my mother daily, helped her coordinate appointments, came to our home to help both my parents, spent endless hours of her off time with my parents, made food and brought it over to my parents when she knew my mother was exhausted, and many many more acts of kindness. Last week she came over on her own at 5:00 A.M. to help dress my father for a doctor's appointment, when my mother was just thinking how would she get dad dressed and in the car, there was K.V. like a guardian angel.

My father has done well, however, the cancer has taken over now and he is going to die soon. K.V. spoke to all of us children this past week as we were home, again when she leaves our home, we look at one another and say "what would we do without K.V.?"

My mother insisted that I return home to take care of my family, it was the hardest thing I've ever done to leave today, but I was comforted by the thought that K.V. is still there for my parents.

Even through this letter I can't begin to have you realize what a major role K.V. has played in our lives. Without her this tragedy would have been so much harder. Thank you for having K.V. assist . . . clients and their families. So many times in Denver I've spoken to my peers and said, "Why don't we have someone like her at our Medical Center? Why doesn't every specialty have someone like her to help them through . . . any medical condition that is so devastating to the client and family?" I thank God she was there for us! . . .

Sincerely,

Daughter

THE CARE CONTINUUM

The acute care bedside nursing delivery system provides the foundation to implement nurse case management. Professional nurses at the bedside must balance responsibility, authority, and accountability to impact health-care costs and quality. The importance of the role cannot be minimized. As lengths of hospital stays shorten, the opportunities to interact and engage in caring behaviors diminish within the acute care setting. Caring or the care rendered must be relevant, effective, and creative. Otherwise, clients and families will perceive that they have been shortchanged or cheated and thereby become mistrustful of the health-care system.

Traditional authoritarian bedside nursing delivery systems that are highly prevalent in nursing divisions found across the country do not offer the professional nurse the opportunities to engage in participatory management (Manthey, 1980). Until professional nurses are given the freedom to make decisions and resolve conflicts, they cannot truly be effective at the bedside. Nursing process promotes critical thinking and synthesis of information given by clients and families and is enhanced by a decentralized delivery system. In this system, nursing leadership's role is one of facilitator rather than director. Nursing leadership must see their own practice as an art which means attending to the beauty of each artistic nursing act of self and others (Brown, 1991). The environment in which the professional nurse practices is the responsibility of nursing leadership. Caring is a finite resource that needs to be replenished. The creation of a nurturing supportive work environment for nursing is essential to the quality of care a client and family receive (Brown, 1991).

Case management is a collaborative process that develops options and services to meet an individual's health needs through communication and through resource allocation that promotes quality, cost-effective outcomes (Case Management Society of America, 1994).

The Primary Nursing Delivery System facilitates individualized commitments of continuing care. It allocates 24-hour responsibility, accountability, and authority for each client's and family's care to one nurse who facilitates, coordinates and directly provides the care when appropriate. The primary nurse coordinates information and instructions for the client's care so that the nurses delivering care during the primary nurse's absence know about the client as a person and exactly how specific interventions should be administered and delivered. The primary nurse also has the majority of responsibility and accountability for preparing the client and family for discharge (Manthey, 1980). Collaboration between the primary nurse and NCM helps to develop a "seamless" continuum where the client and family can move between health-care settings without fragmentation and duplication.

The Primary Nurse Delivery System becomes the foundation for case management. The primary nurses manage inpatient stays to achieve identified outcomes within specific time frames by using an integrated *care path* together with appropriate resources. Hospital stays are without a doubt the highest expense incurred along the care continuum. Because of this, every client needs to have care managed within the hospital setting and assessed for aftercare services.

The NCM serves as a gatekeeper, brokering appropriate services along the care continuum. A NCM needs to possess negotiation and conflict resolution skills. To be successful, the NCM understands and respects peoples' values and incorporates those values into a plan of care as communicated to the members of the health-care team. NCMs create independence through teaching clients and families ways to prevent illness (Wolfe, 1993). Warning signals of impending deterioration are taught (Redford, 1992). Earlier pattern recognition enables clients to see health alternatives, not just episodic illness services. Earlier interventions reduce the incidence of more costly interventions, and thereby enhance the quality of life. Pattern recognition is best accomplished over time by seeing clients in their homes and in relation to their family's interactions and dynamics (Ethridge, 1990).

Figure 12-1 demonstrates a delivery system that has a regionally focused continuum of care. It depicts a hospital-based case management model. The *inner circle* represents the continuum of care and includes access points within the community and region. Case management encompasses the continuum and links community and regional services. The *pyramid* represents acute care and has four essential components. The first component is effective relationship management, which includes communication and negotiation skills. Effective relationship management is key to any client care delivery system. Effective relationship management is the fulcrum that balances case management and the acute care system. Case managers, nursing staff, physicians, and other members of the health-care team combine their expertise to create a "seamless" continuum of care for clients. Effective relationship management is critical to the development of a successful collaborative practice. It is just as important among members of the health-care team to have effective relationships as it is among the nurse and the client group. Relationships build trust. It is in the context of relationships that trust is built, that freedom is found, and that care is delivered.

Interdisciplinary care paths are key road maps in providing cost-effective quality care in a managed and/or capitated environment. Client progress is documented

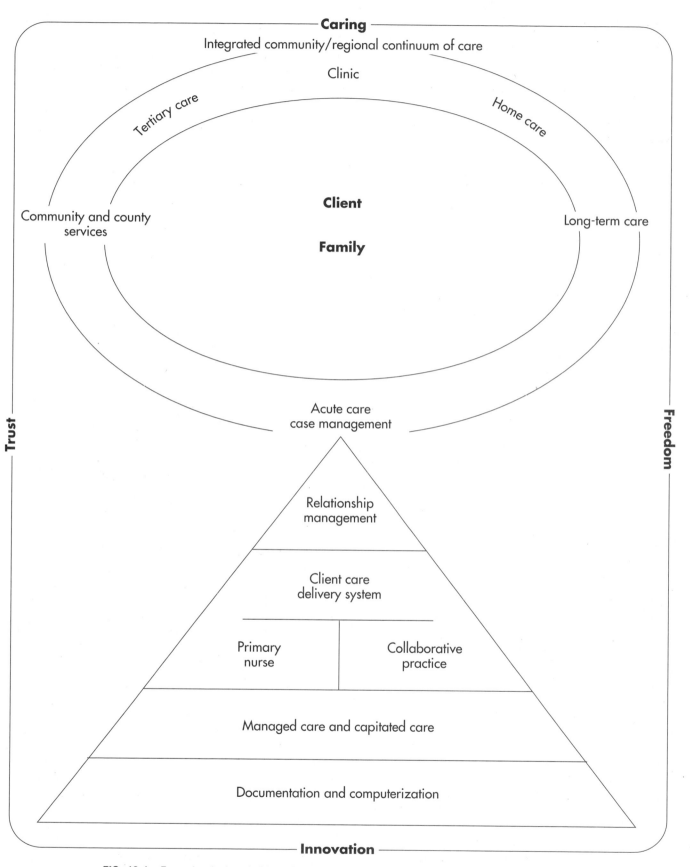

FIG. 12-1 Example of a hospital-based case management model, a regionally focused continuum of care. The inner circle represents the continuum of care, and the outer circle, case management. The pyramid represents acute care. Effective relationship management is the fulcrum that balances case management and the acute care system.

via the computerized integrated client record with variance tracked to identify opportunities to enhance clinical outcomes in a cost-effective manner.

COST AND QUALITY OUTCOMES

The health-care industry is being challenged to provide high-quality accessible services at a reasonable cost to all United States citizens. Health-care reform demands that the current health-care system be restructured with different incentives to provide and to receive services (Madden & Ponte, 1994; Pepper Commission, 1991). Our traditional fee-for-service model needs to shift to a health-outcome-oriented model.

It was not until the 1930s that health care was viewed as a right for United States citizens. As a result of the Depression, people began looking to the government to help ensure that health-care services would be available to everyone regardless of ability to pay. What has evolved in the last 60 years is a multibillion dollar industry that has exceeded 12% of the gross national product. In 1991, health-care costs topped 761 billion dollars. If no controls are put in place, health-care spending is expected to reach 1.2 to 1.3 trillion by 1995. By the year 2000, between 2.1 and 2.7 trillion will be spent on health care if the current system remains unchanged (National League of Nursing, 1991).

Health-care providers are being held accountable for their performance and for overall outcomes by consumers, by third-party payors, by legislators, and by their peers in a way never known to the health-care industry. To be outcome oriented and cost effective is no longer a goal but a mandate (Bowers, 1992). Solutions are being sought to bridge the gaps in health-care services, to decrease duplication, to avoid unnecessary treatment or interventions, to control escalating costs, to improve outcomes, and to increase client and provider satisfaction (Healthy America: Practitioners for 2005, 1991).

Americans profit daily from the health-care system's technological excellence, well-educated health-care professionals, extensive medical research, and a diverse group of providers and facilities. Nevertheless, with escalating health-care costs, inconsistent quality, and health-care benefits unequally distributed, the American Health Care System is in crisis (National League of Nursing, 1991).

As costs have escalated, consumers have become increasingly dissatisfied with the cost and the quality of health-care services. Public trust and confidence has been eroded as the existing health-care system's ability to meet consumer needs has declined. Hospitals and physicians are being perceived as profit motivated instead of being client centered. Researchers and practitioners recognize that public relations campaigns and refurbishing of the hotel-like services hospitals provide fall short in meeting consumer expectations (Stevens, 1989).

A panel of senior health-care executives predicts that within three years, client satisfaction will emerge as the single most important criteria for assessing outcomes. This is to the amazement or dismay of health-care professionals, and the delight of clients (Trend Watch, 1993).

There is a relationship between expectations, perceptions of excellence, and satisfaction. What the health-care industry has failed to recognize is the consumer's perception of the health-care experience. In some instances, the consumer may not even be qualified to make a true judgment. Health-care providers must, however, understand the consumer's values to make recommendations and initiate treatment if consumer satisfaction is to be achieved (Maloney & Paul, 1993).

Studies relating cost reductions and increased client satisfaction to nurse case management are encouraging. Nurse case management focuses on problems and needs of clients and their families and friends who support them, through the enhanced coordination of the care and the services provided to the clients and their families. It is the coordination of care that improves outcomes and that reduces fragmentation, duplication, and ultimately costs. "Nurse case managers have a broad vision of client needs, especially related to desired outcomes and how to support clients in moving them toward those outcomes, as well as the continuum of care represented by the client populations, and the issues of costs of care for the client and for the institution within which they function" (American Nurses Association Congress of Nursing Practice Report on Case Management by Nurses, 1991). Health-care reform will change the reimbursement structure. Fee-for-service models will no longer exist and a new emphasis on cost and quality will emerge.

Capitation is predicted to be the reimbursement method of the future. Capitation—a preestablished reimbursement amount per enrollee for a given period of time—does not vary by the volume or complexity of the services provided. Capitation will have many aberrations until a standardized process has been selected. It will force hospitals, physicians, insurers, and consumers to have interlocking interests. Capitation could help change aligned incentives to keep clients well or at a higher level of functioning than reaching a compromised health status (Holloway, 1993). Again, the capitated Hospice Medicare model has the demonstrated elements to achieve client and family satisfaction cost effectively. In this model, consumers assume more responsibility for their own care and become better informed about the range of providers and potential options for services. The end result is that consumers make informed choices—a situation that leads to empowerment—thereby impacting quality and cost outcomes. Partnerships between providers and consumers must be developed so that choices can be presented that best meet consumer's needs (National League of Nursing, 1991). A nation-wide survey of nursing case management programs responded that the nurse case manager was key as the gatekeeper for the multidisciplinary client care team, thereby playing a significant role in cost containment, quality control, appropriate resource allocation, and reduction and prevention of fragmentation and duplication in care provided (Tahan, 1993).

Clients and families express a sense of security in having a familiar individual, the nurse case manager, educating and supporting them. Clients have demonstrated improved behavior simply because they are being monitored. To date our experience in influencing improved client and family satisfaction at reduced system cost is highlighted in the ensuing two examples (Box 12-1 and Box 12-2).

These two studies identified that one of the key roles of the nurse case manager is that of teacher. The teacher creates a connection rather than a separation, understanding and acceptance rather than judgment, collaboration rather than competition, and a pattern of evaluation rather than setting expectations. Evaluation of learning is most effective when done in collaboration between the learner and the teacher. In nurse case management, this collaboration occurs between the client and the nurse case manager (Bunkers, 1990). To be successful, the nurse case manager must understand and respect the individual's values and incorporate those values into a plan of care that is communicated to all members of the health-care team.

CONCLUSION

Nursing's challenge is to be stewards of resources. Currently, there are enough financial resources within the health-care system to meet the *health* needs of our society. Nevertheless, a paradigm shift needs to occur to divorce ourselves from the traditional thinking of our present system (Figure 12-2).

The shift in thinking involves empowering people and communities to take more responsibility in addressing health holistically. When the concepts of

freedom, trust, and caring become the basic foundation to build a delivery system, people experience the freedom to discuss what their feelings and thoughts are about the process of care being delivered. As a result, trusting relationships evolve which create a synergistic environment whereby we can mutually build on what it is we collaboratively know. *Caring is the nonjudgmental ability to internalize the experience of the client and family and to communicate that experience back to the client and family.* It is a validation of the experience.

As collaboration is emphasized, the caring approach is carried into the community. Caring tears down turf barriers and allows people with like concerns to join forces and resources in helping solve health-care issues. Nursing leadership's role is to pave the way for this to happen through searching "for meaning of caring within their institutions, by listening to nurses and clients, hearing what they need and responding with caring concern, by organizing structures and processes to support the art of nursing" (Brown, 1991). Case management addresses the entire continuum of care with an emphasis on clients together with their support systems accepting responsibility for their own health (Ethridge, 1990). Understanding clients and their support system values is vital to developing mutually set health-care goals. It is our belief that case management facilitates a trusting relationship between the case manager and the client that fosters client independence and the development of the freedom to make informed choices.

A major role of nursing is that of *leadership*. It is imperative that nurses develop the framework which allows enough freedom for individuals to take responsibility for their health and provide the environment and information so that this can occur. In the words of Florence Nightingale, "All the results of good nursing . . . . may be spoiled or utterly negated by one defect, viz: Petty Management or in other words, by not knowing how to manage so that what you do when

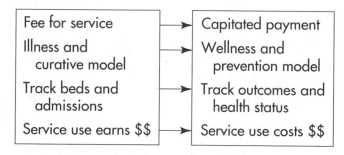

Fee for service	→	Capitated payment
Illness and curative model	→	Wellness and prevention model
Track beds and admissions	→	Track outcomes and health status
Service use earns $$	→	Service use costs $$

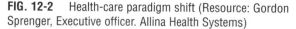

FIG. 12-2   Health-care paradigm shift (Resource: Gordon Sprenger, Executive officer. Allina Health Systems)

BOX 12-1

INTERREGIONAL CARDIOVASCULAR COLLABORATION PROJECT—PHASE I & PHASE II*

This project was funded in part by the Robert Wood Johnson Foundation/Pew Charitable Trusts "Strengthening Hospital Nursing, A Program to Improve Patient Care." Representatives from a rural area (three hospitals, associated medical practices, a state university nursing program) in South Central Minnesota and an urban tertiary medical center in Minneapolis, Minnesota, began collaborative work together in the spring of 1992. This collaborative team began to examine the current reality for cardiovascular patients transferred from southern Minnesota to the tertiary center and home again. They defined the purpose of this collaborative interregional project to: "Improve the process of health care (continuity, quality and cost) through the entire episode of illness for patients having a cardiovascular event necessitating interregional (primary and tertiary) care." The Mission Statement for this interregional project states "Patients are the reason health care exists. Realizing that an acute illness requiring hospitalization is but one point in the overall episode of illness experienced by the patient, our mission as health team members is to provide the integrated and holistic health services needed to assist the patient in reaching their optimum level health in the most efficient manner."

The Research Design and Data Analysis has been divided into two phases. (April 1992-1993)

Phase I: Qualitative descriptive study to identify the current interregional cardiovascular health-care process through patient interviews and chart reviews. (Data collection currently in process.)

Phase II: Quasiexperimental study to test nursing coordination of an interregional process of cardiovascular health care, using a one-year clinical progression, informed by Phase I, the literature, team members, and stakeholders.

Phase I data gathering about the patients' current reality was initiated in 1992. The methodological framework involved collecting information from medical records, client interviews, and input from nurse care providers. The two questions to be answered by Phase I were:

1. What factors (client/demographic, diagnosis/complications, numbers of unit/agencies traversed, duplication of techniques, type of documentation between agencies, and discharge status) characterize this interregional cardiovascular health-care experience?

2. What are the themes in the stories of clients who experienced an interregional cardiovascular episode of illness?

Results from a sample of 27 clients indicated test duplications, provider communication and documentation issues, concerns about continuity of care after tertiary center discharge, concerns about client and family ability to manage the therapeutic regimen and the effectiveness of education as presently delivered. The outcome of the dissemination of these data and discussions with physicians at all four sites has resulted in test duplications being greatly reduced. Secondly, nurse-coordinated interregional health care is currently being tested in Phase II.

Recent research has suggested that health-care provider communication is vital to optimal health-care outcomes (Knaus, Wagner, & Zimmerman, 1986; Shortell, et al., 1992). In situations where clients must be referred or transferred from their rural community care center to an urban tertiary care center, providing consistent, timely communication and coordination of care is a challenge.

The redesign process in Phase II incorporates a *research design* of two group quasiexperimental design with a purposive sample of 200 clients (100 intervention subjects and 100 comparison subjects). The hypothesis for Phase II states:

1. Clients receiving case management will have improved health status and risk behaviors.
2. Clients receiving case management will have higher satisfaction with health care than those who do not.
3. Clients receiving case management will have a decrease in health-care cost, rehospitalization, and acuity at rehospitalization.
4. Providers caring for clients receiving case management will have higher levels of satisfaction than those who do not.

Three interventions that have been implemented as a result of the Phase I data are:

1. A 12-month *clinical progression care path* which is in the possession of each client and family member as they journey through present-day systems of care.
2. *Interregional case managers* whose role is to coordinate triage, communication, interdisciplinary collaboration, education, and ongoing analysis.
3. Implemented health-care patterns utilizing the Omaha System as the framework.

Dr. Thomas W. Langfitt states in the forward to *Healthy America: Practitioners for 2005*, "No one is managing the client's transition through the (health care) system." In this project, the nurse advocates are currently analyzing the outcomes of coordinating the transition of a defined population by NCMs through an interregional health care system.

---

*See acknowledgments on p. 116.

BOX 12-2
INTEGRATED COMMUNITY MENTAL HEALTH CASE MANAGED POPULATION

Co-author Alice Weydt conducted a six-month retrospective descriptive study of 28 clients with mental health diagnoses who were nurse case managed in order to determine differences in cost and client satisfaction. Financial information was obtained through the hospital's and the psychiatric clinic's computer systems. Client satisfaction information was collected by the hospital's client satisfaction monitor and by ancedotal information. Data were compiled for each client for six months before implementing nurse case management and then compared to the subsequent six months after case management was implemented.

The data elements for cost and satisfaction were as follows:

> Number of inpatient hospital days
> Length of stay
> Admission acuity
> Hospital inpatient charges
> Number of emergency room visits
> Emergency room charges
> Recidivism
> Physician/clinic charges
> Client satisfaction

The results indicate significant decreases in the number of inpatient hospital days, length of stay, hospital inpatient charges, emergency room visits, emergency room charges, and recidivism (see table below).

There were no significant changes in physician/clinic charges. Admission acuity significantly increased. Changes in client satisfaction could not be determined because only three client satisfaction surveys were returned out of the eleven inpatient admissions reviewed. However, anecdotal information from the case managers was obtained.

The following is one of those anecdotal stories:

"I believe that some of my client contacts have prevented readmission. This is primarily because once we have established a trusting relationship, a client may call me before their situation reaches crisis proportions. I can help them through and/or facilitate quicker access to their physician. One client has had numerous situations like that and yet twice ended up as an inpatient, which is still less than last year. She is pleased that she has not been in the hospital so often."

This retrospective descriptive study concludes that nurse case management can significantly decrease hospital inpatient and emergency room charges without increasing physician and clinic fees. The mean admission acuity was significantly higher because of fewer lower-acuity admissions. Future admissions acuities will probably rise as other available alternatives to manage client needs are developed; however, the authors believe that there will be fewer admissions to the critical care unit because of nurse case management early intervention.

The preliminary findings are very encouraging, however, this study needs to be replicated in other settings with different groups of clients. Another method to measure mental health client satisfaction must also be developed. A key finding is that a streamlined process for data collection and analysis is needed for individual nurse case managers to concurrently collect and analyze their own data. Computer systems need to be integrated to support the continuum of care, replacing current systems, which are episodic based. A three-pronged integrated approach to evaluation, which includes clinical outcomes, client satisfaction, and cost must be developed across the entire care continuum. Our present mechanisms do not evaluate and integrate all three indicators.

Results from the Integrated Community Mental Health Case Managed Population Study

Outcome indicators (N = 28)	Before case managed (6 months)	After case managed (6 months)
Number of inpatient hospital days	357	89
Length of stay	9.64	8.09
Admission acuity	6.25	6.30
Hospital inpatient charges	$247,492	$56,473
Number of emergency room visits	29	19
Emergency room charges	$13,179	$4,782
Recidivism (readmission)	30	9
Physician/clinic charges	$38,225	$41,335

you are there is done when you are not" (Nightingale, F., 1869). Additionally, Florence Nightingale writes, "It is fundamental that the hospital shall do nothing to harm the patient. My view is that the ultimate destination of nursing is the nursing of the sick in their own homes. I look at abolition of all hospitals and work infirmaries. But it is of no use to talk about the year 2000" (Nightingale, F., 1860). Your authors believe we are here! We are challenged as providers to be innovative as we collaboratively facilitate the future of health care. It is our belief that this innovation is linked to the three concepts of *freedom, trust,* and *caring.*

ACKNOWLEDGMENTS

Health Bond and Abbott Northwestern Hospital Interregional Collaborative Cardiovascular Project team representatives include:

Annette McBeth, Vice President
    Immanuel-St. Joseph's Hospital, Mankato, MN,
    Nurse Executive
D. A. Nordquist, Nurse Clinician
    Immanuel St. Joseph's Hospital, Project Director
    and Care Manager
Cathy Ahern, Cardiac Rehabilitation Coordinator
    Immanuel-St. Joseph's Hospital, and Care
    Manager
Trudy Thomas, Home Care Supervisor
    Immanuel-St. Joseph's Hospital, and Care
    Manager
Donna Schiro, Nursing Services Director
    Arlington, MN, and Care Manager
Mary Fette, Cardiac Rehabilitation
    Waseca Area Memorial Hospital, Waseca, MN, and
    Care Manager
Sharon Aadalen, Health Bond Consortium Director
    Associate Professor, Mankato State University, and
    Methodology Resource Person
Abbott Northwestern Hospital representatives
    include:
Carol Huttner, Director Client Services
    Abbott Northwestern Hospital, Minneapolis, MN,
    and Nurse Executive
Pam Van Hazinga, Nurse Manager
    Abbott Northwestern Hospital, and Project Director
Karen Doran, Clinical Nurse Specialist
    Abbott Northwestern Hospital, and Care Manager
Elaine Hogan-Miller, Clinical Nurse Researcher
    Abbott Northwestern Hospital, and Methodology
    Resource Person

REFERENCES

American Nurses' Association. (1991). *Case management by nurses.* Kansas City, MO: American Nurses' Association: 1991.

Bunkers, S. S. (1990). The healing web: A transformatic model for nursing. *Nursing and Health Care, 13* (2), 68-73.

Bowers, K. (1992). *Case management by nurses.* Washington: American Nurses Publishing.

Brown, C. L. (1991). Aesthetics of nursing administration: the art of nursing organizations. *Nursing Administration Quarterly, 16* (1), 61-70.

Case Management Society of America (1994). *Standards of practice.* Washington, DC: Case Management Society of America.

Erickson, H. C., Tomlin, E. M., & Swain, M. P. (1983). *Modeling and role-modeling.* Englewood Cliffs, NJ: Prentice Hall, Inc.

Ethridge, P. (1990). A nursing HMO: Carondelet St. Mary's experience. *Nursing Management, 22* (7), 22-27.

Healthy America: Practitioners for 2005 (1991). *An agenda for action for U.S. health professional schools.* A report of the PEW Health Professions Commissions.

Holloway, D. C. (1993). *Implications of capitation for Stanford University Hospital: criteria for success under prepayment.* Palo Alto, CA: Stanford University Hospital.

Knaus, W. A., Wagner, D. P., Zimmerman, J. E. Interregional Cardiovascular Collaboration Project (1986). An evaluation of outcome from intensive care and major medical centers. *Annals of Internal Medicine, 104*: 410-418.

Lamb, G. S., & Stempel, J. E. (1994). Nurse case management from the client's view: growing as insider-expert. *Nursing Outlook, 42* (1), 7-13.

Langfitt, T. W., *Forward to healthy America: practitioners for 2005.*

Madden, M. J., & Ponte, R. P. (1994). Advanced practice roles in the managed care environment. *Journal of Nursing Administration, 24* (1), 56.

Maloney, T. W., & Paul, B. (1983). Rebuilding public trust and confidence. *Through the client's eyes* (pp. 280-296). San Francisco: Jossey-Bass Publishers.

Manthey, M. (1980). *The practice of primary nursing.* Boston: Blackwell Scientific Publications, Inc.

Nightingale, F. (1860). *Notes on nursing.* London: Harrison & Sons.

Nightingale, F. (1869). *Notes on nursing.* New York: Dover Publications.

National League for Nursing. (1991). *Nursing's agenda for health care reform.* New York: National League of Nursing.

Pepper Commission (1990). *A call for action,* Washington, DC: Pepper Commission.

Redford, L. J. (1992). Case management the wave of the future. *Journal of Case Management, 1* (1), 5-8.

Shortell, S. M., Zimmerman, J. E., Gillies, R. R., Duffy J., Devers, K. J., Rousseau, D. M., & Knaus, W. A. (1992). Continuously improving client care: practical lessons and an assessment tool from the ICU study, *Quarterly Review Bulletin,* May: 150-155.

Stevens, C. E. (1989). *In sickness and in wealth: American hospitals in the twentieth century.* New York: Basic Books.

Tahan, H. (1993). The nurse case manager in acute care settings. *The Journal of Nursing Administration, 23* (10), 53-61.

Trend Watch. (1993). Outcomes management: the new yardstick. *Trend Watch, 3* (3), 1-4.

Westberg, Granger. (1990). *The three acts of illness,* Video. National Parish Nurse Resource Center.

Wolfe, G. (1993). Convincing planners of CM benefits. *Case Management Advisor, 4* (8), 113.

Part Three

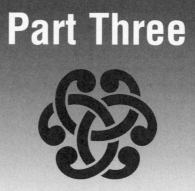

PARTNERS IN HEALTH: NURSES AND CLIENTS

A crucial factor in the theory of practice is the nature of the nurse-client relationship.

Margaret Newman

Part Three is client focused. Chapters 13 through 17 describe not only the crucial elements in the client-provider relationship but also the process of developing such relationships. Several authors identify outcomes of the development of successful partnerships, using a case study approach to deal with a variety of patient populations. These case studies demonstrate the nurse case manager interventions that respond most closely to client and family needs and at the same time strengthen the professional-client partnership.

Chapter 13

Theory of the Nurse-Client Partnership

Margaret A. Newman, PhD, RN, FAAN

OVERVIEW

*In professional partnerships between nurse and client,
the nurse's knowledge is important, but the nature
of the relationship is paramount.*

Nurse-client partnerships are the natural outgrowth of nursing theory. This chapter describes a model of practice designed to integrate nursing's role in administering medical technology within a broader context of nursing's view of health and commitment to caring. The application of nursing theory occurs as nursing practice is transformed by understanding of the theory.

The theory underlying nursing case management is a natural outgrowth of the development of nursing theory and practice . A concept of health as expanding consciousness (Newman, 1978; 1979; 1986; 1994) has emerged from the nursing paradigm of science introduced by Martha Rogers (1970). This view of nursing and health is distinct from the medical paradigm of health in which most nursing practitioners have functioned. The difference lies in two crucial perspectives: (1) how disease is regarded, and (2) the nature of the whole. In the medical paradigm, health is the absence of disease, which can be viewed as a separate and isolatable phenomenon. In the nursing paradigm, health encompasses disease as a manifestation of the underlying pattern of the person—a unitary, indivisible pattern of the whole.

The demands of these paradigms are often in conflict. To resolve the conflict a model of practice was developed to honor the differences and at the same time attempt to integrate them (Newman, 1990). At first, the model of practice and the theory of health as expanding consciousness seemed to represent two parallel lines of thinking, but the connection between the two has become apparent in the practice of the clinician/case manager and will be described later in this chapter.

The motivation for proposing the tri-level model stemmed from the intense awareness that the arena in which most nurses practiced was dominated by the medical regimen. Nursing had little or no arena that supported the actualization of practice grounded in nursing theory. The prevailing paradigm guiding practice by nurses, both in the hospital and in the community, has been and still is a medical model, which embraces a concept that health is the antithesis of disease. The activities of nurses functioning within this paradigm are derived from the medical paradigm, aimed at the prevention and treatment of disease.

Before the advent of the DRG-related prospective payment system (in 1983) and Medicare regulations regarding home care, there was enough slack in the system to allow nurses the time to pursue their practice stemming from the nursing perspective of person-oriented care in an all-encompassing program of both nursing and medical care. The cost factors that have preoccupied health-systems management the past decade, however, have squeezed that which is truly nursing practice out of the picture. Clinical nursing specialists increasingly have been considered costly extras unless they devote their expertise to enhance the medical program of treatment.

This situation is characterized by dissatisfaction on the part of consumers and nurses, and by confusion and compromised vision on the part of nursing leaders (Newman & Autio, 1986). The public has become increasingly aware of the lack of access to appropriate health services, lack of information to assist them in making decisions about their own health care, and general depersonalization that characterizes the service they receive. Nurses are dissatisfied because they lack control over their practice and their time. There is little time available to attend to the vital aspects of nursing. (vis à vis medicine). Nursing service directors find it difficult to extend their vision beyond the parameters of care established by medically dominated hospital authorities.

A MODEL OF PROFESSIONAL NURSING PRACTICE

·Thus, it seemed critical to develop a model of practice that focused on *professional* nursing practice as the *centerpiece* of nursing practice; that is, a professional role in direct relationship to the client *whenever and wherever* the client is in need of nursing consultation and service.· Without nurses functioning in this kind of direct relationship to clients, nursing is not fulfilling its mission to society for personalized, supportive care throughout the client's health experience.

What is needed is a role of *professional partnership*, also referred to as "insider expert" (Lamb & Stempel, 1994) and "instrumental friendship" (Rawnsley, 1990). The knowledge brought to the relationship is important, but the nature of the relationship is paramount.

In the zeal to establish nursing's professional status, many have tended to ignore the need for the caring, competent nurse partner. Although there is a significant body of work related to caring as the essence of nursing, the extent to which that work has pervaded the general practice of nursing in a significant way is not

clear. Physicians and hospital administrators, as well as nurses, are now beginning to recognize the compassion gap existing in health care and are calling for greater emphasis on human caring. How could the basic mission of nursing have been neglected to this extent?

So the theoretical basis for the tri-level model of differentiated practice starts with the paradigm guiding practice. The paradigm guiding the practice of the nursing clinician/case manager is the nursing paradigm of person-oriented care. It embraces caring as a moral imperative and health that focuses on the evolving pattern of the whole of PersonFamilyEnvironment.

If nurses are to continue to function within a context dominated by medical care, there is a need for two other roles: (1) one devoted primarily to assistance with daily living tasks and implementation of the medical regimen and (2) one whose responsibility it is to transmute technology into an individualized nursing perspective, facilitate the work of associate nurses (whose preparation and role address a circumscribed application of medical and nursing technology), and act as a pivotal point of information and interface with the multiple professionals involved in the patient's care. The first role is carried out by an associate nurse (a minimum of associate degree preparation) and the latter by a nurse prepared at the baccalaureate level, variously referred to as team leader, patient care coordinator, liaison nurse. This latter role requires sufficient knowledge of both nursing and medical models to be able to translate medical technology into the perspective of individualized nursing care, as well as leadership ability and communication skills.

THEORY GUIDING PRACTICE

·The theory that guides the practice of the nursing clinician/case manager addresses the *caring relationship* in which the nurse engages the client and the process of *pattern recognition* in which the nurse and client participate mutually as they seek to reach a point of insight that illumines the action appropriate for the health of the client.·

As background to the theory and knowledge germane to this process, some of the assumptions set forth by Rogers are relevant. First, pattern is basic. Pattern identifies the unique wholeness of a person and is in constant flux as the person coevolves with the environment. The phenomena commonly called health and illness are expressions of this evolving pattern of the whole.

Health dealt with within the nursing paradigm is the health of the whole (both words stem from a root meaning). This is a unitary process, one that cannot be segmented, such as in healthy versus unhealthy. For example, when body temperature is being addressed, one does not consider the points of measurement as separate entities but rather looks at the cycles of peaks and troughs. The meaning lies in the pattern of the whole. Similarly, the whole of a person's health experience is the focus of the discipline.

Bohm's fish tank example helps to illustrate how what is seen is a reflection of a larger whole. Bohm suggested that one imagine two television cameras (labeled A and B) focused from different angles on a tank of fish and flora. Then imagine the pictures being portrayed on screens A and B. The pictures would portray the same phenomena from different perspectives. They would be two-dimensional, dynamic portrayals of a phenomenon of greater dimensions. They represent a limited view of things. Although the movements are somehow correlated, there is no force of interaction between the two screens. One does not cause the other (Bohm, 1980).

Now if this illustration is applied to the way in which Body is singled out from Mind, imagine that one could capture Mind on one screen and Body on the other. Each is a reflection of an underlying pattern of greater dimensions, and although there is often a correlation between them, one does not cause the other. Each is a reflection of the larger whole.

Stretch the analogy one step further. Imagine the two screens as portraying Disease and Non-disease (health in medical model terms). Each is a reflection of a larger whole, a pattern of infinite dimensions. Each is a limited portrayal of the larger phenomenon.

Theories emerging from many different disciplines indicate that the life process is evolving toward higher levels of consciousness. Think of consciousness as the total information of the pattern of the field. With that as an assumption, all manifestations of the field, including illness, (or in medical terms, pathology) are manifestations of the process of expanding consciousness. Hence, the designation of the theory of health as expanding consciousness.

The interrelatedness of the concepts of *health* and *caring* can be captured in the phrase, *caring in the human health experience*, which has been designated as the focus of the discipline of nursing (Newman, Sime, & Corcoran-Perry, 1991). This focus incorporates all manifestations of the evolving pattern, including but not making primary the pattern and evolution of disease. It includes, for instance, all those other experiences of health not characterized by disease, such as growing up, establishing intimate relationships, having babies, developing families, family violence, workplace abuse, and so on. Further, caring is not just a feeling or an attitude but is the highest level of human development. This level of development is needed by practitioners as they engage with clients. Some theorists (Boykin & Schoenhofer, 1993) consider caring as a

defining human characteristic, and that the intent of the nursing process is to bring about the experience of caring in those served.

NURSE-CLIENT RELATIONSHIP

A crucial factor in the theory of practice is the nature of the nurse-client relationship. It is a coming together of nurse and client (which may be a family or community as well as an individual) and moving apart in a rhythmic fashion during which their patterns interpenetrate. In the process, the clients center and recognize their evolving pattern. The recognition is insight regarding the meaning of the pattern and the action that is needed.

Intervention derived from the instrumental paradigm of medical science requires that the professional identify the client's "problem" and take steps to remedy it. Intervention derived from the relational paradigm of nursing science directs the professional to enter into an authentic relationship with the client with the mutual goal of gaining insight into the process and thereby evolving to a higher level of consciousness. According to Lamb and Stempel (1994), the nurse case manager does both: identifying and taking steps to remedy the client's acute problem (usually one of pathophysiology) in the early stage of the relationship and continuing in the process of pattern recognition and insight as the nurse-client relationship deepens.

The nurse-client relationship proceeds in cycles of coming together and moving apart. The nurse and client come together often at a time of disorganization, crisis, or chaos. Clients have reached a critical point in their health experience when they do not know what to do. Things that have worked in the past no longer work. They need a professional partner to help them see beyond the present, seemingly hopeless, situation: The nurse enters into this experience with the client and provides a kind of organizing force that supports the client's journey through the chaotic period until the client emerges at a new level of order. This process is analogous to the process of dissipative structures described by Prigogine (Prigogine & Stengers, 1984), namely, the system moves from normal repetitive patterns to disorganized, unpredictable patterns and then elects another repetitive pattern at a higher level of organization.

The nurse-client dialogue centers on the unfolding of the clients' stories of the most meaningful persons and events in their lives. Pattern recognition occurs as revelations regarding the meaning of the evolving pattern become apparent in actions such as changes in movement patterns within the family and in relation to the community.

Litchfield's (1993) work illustrates this theory. She has characterized the nurse-client relationship as extending from a period of disruption characterized by uncertainty and unpredictability to a point at which the client moved from relative disorder to order at a higher level. The process by which this occurs is one of dialogue and pattern recognition, unfolding increasing alternatives and connectedness with others and the environment. In her study of families who were experiencing frequent illnesses and hospitalizations of their young children, the families moved from a present without vision (no tomorrow) to the integration of both past and future in a vision of possibilities. The present without vision was a kind of treadmill experience of survival without connection to the past or the future. Through the reflective process of the dialogue, they were able to envision an expanding horizon with plans for the future and intentions to act. In addition, they were able to look beyond their own situation to what they could contribute to the larger community. The previous concentration on the child, the designated patient, was broadened to an integrated pattern of connectedness within the family and with the wider world—a process of expanding consciousness.

Lamb and Stempel (1994) examined the nurse case manager's role from the standpoint of their clients and found a similar process of coming together with the client during a time of disruption, a resolving of the immediate crisis, and then moving on to the meaning of family patterns in relation to health. They used the term "insider expert" to describe the role. This designation was derived from both the client's feeling of intimacy with the nurse in being really known and cared for and also the confidence that the nurse was knowledgeable regarding the medical-physiological crisis being experienced by the client and was taking appropriate action:

> Initially, clients see the nurse case manager in the role of expert, someone who can monitor their physical status and teach them ways to take care of themselves. Over time, bonding occurs between nurse and client which allows the client to feel known and cared about as an individual. In the context of this bonding, clients begin to think differently about their situations, develop confidence in their ability to care for themselves and take on greater responsibility . . . (Lamb & Stempel, 1994, p. 9).

The situations that Lamb and Stempel describe illustrate bringing order out of chaos and light out of darkness. One client described the experience of having the nurse "pull her out of a dark hole."

The important point is that the nurse be accessible at such critical choice points in the client's life and be fully present with the client in the experience until a new pattern emerges. Litchfield's experience in this regard convinced her of the need for what Heron (1988, p. 52) has described as a "collapse into confusion, uncertainty, ambiguity, disorder and chaos . . .

feeling lost to a greater or lesser degree." The nurse must have tolerance for finding no outcome in the present and be able to wait for the order that will emerge from the chaos.

The nurse enters into the client's experience. This means letting go of predetermined agendas regarding what a nurse should do in such situations and waiting, being fully present until the client's pattern emerges. As the pattern reveals itself, the needed action (the action potential) will become apparent, and the client will know what action is needed. Lamendola described his experience in letting go:

> I . . . realized that all I had to do was "Be there" and listen . . . I needed to let go of thinking. I had to lead the interview in a direction or make the pain better or fix a problem. The purpose . . . was to allow a sense of the whole to emerge (Lamendola & Newman, 1994).

Getting in touch with what is meaningful to the client (meaning is pattern) may or may not occur immediately. The nurse must be able to continue with the client until the insight or action occurs.

Lamb and Stempel (1994) observed that clients with greater perceived need and greater comfort with intimacy seem to move through the nurse-client process of bonding, working, and changing more rapidly and with greater intensity. In contrast, the conditions described by Mishel (1990) as blocking the growth opportunities emerging from uncertainty include the client's delayed response to their diagnosis and isolation from social interaction. These findings help to explain why some clients, whose patterns depict denial of their disease and isolation from others (Jonsdottir, 1994), do not manifest behaviors associated with expanding consciousness.

CONCLUSION

An area of needed study is the timing of the nurse-client relationship—when to come together, when to move apart, when something is helpful, when it is not, when learning is optimal, and so on. Rhythm is an essential characteristic.

The way in which nursing theory is applied is by virtue of the theoretical transformation that is taking place in the person of the nurse. The nurse's field of consciousness (informational capacity) is transformed and through the interpenetration of the nurse-client field, the client's field is transformed.

REFERENCES

Bohm, D. (1980). *Wholeness and the implicate order.* London: Routledge & Kegan Paul.

Boykin, A., & Schoenhofer, S. (1993). *Nursing as caring: a model for transforming practice.* New York: National League for Nursing.

Heron, J. (1988). Validity in co-operative inquiry. In P. Reason (Ed.). *Human inquiry in action: Developments in new paradigm research* (pp. 40-59). London: Sage.

Jonsdottir, H. (1994). *Life patterns of people with chronic obstructive pulmonary disease.* Ph.D. dissertation, University of Minnesota, Minneapolis, MN.

Lamb, G. S., & Stempel, J. E. (1994). Nurse case management from the client's view: growing as insider-expert. *Nursing Outlook, 42,* 7-13.

Lamendola, F., & Newman, M. A. (1994). The paradox of HIV/AIDS as expanding consciousness. *Advances in Nursing Science, 16* (3), 13-21.

Litchfield, M. C. (1993). *The process of health patterning in families with young children who have been repeatedly hospitalized.* Master's thesis, University of Minnesota, Minneapolis, MN.

Mishel, M. H. (1990). Reconceptualization of the uncertainty in illness theory. *Image, 22* (4), 256-261.

Newman, M. A. (1978). *Toward a theory of health.* Paper presented at Nurse Educator Conference, New York, NY.

Newman, M. A. (1979). *Theory development in nursing.* Philadelphia: Davis.

Newman, M. A. (1986). *Health as expanding consciousness.* St Louis: Mosby.

Newman, M. A. (1990). Toward an integrative model of professional practice. *Journal of Professional Nursing, 6* (3), 167-173.

Newman, M. A. (1994). *Health as expanding consciousness* (2nd ed.). New York: National League of Nursing.

Newman, M. A., & Autio, S. (1986). Nursing in the world of DRGs and prospective payment. *CURA Reporter* (University of Minnesota Center for Urban and Regional Affairs), *16* (5), 1-7.

Newman, M. A., Sime, A. M., & Corcoran-Perry, S. A. (1991). The focus of the discipline of nursing. *Advances in Nursing Science, 14* (1), 1-6.

Prigogine, I., & Stengers, I. (1984). *Order out of chaos.* Boulder: Shambhala.

Rawnsley, M. (1990). Of human bonding: the content of nursing as caring. *Advances in Nursing Science, 13* (1), 41-48.

Rogers, M. E. (1970). *An introduction to the theoretical basis of nursing.* Philadelphia: Davis.

Chapter 14

Working in Partnership

Joan Stempel, MS, RN, CCM
Arlene Carlson, MA, LPN
Cathy Michaels, PhD, RN

OVERVIEW

Partnership is the essence of nurse case management.

This chapter describes the partnership process that occurred at Carondelet St. Mary's Hospital and Health Center (Tucson, AZ) between high-risk chronically ill clients and professional nurse case managers (pncms).[1] This process focused on a holistic approach to client interactions which was based on a relational rather than a medical paradigm. Clients were assisted by recommendations from their pncms, who identified health-care concerns and interventions these clients were willing to implement. Key concepts such as viewing the client as the expert, facilitating readiness, and identifying triggers of exacerbation are discussed together with pncm actions that clients reported helpful in supporting them through their process of change.

Professional nurse case management is a service of partnership for people whose health and functionality is declining because of serious, persistent, or chronic illness and disability. Begun in 1985, through Carondelet St. Mary's Hospital and Health Center, Tucson, Arizona, professional nurse case managers (pncm's) have partnered with over 6000 people who have used the Carondelet Health Care system. Originally, the service was targeted toward the elderly. Today, the program also includes adults and children and their families, but because of their higher inci-

dence of serious, persistent or chronic illness and disability, the elderly remain the largest case managed group.

Individuals are considered to be at high risk when a mismatch exists between their state of health and their self-care ability. Often profiled as cognitively or emotionally challenged, these people tend to have inadequate caregiving support and frequently use hospital and emergency room services.

---

[1]The authors have intentionally written pncm in lower rather than upper case letters. The partnership described in this chapter, that between pncm and client, is between two equals. Identifying both partners in lower case denotes the equality of this relationship.

Special thanks to Nancy Mairs for her assistance in editing this chapter and to the National Multiple Sclerosis Society for providing a grant that partially funded this research. We also acknowledge the work and insights of other project members, including Gerri Lamb, PhD, RN, Principal Investigator, Donna Zazworsky, MS, RN, Professional Nurse Case Manager, and Dory Martin, MSW, Social Work Case Manager.

From the health-care system perspective, the purpose of pncm service is to:
- Monitor clients,
- Offer illness prevention strategies,
- When needed, help them access primary, acute, transitional, or long-term care appropriately.
- From the clients' perspectives, the pncm services:
  - Foster confidence,
  - Help them acquire the knowledge and skills which allow them to manage their illness more effectively,
  - Connect them to community services for which they may be eligible,
  - Obtain equipment to enhance their self-care ability,
  - Familiarize them with their personal and medical options, and
  - Advocate for them within the health-care arena. •

Perhaps the best description of the pncm-client partnership comes from Margaret Newman (1994):

> Nursing intervention is derived from a relational paradigm that directs the professional to enter into a partnership with the client, often at a time of chaos, with the mutual goal of participating in an authentic relationship, trusting that in the process of its unfolding, both will emerge at a high level of consciousness. . . . The thing that brings people to the attention of a nurse is a situation that they do not know how to handle. They are at a choice point . . . We come to a point when the old rules do not work anymore . . . and the task of life, the crux of life is to learn the new rules. . . . This means learning how to transcend a situation that seems impossible, to find a new way of relating to things, and to discover the freedom that comes with transcending the old limitations. The necessity of "hanging in there" in the midst of the uncertainty and ambiguity of the chaotic situation is an import factor in the healing process. . . . We as nurses enter into the process with a client to be present with it, attend to it and live it, even if it appears in the form of disharmony, catastrophe, or disease.

In their partnership endeavors, many pncm's are guided by a holistic nursing model based on principles introduced through the Traditional Indian Medicine Program directed by Edgar Monetatchi, Jr. These principles include viewing the client as his own expert on his health and as the one responsible for management of his condition, developing a working partnership with each client, facilitating readiness, helping to identify exacerbation triggers and developing strategies to cope with them. All pncm's seem to embrace a basic tenet of respecting each person's right and responsibility for individual choice and consequence. Through their work, pncm's have come to view illness as a process that offers the individual and family the opportunity to learn more about themselves and their situations.

VIEWING THE CLIENT AS THE EXPERT

The pncm partner sees clients as the "experts" on their disease process because they have a wealth of information and knowledge about their condition and situation. For example, if clients have chronic obstructive pulmonary disease (COPD), *they* are the *only* ones who know what symptoms usually occur when they are experiencing an exacerbation, and what situations are apt to trigger one. They know how they use the health-care system when an exacerbation occurs, what makes them feel better or worse, how they care for themselves between hospitalizations, what kind of self-care behaviors they are willing to attempt, and how the illness is affecting the mental, emotional, and spiritual aspects of their lives.

At the start of their partnerships with pncm's, clients may not view themselves as the experts. Often, health professionals perpetuate this belief by not asking clients to share their knowledge and experience or by only giving lip service to it, not incorporating their information into services and plans of care. The authors' experiences, however, with partnership has shown that over time and with encouragement, clients frequently come to realize that they know themselves better than anyone else and learn to trust their own knowledge and judgment. The pncm's trust in clients' abilities enhances this process and helps clients build confidence in their medical self-care abilities.

Health Care Outcomes— the Client's Responsibility

Under this holistic model, not only are clients seen as the experts, but they are also seen as the people responsible for their own health-care outcomes. Acknowledging the responsibilities of the clients requires a shift in perspective for many nurses who have been taught to "take charge" and "take care of" but not to "take a back seat." In the experiences of the authors, true caring means acknowledging clients as the drivers and the pncm as the one helping them find the signposts.

Often, when working with clients, pncm's become aware of their own personal issues—fear of giving up control, perhaps, or anger at having excellent advice ignored—rising to the surface. Pncm's are challenged to become aware of their own personal agendas for clients and resolve these issues as they occur.

Identifying Exacerbation Triggers

Unlike other health-care providers, whose involvement is generally limited to the acute phase of an illness, pncm's follow clients for as long as both feel these services are beneficial. When clients are first seen by their pncm's, most of their attention and energy is usually focused on stabilizing physically and regaining as much of their former lifestyle as possible. As these clients become stronger, they often become willing to take the next step and explore the physical, emotional, and spiritual stresses or "root causes" that may have contributed to triggering their exacerbations. Many times, physical symptoms of illnesses are affected by unresolved emotional and spiritual issues. For example, exacerbations of multiple sclerosis (MS) sometimes seem related to stressful family dynamics. As pncm's and individuals develop ways to lessen these triggers, close therapeutic relationships are often forged.

Modalities that many have found helpful in identifying and working with these triggers include active listening, therapeutic touch, relaxation, breathing, physical exercises and other body awareness therapies, mutual story telling, life review, and imagery.

Facilitating Readiness

Readiness, as defined in the pncm model, refers to a person's willingness to become aware of behavioral, cognitive, or attitudinal patterns and eventually to consider changing them. Recognizing and acknowledging the choices they have made in the past, regarding their health behaviors, is often the first step. Once recognition of these behaviors occurs, clients begin the process of linking their choice of health behaviors to their consequences. If these consequences have been experienced as detrimental *by the client*, they often are ready to reconsider the choices they are making and change their behavior. The pncm's trust in the client as the responsible one seems to boost his confidence during this process. Learning to shift health behaviors may be facilitated in a step-wise process often requiring experiential learning.

Developing a Plan of Care That Reflects a Nurse-Client Partnership

Rather than adopting nurse-developed plans of care, clients and pncm's working together in the clients' residences, develop plans based on ways these clients wish to deal with their health challenges. During these processes, clients share their health concerns and the knowledge they have regarding their condition. How clients perceive bodily changes, what knowledge exists about initiating and following up with self-care strategies (such as relaxation), or those prescribed by the physician or other health-care professionals are explored. The pncm also learns how these individuals have managed their illnesses in the past and how they respond to exacerbations. Do they identify an exacerbation when one is occurring and immediately seek medical attention or do they ignore the symptoms until a crisis arises? The intensity of focus clients place on their illness and the extent to which other impor-

tant aspects of their lives are being set aside is also key information when developing a plan of care.

One of the major elements in developing client competencies and implementing plans of care is the formation of authentic, caring relationships between pncm's and clients. Relationships in which clients experience the pncm as someone who . . . "knows me," "cares about me," "I can count on to be with me," and "is interested in *all* of me" are interpersonal relationships in which clients feel motivated and safe to try out new ways of thinking and acting . . ." (Lamb & Stempel, 1994).

MULTIPLE SCLEROSIS RESEARCH STUDY

In 1990, Carondelet St. Mary's Hospital received a grant from the National Multiple Sclerosis Society, which was matched by funds from Carondelet St. Mary's, for a one-year experimental study. The purpose of this study was to determine the impact and the benefit working with a pncm might have for people with progressive MS who were at high risk because of their fluctuating or deteriorating health status.

Known as a neuromuscular disease, recent research has shown MS eventually impacts cognition, memory function in particular. Those people with MS who are cognitively challenged are at even greater risk for mismanaging their health concerns than those with neuromuscular dysfunction alone. Moreover, the rapid change in functional status which can occur magnifies the risk. One day, the person may be able to walk and the next day be wheelchair bound.

Under this study, 25 people with progressive MS received pncm services for one year, while a control group of 26 similar people received no case management. Both groups were assessed at the beginning of the study, six months later, and again at twelve months. Such items as quality of life, symptom management, care giving, empowerment, use of health services, and ability to perform ADLs (activities of daily living) were measured quantitatively; clients' records and subjective narratives were also analyzed by using qualitative methodology. Upon completion of the study, subjects in the control group were offered the opportunity to receive pncm as well, and 12 subjects accepted.

This study afforded pncm's a unique opportunity to work with clients with MS and their families over a long period of time, thus allowing them to know the individuals, form strong relationships, and assist with the setting of long-term as well as short-term goals. Early analysis of anecdotal data seems to indicate that pncm's have the greatest impact on clients who see themselves as being in crisis and also have an authentic and caring relationship with the pncm.

The dynamics that occurred in the partnership between MS clients and pncm's are similar to those experienced when working with all populations. This chapter will focus on the experience of these clients and the pncm's who worked with them. Attitudes and patterns of behavior of clients and pncm's which assisted care or created barriers will be described, together with strategies clients reported useful. Because the number of women experiencing MS exceeds the number of men with the disease, for the purpose of discussion clients will be referred to in the feminine.

Beginning the Process

Most clients and families had weathered a wide variety of situations caused by the impact of MS upon their lives before meeting and working with their pncm. These clients had developed various individual patterns of coping, influenced by their symptoms as well as their family dynamics, previous experiences, values, beliefs, and available resources. Some strategies, such as attending support groups or redistributing household chores, worked well, whereas others, such as isolating oneself, appeared less beneficial.

The pncm and each client began their relationship by identifying and using the client's knowledge of herself to complete a client-family assessment and develop a plan of care. Impaired mobility, symptom management, self-care deficits, safety, unavailability of a support system, caregiver burnout, lack of knowledge, isolation, depression, fear, equipment needs, and lack of medical and supportive care were the most frequently identified problems needing intervention. Once these problem areas were identified, available options to deal with each were explored.

During the next stage of the process, clients and their pncm's began implementing interventions each client felt ready to pursue. Clients usually chose to begin with interventions they valued and believed would be helpful and ones which necessitated behavioral or lifestyle changes they felt ready to pursue.

Readiness

Readiness, as previously stated, is used by pncm's to describe a person's ability to alter behavioral, cognitive, or attitudinal patterns and to make lifestyle changes. Readiness, or reaching a choice point in this population is influenced by many factors, including the past and present impact of MS on the person's life and how much this impact is felt as crisis. Previous experiences with lifestyle changes influence a person's readiness, because someone who has successfully modified her lifestyle in the past often has less difficulty with change than someone whose patterns have been more fixed.

Not only does readiness, or willingness, to change vary from individual to individual, the ability to make specific changes also varies *within* each individual, depending on the meaning a given change has for each person. Changes that challenge the image a person has of herself, or involve giving up things she values, are more difficult to make and require a higher degree of readiness than changes she views as trivial. For example, a person with MS who has changes in walking and gait and values "looking normal," is often willing to adopt an exercise program but less willing to accept the need for a cane or Canadian crutches.

How much pncm support is accepted by the individual during the process of attaining readiness is affected by several factors. Past encounters with the health-care system, whether the nurse is viewed as knowledgeable, and how valuable the individual with MS believes the suggested changes will be in improving her situation are all major influences (see Case Study).

CASE STUDY

Forty-two-year-old Jenny was diagnosed with MS 20 years ago. In the initial interview with her nurse, it became apparent that during these years, Jenny had learned very little about MS. She was experiencing numerous exacerbations accompanied by extreme fatigue, difficulty walking, frequent falls, urinary incontinence, muscle spasms, and headaches. When these symptoms occurred, Jenny felt she had no control over her MS, fearing her disease was progressing and soon would cause her to become totally bed bound. Her pattern of coping with the emotions raised by this belief was to throw herself into her work. As her exacerbations became more frequent and she became increasingly frightened, she worked 8 to 12 hours a day, ignoring her fatigue. This exhaustion then triggered more symptoms.

Gradually, over a nine-month period, Jenny confided her fears to her pncm and became willing to explore the connection between overdoing and increased symptoms. When experiencing an exacerbation, she learned to ask herself how much she had done in the previous 48 hours. After many repetitions of the exacerbation/overworking/exacerbation cycle, Jenny was able to see a connection. She tried limiting her activities to four to six hours a day for two weeks and to stop working when she became tired. Much to her delight, she found her spasms, incontinence, and headaches greatly decreased and her walking improved. Once she understood the connection between exhausting herself and increased symptoms, she became less fearful and felt a sense of control over her illness. She stated, "Now when I get the urge to work late into the night, I ask myself do I want to pay the consequences. Usually I don't. By making my days shorter, I actually get more done because I'm not having to spend three to four days a week in bed recovering."

Enhancers of Relationships

Several clients identified themselves as medical experts. Diagnosed with MS several years before meeting a pncm, they had become very knowledgeable about their disease and had developed excellent disease management skills. Their pncm's, somewhat intimidated by the new and difficult experience of working with people who knew more about their illnesses than their pncm's did, felt challenged when forming relationships with these clients. Initially, when these pncm's reacted to their own feelings of insecurity and loss of control by attempting to prove *they* were the experts in MS management, several clients became somewhat hostile and withdrawn. Many of these client experts, finding it hard to believe that suggestions made by the pncm would improve their situation, were reluctant to share either their physical or their emotional difficulties with her. As one commented, "Unless you have multiple sclerosis yourself, you don't know what it is like to live with it day in and day out." These clients often took longer than more recently diagnosed individuals to begin trusting and confiding in their nurse case managers and entertaining suggestions from them.

Gradually, pncm's became aware of their own agenda and its basis in feelings of insecurity and need for control. As a result of this shift in consciousness, the pncm's changed their behavior, validating clients' knowledge rather than challenging their expertise. As clients realized that their knowledge was respected and valued, they became less defensive and more willing to share their concerns and try new interventions.

Accessing Health Care

Often, during a client's assessment, symptoms that needed medical intervention requiring contact with a physician were identified. Many clients were reluctant to make this contact. Some stated their reluctance directly, whereas others displayed their hesitation through their behavior—repeatedly forgetting to make the appointment or to keep it, failing to find a ride, or canceling the appointment because "I didn't feel up to going."

Pncm's and clients explored these behaviors and discovered a variety of causes. In some instances, individuals who had very little income and no medical insurance simply lacked the resources needed to seek medical attention. Pncm's assisted willing and eligible clients to apply for state- and county-supported medical programs and negotiated with receptive physicians to see ineligible clients for a reduced fee or free of charge.

Usually, however, the client's hesitation was due to negative encounters she had experienced with the health-care system in the past. Several people described feeling angry and frustrated when told their symptoms were psychological rather than physically based, thereby delaying diagnosis of their MS. Others recounted the insensitive manner with which they were informed they had the disease. A young woman related how furious she felt when she received her diagnosis. One moment she was told, "You have MS." The next moment, she and her husband were informed that most marriages of individuals with MS ended in divorce. "That's the last thing I needed to hear right then, as if I wasn't frightened enough already."

Individuals who experienced difficulty relating to their physicians were encouraged to resolve this situation. Annie, a warm, caring woman, described how emotionally distant her physician was when talking to her. His detached attitude made her feel uncomfortable and unsupported. She confronted her doctor with her feelings and described the type of relationship she wanted them to develop. She was very pleased when her doctor admitted she was the first person he had ever treated with MS and said he welcomed the opportunity to learn how to relate to her. When clients were unable to develop a comfortable relationship with a health-care provider, they often changed providers. In these instances, they were encouraged to get recommendations from the MS Society or others who had MS.

Frequently, clients had been told at the time of diagnosis, "There is nothing that can be done for MS so go out and learn to live with it." Because of these experiences, many individuals concluded that they had no reason to obtain conventional medical attention for any reason. Often, they went several years without seeking even such basic preventive medical care as physical examinations or pap smears. Some explored alternative medical therapies such as acupuncture or vitamin therapy, as a way to control symptoms or slow the progression of MS. Pncm's learned to wait until they discovered how a particular client viewed the health-care system before suggesting that she seek medical attention. When the client held a negative view, trust needed to be established between the person and her nurse before interventions requiring physician contact were discussed. If such a proposal was made before this relationship was established, the suggestion was often ignored or met with anger. Building a rapport with the client became more difficult under these circumstances.

Implementing Interventions— Variations in Adjustment

Reactions to living with MS varied widely among individuals. Some clients accepted the fact they had MS, whereas others denied the disease was causing permanent changes in their physical or cognitive abilities. One group had a history of making successful changes and appeared pragmatic in their approach to the illness. As each symptom developed, these individuals made the adjustments needed to maintain a lifestyle they valued.

Lucy was an example of this group. A 30-year-old woman who used a motorized scooter, Lucy lived alone and continued to hold a full-time job. When asked about learning to live with MS, she stated, "There is nothing MS has taken away from me that I can't replace if I'm willing to pay the price, but sometimes it takes me a while to decide if I want to pay the price." The high value Lucy places on autonomy is reflected in the way she chooses to manage her illness. When her physical limitations increased to the point where she needed help with ADLs, she moved into an assisted-living apartment rather than live with her family. When urinary incontinence became a problem, she chose a surgical procedure rather than constantly ask willing friends to help her to the bathroom.

Such individuals as Lucy were adept at minimizing the impact MS had upon their lifestyles. Unlike the individuals who identified themselves as experts, however, they bonded easily with their nurses and actively sought suggestions. Whatever the challenge, Lucy and individuals like her emphasized finding solutions over emotional processing.

A number of individuals, although not denying they had MS, did not adapt their lifestyles to accommodate the changes they were experiencing. Many had been diagnosed with MS for several years but, unlike Lucy, they had chosen to learn little about MS and viewed their symptoms as temporary. All were expecting some kind of reversal that would cause limitations to disappear. Beliefs about how this would happen took different forms.

Usually, patterns of denial persisted unchanged until some form of crisis occurred. Crisis forced many clients to explore their patterns and the consequences of their choices. Often they reevaluated decisions they had made or deferred. As their resistance to change diminished, they moved toward suggested lifestyle changes that they had previously rejected.

Lisa was diagnosed with MS 13 years earlier, after the birth of her son Jeff, and had learned very little about MS since. During her first six months of working with the pncm, Lisa described her symptoms as temporary; an exacerbation not requiring any management interventions. Over time, Lisa's ability to ambulate continued to decrease and she became dependent on an Amigo. She experienced fatigue, muscle spasms, and urinary incontinence which she kept hoping would subside.

One day, in tears, she confided to her pncm that Jeff was staying out late and skipping school. When Lisa attempted to discuss the situation with her husband Mark, he became angry and told her he was consider-

ing a divorce. She and her pncm explored available options and after much discussion, the family started marriage counseling with a therapist who specialized in dealing with chronic illness.

After several months of therapy, Lisa stated that she'd had no idea she had been so angry or that she took her anger out on Mark and Jeff. With the help of the therapist, the family was able to discuss their feelings and address many of their differences. Now, rather than disagreeing about Jeff's curfews and household responsibilities, Mark and Lisa are learning to negotiate agreements with him, a method that is more satisfying to all.

This crisis motivated Lisa to reevaluate some of the decisions she had made regarding how she was choosing to manage her MS. Because she'd had several negative encounters with physicians, Lisa had not seen a doctor for several years. She did not know what type of MS she had and had little information regarding symptom management. During a visit with her pncm, Lisa announced she would like to see a doctor. Both she and Mark, now ready to learn more about her illness, met with a neurologist who was highly recommended by others with MS. Later, when describing the visit to her pncm, Lisa stated she was saddened and shocked to learn that she had a rapidly progressing form of MS. At the same time, she was touched by the physician's compassionate sharing of this information with her and Mark. "It was just like he could step inside my body and know how I was feeling," she said. Difficult as it was for her to hear his prognosis, Lisa was relieved to find a doctor she felt understood what she was experiencing and who was able to support her.

Isolation

Another of the challenges faced by pncm's was partnering with clients who, once they received their diagnosis of MS and experienced physical limitations, isolated themselves at home. Often these individuals worked until forced to go on disability and sought out little interaction with others who had the disease. Usually, they chose not to attend support groups, stating they did not want to "sit around and listen to other people complain." They preferred to be relatively home bound rather than use ambulatory devices. Depressed by the feeling that MS was completely dominating their lives, they often identified themselves as having few choices.

Pncm's found these individuals benefited from networking with others. Although the majority preferred not to attend support groups, many expressed an interest in attending an exercise program, and so an exercise group was formed, funded by monies from a state disabilities program. These clients, usually unwilling to leave their homes, did attend the classes.

Along with learning exercises and relaxation techniques, they shared their stories with each other, often talking to someone else with MS for the first time. Through sharing fears and frustrations, they realized that their experiences were not unique. They offered each other encouragement and support, forming friendships that continued beyond the classes.

When isolation was compounded by depression, pncm's encouraged clients to seek medical attention or counseling. Formal counseling and antidepressant medication brought relief to several individuals.

Mobility as a Metaphor

The ability to accept and use mobility devices is often pivotal to reconstructing a life affected by MS. Clients needed a great deal of support and encouragement to take this step.

A past program director of our local MS chapter, Nancy Keller, introduced the pncm's to the following metaphor, "The manner in which someone with MS handles mobility problems is a metaphor for where that person is in the process of adapting to her illness and how ready she is to move in other areas of her life." As one woman stated, "When I have to use a cane, I can no longer pretend I'm normal."

Jenny realized she needed to use an Amigo or a wheelchair during exacerbations as her gait became unsteady and her legs would not support her. Her financial resources were very limited and she did not have medical insurance. Luckily, she was able to obtain an electric wheelchair from a community equipment loan chest. Her pncm arranged to have a ramp built free of charge in front of her mobile home. Jenny cried when she saw the completed ramp, saying, "I know I have to have the ramp to get in and out of my house, but I hate it. It looks ugly and it marks my house. It tells everyone I'm crippled. Now every time anyone goes by they will see that ramp and think, a cripple lives there."

Allowing clients to express feelings of anger and despair and offering them emotional support was key to their process of redefining who they are and to developing their ability to make changes. Often, when a change such as Jenny's evoked strong emotions, the pncm would arrange for a peer counselor, a volunteer who also had MS, to visit. As in many other situations where a change in health status evokes strong personal feelings, talking with someone else who has dealt with these issues proved helpful. Once an individual was able to work through her reluctance to accept a mobility aid, her options increased and the quality of her life improved.

Working with Families

MS impacted the lives of children, parents, and spouses in a variety of ways, offering individuals and families an opportunity to learn more about themselves. Some people responded to the challenges presented by caring for a family member with MS by developing abilities and strengths they might not have otherwise experienced. Others found their emotional and physical resources exhausted when attempting to provide the care or needed support.

Clients participating in the study were cared for and supported by several kinds of caregivers: spouses, parents, children, friends, members of their church, and paid attendants. The most common situation involved husbands caring for wives. Several husbands gave up their jobs to devote themselves to full-time caregiving. A few husbands displayed controlling behavior patterns, making most of the decisions, usually without consulting their wives. Often, they established strict regimens, resisted changes, and were reluctant to let the pncm visit.

As each client's increasing physical disabilities forced her spouse to provide greater amounts of care, her feelings of frustration and powerlessness increased. Alcohol abuse on the part of the husband contributed to creating a crisis situation in several instances. Feeling physically helpless, many wives found it difficult to set boundaries with their spouses. Often, they looked to the pncm to "fix" the husband and were disappointed when this did not occur. Some exacerbations seemed to be connected to increases in emotional tension created by these dynamics (see Case Study).

Few people with patterns of dependency accepted counseling. Several couples who lived in the same neighborhood, however, agreed to regular meetings,

---

CASE STUDY

Jerry was a successful architect when he decided to retire to care for his wife Mary. Because he felt guilty that she was sick and he was well, he decided to make it up to her by devoting himself to caring for her full time. Refusing to leave her, he soon began to feel "like a prisoner in my own house." Mary, in turn, felt controlled by what she considered a domineering husband. Jerry handled the growing tensions by escalating his drinking. When first contracted by the pncm, Mary was delighted to have someone else to talk to, but Jerry was reluctant to let the pncm visit and refused to leave the pncm and Mary alone together. As the pncm-client-family relationship developed, the pncm encouraged Jerry to use her visits as a respite. After visiting for six months, the pncm felt she had established a strong enough relationship with the couple to discuss with them the dynamics she was observing. Gradually, as the result of these discussions, Mary began reading Al-Anon literature, and she and the pncm attended several meetings together. Some months later, Jerry's drinking subsided, although his basic pattern of doing everything for Mary continued.

first facilitated by their pncm, then gradually on their own. The men felt particularly supported by interacting with other males who were also caregivers.

Parents caring for children with MS had difficulty reconciling themselves to their child's illness and not becoming overly protective. Jenny's mother, heartbroken at her daughter's deterioration, needed encouragement and support from the pncm. She had difficulty letting Jenny discover her own limits, wanting to take over and "make it easier."

Parents of teenagers experienced trouble distinguishing between normal parent-teen dynamics and tension related to children's reactions to parental MS. Parents like Lisa and Mark assumed that without the disease, their children would not misbehave and talk back and would do homework, spend less time with peers, do chores without prompting, and so on. Pncm's encouraged these parents to learn more about adolescent development by reading literature or attending classes on normal teenager behavior. Some children, particularly teenagers, did feel embarrassed when friends saw their disabled parents. Often when one of these teens preferred to spend time at the home of a peer, the parent felt rejected.

Families, like individuals, reached a certain stage of readiness, usually produced by a crisis, before they were willing to make changes in their patterns. Until this point, change was difficult to accomplish.

CHALLENGES OF PNCM'S

Working with individuals with MS provided intense emotional experiences for their pncm's. Interacting with people their own age with severe physical impairments created an immediate sense of their own vulnerability to disease. The pncm's also experienced feelings of powerlessness and helplessness because of the uncertain course and incurability of MS. Supporting someone through episodes of severe emotional pain and disappointment or during periods of rapid deterioration was deeply challenging.

Clients sometimes mirrored issues, such as dependency, which the pncm had not resolved within herself, triggering emotions she needed to assess continually while interacting with clients. When a pncm sensed that her relationship with an individual was not going well, as in the case of the "expert" client, she sat down with coworkers, clarified her reaction to the client and family, and explored whether she was hindering the client's process and what she could change.

Pncm's discovered they could be most helpful simply by listening, that is, allowing clients and family members to verbalize privately all their feelings of anger, fear, frustration, resentment, despair, or self-pity. As one individual expressed it, "If I said these things to my husband, he would feel devastated knowing how depressed and resentful I feel. It would take him days to recover. But I feel its okay to say it to you [the pncm] because I don't worry about whether or not you can handle it. You have volunteered to and you deal with your reactions on your own time. My feelings will go out the door with you."

At times, pncm's had difficulty putting aside their own goals and desires for a client and remaining non-judgmental. Self-understanding is needed as well as empathy when partnering with a client like Jenny as she moves through her process at her own pace, experiencing the consequences of her choice to overwork, and setting her own goals, until she recognizes the need for change. Often, nurses struggled to express their feelings respectfully about choices they did not agree with, as when Lisa ignored her symptoms hoping they were temporary and her functional ability would soon improve.

Pncm's felt angry and disapproving when confronted with such issues as alcoholism and dependency: "At times I just wanted to shake both Jerry and Mary," their pncm confessed. By recognizing their feelings of anger, judgment, impatience, and control, and by working through issues being mirrored, pncm's grew emotionally along with their clients.

Working in partnership from the perspective of the pcnm's has been discussed in this chapter, but how was this process experienced by clients? To explore this question, one of the clients who participated in the study agreed to write of her experience (see Client's Perspective).

CONCLUSION

This chapter discusses the partnership process that occurred between pncm's and individuals with progressive MS, from the perspective of a relational paradigm rather than a medical one. Using the holistic approach described here, clients assisted by recommendations from their pncm's identified health-care concerns and interventions each client and family felt that they wished to address. Such group interventions as the exercise programs or the couples support group were presented. Interventions of this type were not only a cost-effective way to provide the needed service but a means through which clients received support and encouragement from their peers. Although the case studies depicted in this chapter focused on case managing individuals with MS, many of the situations described characterized situations that commonly occur in most case managed populations.

• Readiness was identified as an essential factor in a client's implementation of self-management strategies and lifestyle changes.• Pncm actions that clients reported helpful in supporting them through their process of change were addressed.

The Client as Control and Subject

By Nancy Mairs

At the end of our first interview, Gerri Lamb took out the sealed envelope that would decide my fate. We had hit it off from the start, and I was really eager to be a subject in her study. Alas, the slip inside the envelope read *control.* I would be interviewed halfway through the study, and again at the end of the year, but otherwise I would have no contact with the research team.

"Oh, Gerri," I wailed when she called to schedule the midpoint interview, "you have no idea how much I've *needed* a nurse case manager!" In the months since our first contact, my husband's melanoma had recurred, necessitating extensive abdominal surgery, and he was now undergoing a wicked course of chemotherapy. My MS was progressing at an alarming pace, and my caregiver, who had also been my beloved companion for nearly 30 years, seemed likely to die quite soon. I felt panicky, disoriented, abandoned.

Of course there was nothing Gerri could do, except to express her sympathy as she did very warmly. Nor did I expect her to, knowing that controls are every bit as essential to authentic research as subjects are. Imagine my delight, however, when at the end of the year the controls were invited to participate in the program. I was on the telephone instantly saying, "Sign me up."

And so I got my nurse case manager at last. My nurse case manager met my needs perfectly, because before working with MS clients she had spent several years with Hospice and was thus familiar with the stresses cancer places on every family. With her encouragement, I began to look into my finances, which George had always managed, and to think about living arrangements. By putting me in touch with others as severely disabled by MS as I am, and by arranging for a consultant from the state to inspect my house and suggest modifications to maximize my independence, she enabled me to hope that, with home help, I might be able to stay out of a nursing facility. She suggested and supervised a meeting with George and me, our two children, and their spouses, which gave us a chance to discuss our anxieties, options, and expectations.

Practical expertise of this sort is invaluable. Harder to convey, though even more vital, has been the nurse case manager's support of my spirit. One day she listened, unruffled, while I bemoaned the miseries of MS at wearisome length. Unlike people for whom chronic illness is unfamiliar and unnerving, she didn't try to leap in with reassurances, but after a while she asked in her light, quiet voice, "But Nancy, who would you be if you didn't have MS?" There is, after all, no other Nancy. Most of what I like about myself, as well as most of what I don't, is related to my condition. Her question, which has resounded in memory ever since, was a kind of gift of my self to me.

About three years have passed since I met my case manager. Miraculously, George's melanoma has remained in remission, but I am still terrified of losing him, and she fathoms my fear as few others can. With the end of the research project, we have moved our relationship from a professional to a personal one. But then, what's "professional"? What's "personal"? A study like this reveals how arbitrary the distinction is. People with chronic illnesses—like the rest of humanity—need professionals who treat them as persons. The model of nurse case management fills this lack amply.

The case studies discussed here also suggest ways in which crisis may precipitate readiness in some individuals and the importance of a trusting nurse-client-family relationship for carrying out interventions once a client is ready for them. In fact, recognizing when an individual was at a choice point and assisting him with that process in a respectful manner was identified as a major nursing challenge when working with any case-managed individual.

Pncm's who start out aware of such challenges and strategies may avoid some pitfalls and, by establishing trust and cooperation early in their partnerships with clients, serve their clients more efficiently and effectively. More important, this approach enables a depth and quality of interactive caring that may lead to emotional growth for everyone concerned.

REFERENCES

Lamb, G., & Stempel, J. (1994). Nurse case management from the client's view: growing as insider-expert. *Nursing Outlook, 42,* 7-13.

Newman, M. A. (1994). *Health as expanding consciousness* (2nd ed.). New York: National League for Nursing Press.

RECOMMENDED READINGS

Cleveland, M. (1989). *Living Well: A 12 step response to chronic illness.* New York: Harper and Row.

Coombs, J., & Rusch, S. (1990). Creating a healing environment. *Health Progress, 73,* 38-41.

Hammerschlag, C. A. (1988). *The dancing healers: A doctors journey of healing with Native Americans.* San Francisco: Harper Collins.

LeMaistre, J. (1985). *Beyond rage: the emotional impact of chronic physical illness.* Oak Park: Alpine Guild.

Mairs, N. (1990). *Carnal acts.* New York: Harper Collins.

———. (1986). *Plaintext.* Tucson: University of Arizona Press.

Michaels, C. (1992). Carondelet St. Mary's nursing enterprise. *Nursing Clinics of North America, 27* (1), 77-85.

Newman, M. A. (1986). *Health as expanding consciousness.* St Louis: Mosby.

Newman, M. A., Lamb, G. S., & Michaels, C. L. (1992). Nurse case management: The coming together of theory and practice. *Nursing and Health Care, 12* (8), 404-408.

Strong, M. (1988). *Mainstay.* New York: Penguin Books.

Chapter 15

Nurse Case Management in a Rural Community

Lisa Zerull, MSN, RN

OVERVIEW

Nurse case management produces desired measurable outcomes for a rural health care setting.

Health-care professionals in acute care facilities throughout the United States are challenged to seek innovative ways of providing quality care in a cost-effective manner while achieving positive client outcomes. In an expansive rural setting, where there is a lack of readily accessible health care and where mobility for the population is often an issue, there is the additional need for acute care facilities to reach out into the community to provide care across the continuum. This chapter defines the practice and desired, measurable outcomes of *community nurse case management* in a rural setting.

THE ENVIRONMENT

Winchester Medical Center is a 408-bed tertiary care referral center located in northern Virginia, serving the tri-state area of Virginia, Maryland, and West Virginia. Outside the immediate city and county area, much of the rural population must travel more than 150 miles to see a physician. They often seek health-care services only when acutely ill. The lack of readily accessible health care, as well as the need for cost-effective management of selected individuals with complex needs, has been the motivation for expanding successful acute care-based nurse case management processes "beyond the walls" and into the rural community.

MOVING HEALTH CARE "BEYOND THE WALLS"

Community nurse case management (C-NCM) grew out of an acute care need to continue contact with a select group of chronically ill clients in our rural service area. Most of these clients had complex discharge needs with frequent admissions to the medical center. In early 1992, nursing administration began analyzing this population and found that the majority of clients were Medicare age and were costing the medical center two to three million dollars each year in nonreimbursable costs. They also identified patterns that emerged with this population, such as crisis-based readmissions (the average number of hospitalizations per client was once per month); lengthy hospital stays frequently requiring critical care days; and frustrated clients and families who, perhaps could not understand why hospitalization was needed yet again. It was further discovered that this population did not qualify for skilled home health nursing care for various reasons. For instance, clients were not homebound, or their needs did not require skilled intervention. These identified patterns, coupled with the need for the medical center to provide quality health care and contain costs, especially those associated with nonreimbursable hospital stays, were the motivation to develop a plan for better management of these individuals discharged with chronic and complex needs.

It was clear to nursing administration that traditional health-care delivery, with a focus on treating illness or providing episodic care, must be transformed into a model focused on individuals and how their "choices" at home affect their health. For example, before implementation of C-NCM, an indepth discharge plan was developed with clients and their families, and the client was sent home attempting to manage their complex needs alone. Often there was no community agency or other resource available to assist them, so many of these clients frequently "fell through the cracks," and within a short period presented in the emergency department in acute crisis. Thus, the development of C-NCM needed to address the needs of this high-risk population after hospitalization and to provide for cost-effective use of staff and resources. The pilot project of C-NCM was designed to address these special needs.

THE PILOT PROJECT

After a review of the literature to identify best practices in C-NCM, a pilot project was initiated in August, 1992. Initially, one registered nurse began to see a limited number of high-risk, problem-prone clients in their homes. Most of the client referrals came from the acute care-based nurse case managers (NCMs) and from social workers who had been a part of the C-NCM pilot project planning team. The clients referred had numerous chronic illnesses, usually in combination. These included diabetes, heart failure, angina, pulmonary edema, cancer, anxiety disorder, and chronic obstructive airway disease.

Because C-NCM is a nursing model, in terms of care provision for the client, physician orders were not required to direct client-nurse interactions. In the Commonwealth of Virginia, as in many other states, a registered nurse may assess, plan, educate, coordinate, and evaluate nursing interventions without medical supervision. The community nurse case manager (c-NCMr) did communicate pertinent client information to the physician, and when warranted, accompanied the client to scheduled physician office visits to clarify prescribed medical regimens. If the client's condition changed such that skilled nursing care was necessary, the c-NCMr would refer the individual to a home health agency where medical supervision was appropriate.

Most of the c-NCMr interventions centered on listening to the client. This enabled the c-NCMr to identify client "choices" in taking prescribed medications, eating certain foods, or accessing health care, to name a few. Interestingly, during many of the home visits, health care or prescribed regimens (e.g., medications, diet) was never mentioned. Rather the c-NCMr had clients lead the interactions, encouraging them to speak about whatever was on their mind. Often the client talked about current events in their lives or shared stories from their past. It was obvious to the c-NCMr that the majority of these clients just needed someone to talk to and follow-up with them after discharge from the hospital. The interactions between the client and the nurse were usually scheduled on a weekly basis lasting about 40 to 50 minutes during the pilot project; however, the duration and frequency decreased over time as clients were better able to manage their own health and wellness.

Initial Results

From this limited C-NCM pilot project, the medical center realized a cost avoidance of $78,000 for 18 clients followed during the first seven months of the project, primarily through working with the client to avoid costly readmissions. The initial quantitative data are found in Table 15-1.

The cost avoidance was determined by comparing clients' use of health-care services during the pilot pro-

TABLE 15-1	Initial results from community nurse case management pilot project (October 1992-April 1993)	
Quantitative data		
OUTCOMES INDICATORS (N = 18)	PRE C-NCM (7 MOS.)	POST C-NCM (7 MOS.)
No. of hospital admissions	39	4
Mean HLOS* per admission	7.8	5.5
Total no. of critical care days	8	0
Total no. of emergency department visits	12	1
Total dollar loss per admission	$102,455.07	$23,572.38
Hospital cost avoidance (Total dollar loss Pre to Post)		$78,882.69
Percent change in health care dollar utilization (Pre to Post)		77%

*HLOS, Hospital Length of Stay.

ject to the prior seven-month period. These initial quantitative findings, coupled with the medical center's mission to "promote and improve the general health of the population in its service area" convinced Administration to fund one full-time nurse position halfway through the fiscal year, with the promise of adding additional personnel the following year. To date eight additional c-NCMrs have joined the staff going beyond the walls of the hospital to ensure positive client outcomes.

OBSTACLES TO IMPLEMENTATION OF COMMUNITY NURSE CASE MANAGEMENT

Often, there is a reluctance of hospital administrators to embrace innovative programs because of additional costs associated with resources or personnel. In this case, however, there were few obstacles to the implementation of C-NCM at the medical center.

The first obstacle that had to be overcome involved the technical issue of neutral budget decisions, which made it difficult to gain approval for additional nursing staff halfway through the fiscal year. The outcomes identified in Table 15-1 were sufficient to convince Administration of the cost effectiveness of at least one nurse to continue the pilot project on a full-time basis.

A second obstacle to be addressed was how best to serve a population in such a large mile radius of the medical center, without incurring excessive travel time. During the initial stages of the pilot, a 35-mile limit within the greater Winchester area was established. Because the new nurse hired into C-NCM lived in West Virginia and traveled greater distances to the medical center, this policy was later changed to a 50-mile limit to include other States in the service area. Client referrals who lived greater distances from the Medical Center were reviewed individually by the C-NCM team for appropriateness and for staff assignment.

Because the C-NCM project was designed to reach clients in their home environment, there was a "turf" conflict with home health agencies that challenged the success of the C-NCM project early on. Many of the home health nurses perceived C-NCM as competition to their role of providing services in the home. To address this conflict, the c-NCMrs were invited to home health staff meetings as a means of educating (and reeducating) staff about differences in services between home health and C-NCM, primarily related to medical direction, reimbursement, and duration of care. Also, to diminish any further turf issues, the c-NCMrs would frequently communicate with the home health staff to discuss potential clients and to request their input in planning care. Home health referrals comprised 15% of all client referrals to C-NCM.

Surprisingly, one group of professionals supportive of C-NCM from its initial implementation were the physicians, although it was anticipated that they might have some concerns about a nurse seeing clients without their specific orders. The physicians were impressed with the fact that their high-risk clients were staying out of the hospital and keeping their scheduled appointments. One of the physicians even commented, "I don't know what you're doing out there, but keep it up. Some of my patients are healthier and happier than they have been for years!" As part of the education process to explain C-NCM services, a brochure was developed to provide information about the program to new physicians and to new clients and their families and has been well received in the community.

One other challenge, rather than an obstacle to C-NCM, came in the form of the Joint Commission on Accreditation of Hospitals which, in the Fall of 1994, surveyed C-NCM under the Home Care Standards (JCAHO, 1992). Winchester Medical Center was the first acute care facility with a C-NCM program to be surveyed. Before 1994, JCAHO did not survey C-NCM programs for several reasons. First, C-NCM does not fall under acute care survey because health-care professionals see clients in their homes. Second, if the acute care facility supporting the C-NCM program does not have a home health agency linked with the facility, C-NCM would not be surveyed by the Home Care Division of JCAHO. Third, many of the C-NCM programs across the country were still in the pilot stages—not formalized programs ready for survey. Finally, C-NCM is nursing driven and does not require physician's orders for intervention, which differentiates it from home health. Nevertheless, care is being provided by a professional in the client's home which follows the JCAHO definition for home care.

Preparation for JCAHO took place nine months before the survey and involved formalizing what the c-NCMr was already doing in practice. A reference manual was created to follow the objectives defined by the Home Care Standards. The manual had six sections:

1. C-NCM mission and plan
2. Standards of care
3. Job description and orientation checklist
4. Policies and procedures
5. Continuous performance improvement and data analysis
6. Documentation forms

Once the mission statement and job description were written, C-NCM policies and procedures were created by revising some of the medical center's home health agencies' policies and procedures. The standards of care came from a combination of acute care and home care standards. Because most of the previous C-NCM documentation was completed on a flowsheet with accompanying nurse's notes, documentation forms were revised, including a formalized plan of care using some of the tools and concepts of the Omaha System (Martin & Scheet, 1992). Data, both quantitative and qualitative, to support C-NCM had already been collected and summarized to be placed in the continuous performance improvement section.

During the survey, the c-NCMrs were interviewed and questioned about their activities and knowledge of content in the reference manual. Additionally, two C-NCM clients received a home visit by the JCAHO nurse surveyor. The favorable outcome of the survey was quite evident during the exit conference, with comments such as: "I've never seen a program (C-NCM) like this before . . . It shows how much you care about your community to be doing this. A lot of very nice mechanisms have been put in place, and I can see where this is a very worthwhile program." The nurse surveyor also noted that as the home care standards change every two years, the medical center should continue to show more evidence of coordination of services. At the time of this survey, it was unclear whether JCAHO will develop separate Home Care Standards for C-NCM programs.

REAL PEOPLE AND REAL OUTCOMES OF COMMUNITY NURSE CASE MANAGEMENT
Expanding Nurse Case Management with Nurse Practitioners

Four months after the C-NCM pilot project began, the medical center, with the assistance of numerous local agencies, completed a community needs assessment. An element of community care found to be severely lacking was wellness promotion among the "well" elderly population. A nurse practitioner (NP) was hired by the medical center to begin another community outreach program offered to the five-county primary service area in Virginia. The NP provides "wellness clinics" in each of the county's senior centers, adult care, and assisted living facilities. Some of the services provided include health screenings, educational programs, nurse consultations, and referral opportunities to a primary physician and/or nearest health-care facility. In just two short years, the NP has had over 2000 client encounters and made more than 350 referrals to health-care providers such as physicians, podiatrists, dentists, audiologists, and ophthalmologists. Clients are also referred to available community agencies and to C-NCM, as appropriate. Several examples of how a nurse practitioner made a difference by "case managing" the high-risk elderly are provided here (see Case Studies on pp. 136-138).

CASE STUDY

Client Choices Impact the Level of Wellness

Gilbert, a 76-year-old man, was referred to C-NCM by a social worker during one of his many visits to the Emergency Department that resulted in a short-stay hospital admission. Gilbert suffers from a chronic esophageal motility disorder with recurrent aspiration and dehydration, as well as osteoporosis with ensuing compression fractures. In discussing Gilbert's case with his physician, the c-NCMr found that the physician was concerned that Gilbert's home environment was contributing to his poor health status. Indeed, the c-NCMr discovered that Gilbert lives in a remote, rural area, in an 8' × 8' shed he constructed 10 years ago for his home, isolated from community transportation and support resources with limited conveniences (e.g., no running water, electricity, telephone, or bathroom). His shed has a wood stove for cooking his food and to heat the shed in the winter. Because there is no source of refrigeration, most of the foods that Gilbert consumes are canned or processed. His water comes from a spring on the property. He refuses assistance from any community agencies, stating that he does not trust anyone—"They'll only rip you off!" He cannot read and does not choose to follow his physician's recommendations for diet or medications, frequently missing his scheduled appointments.

Developing a rapport with Gilbert was a slow and arduous process for the c-NCMr. He was agreeable to have the c-NCMr visit him to "see how he was getting along—but that was all!" He did not want a "bunch of strangers poking around in his business." Most C-NCM visits with Gilbert focused on open-ended questions such as, "Tell me about your day today?" and "If I could do one thing for you, what would that be?" rather than on his prescribed medical regimens. The c-NCMr also explored some possible options with the county social services department. To get Gilbert a better home environment, his shed would have to be condemned, forcing Gilbert out of his home; however, this was not his choice at the time. He kept saying that his "house" was just fine for now.

Outcome. After six months of biweekly interactions with Gilbert, he has kept the majority of his scheduled medical appointments and has only presented to the Emergency Department one time, without requiring hospitalization. Gilbert has said that "he appreciates what his nurse has done for him but doesn't want anyone else meddling in his affairs!" He has grudgingly agreed to receive Meals-on-Wheels three times per week and says that he will "consider living somewhere else come winter."

Measuring the Outcomes

The portraits highlighted in this chapter represent a few of the many successes achieved with C-NCM. Box 15-1 lists the overall outcomes of C-NCM, both quantitative and qualitative. Similar findings have been

CASE STUDY

The Frequent User of the Emergency Department

In a six-week period before being referred to C-NCM by the emergency room director, John had 32 visits to the Emergency Department (ED) with two visits necessitating an overnight hospital stay. His presentation was always the same—angina with resultant shortness of breath. When asked what precipitated each ER visit, his reply was always, "I needed help, so I called 911 to bring me to the medical center."

Once the referral to C-NCM was received, a review of John's medical record was completed. The c-NCMr identified that John was not homebound; that a home health nurse had seen him for a short period of time the previous year after his open heart bypass surgery; and that his medications, including a prescription for nitroglycerine, had not changed in the past year. John's cardiologist was frustrated with this patient and could not identify a physiological reason for the repeated ED visits.

During the first two home visits with John, the c-NCMr asked the question, "What happens or how do you feel right before you call 911?" John's reply was that he usually developed chest pain, couldn't breathe, and became "panicky," immediately calling 911 for assistance. Interestingly, one of John's medications was nitroglycerine, so the c-NCMr asked how and when he took it. John said, "I only put one in my mouth when my chest starts to ache. If that doesn't work, I get upset and usually can't breathe, so I come out to the hospital."

The c-NCMr spent her next visits with John talking about nitroglycerine usage, relaxation techniques, and the benefits of resting when tired. Often, she would simply spend 30 to 40 minutes, once per week with a phone call in between visits, talking with John about his wife (now deceased) and his days in the military service. The c-NCMr also found that since John lived up on the mountain and talked of being lonely, a weekly visit to the Senior center proved to boost to John's spirits.

Outcome. It has now been four months since the c-NCMr started visiting John in his home. He is now being seen every other week. John has had no ED or hospital visits, keeps his scheduled appointments with his physician, and verbalizes that he is better, "because someone cared enough to help me."

CASE STUDY

Addressing Environmental Needs That Impact Health and Wellness

Carol is 84, with a right above-the-knee amputation (14 months previous). She also suffers from elevated cholesterol and chronic obstructive airway disease. She has chosen to continue smoking, but says she follows all of the other advice given her by the physician. Her husband suffered a debilitating stroke soon after her surgery and is now in a nursing home. During the past year, Carol had numerous hospital admissions for infection of her stump, breathing difficulties and what her physician describes as "depression-related illness." Carol lives alone and is 32 miles from the nursing home where her husband resides. She is able to see him only once a week.

Carol was referred to the c-NCMr after her most recent hospitalization. After the first few visits, the c-NCMr found that what Carol really wanted was to be closer to her husband. Her depression was caused primarily by the isolation from her spouse, combined with her physical limitations.

The c-NCMr immediately explored transportation and living options closer to the nursing home. In two short weeks, an apartment was found three doors from the nursing home with easy wheelchair access. Carol immediately moved to her new apartment and a local church member comes to help her with household tasks two mornings each week.

Outcome. Carol has not been admitted to the hospital for more than six months, has expressed complete satisfaction with her living arrangements, and tells the nursing home staff that she is "happier than she has been in a long time." Carol was recently discharged from C-NCM.

one is to establish a trusting relationship with the client; step two is to recognize the health care and life choices each client makes; in step three, the client gets to pass GO when he can independently make health-care choices, and finally, the client wins the game when he feels that he has achieved his highest level of wellness and no longer requires my services."

Additional qualitative data about C-NCM were obtained by a faculty member from a local university who visited clients referred to C-NCM during the previous year. A random sample of 26 clients was chosen. The faculty member, as the objective observer, then asked open-ended questions to obtain the client's perceptions about the role of the c-NCMr and the impact of the c-NCMr and client relationship. A few of the clients' responses, representative of the sample group, are provided here.

1. "I think she (c-NCMr) does all she can for me. I feel I can go to her whenever I have a problem and that makes it convenient for me. There are probably a lot of people who don't have access to her that could use her services. It's good to

documented in the literature by St. Joseph Medical Center in Wichita, Kansas (Rogers, Riordan & Swindle, 1991) and Carondelet St. Mary's Hospital in Tucson, Arizona (Ethridge, 1991).

Each nurse who has chosen to expand her practice by becoming a community nurse case manager feels a great sense of pride and satisfaction with her role for the obvious reason of "making a difference in the lives of clients in our rural community." One C-NCM nurse has been known to say, "I really feel challenged with each of my clients to play, what I call, the 'Wellness Game.' Step

CASE STUDY

Wellness Promotion in One Senior Center

Ethel is a 78-year-old widow who lives in the rural farmhouse that her husband built for her 58 years ago. Her daughter, three grandchildren, and the daughter's boyfriend also reside in the home. At her once-a-week visit to the county's senior center, the NP observed Ethel as being quiet, often sitting alone, and speaking only if the nurse spoke first. During an initial conversation, the NP noted a strong, foul, fleshy odor about Ethel, even though Ethel appeared clean and well-dressed. Once the NP had established a rapport with Ethel, she questioned Ethel about any wound or skin problem. Ethel's reply, "Oh, it's nothing, don't worry about it." Finally, after four weeks, Ethel came to the NP and said, "Would you be willing to go to the ladies room with me and look at something?" That something turned out to be a draining lesion on Ethel's right breast. The NP talked with Ethel about her choices, recommending that Ethel see a physician immediately. Ethel's response was that she couldn't ask her daughter to do anything for her and didn't want to be a bother to anyone—this "thing" would eventually heal.

Outcome. During the following two weeks, Ethel did see a surgeon and had a mastectomy followed by chemotherapy and radiation. The daughter became more actively involved in helping her mother, and Ethel expressed her thanks for having a nurse in the community willing to help her. Had the NP not been available to intervene, Ethel's outcome might have been altogether different. Ethel is now being followed by a c-NCMr.

CASE STUDY

A Student Nurse's View of Community Nurse Case Management

This excerpt was taken from the journal of an associate degree nurse, working toward a bachelor's degree, who had the opportunity to shadow a c-NCMr during a clinical rotation. She had been a nurse in acute care practice for four years before this experience.

"As an acute care nurse, I had no actual concept of what posthospitalization life for a chronically ill and frequently debilitated person was actually like; my focus has always been on getting the patient well enough to go home in the shortest time frame possible. Initially, I was unsure of what C-NCM actually entailed. I was unable, in my ignorance, to differentiate between home health duties and those under the jurisdiction of the c-NCMr. This pioneer (C-NCM) program has been able to conclude a valuable secret in the war to contain our massive health-care costs simply by educating patients about wellness and promoting patients to take charge of their own wellness. This sounds deceptively simple and is completely in opposition to traditional health care which is oriented toward fixing a problem after it occurs. The c-NCMr was able to coordinate interdisciplinary and interagency care to coalesce care in a manner acceptable to the clients. By doing so, patients were empowered to take control of their "wellness" and not allow (chronic) health problems rule their lives."

Courtesy of Theresa Thomas, RN.

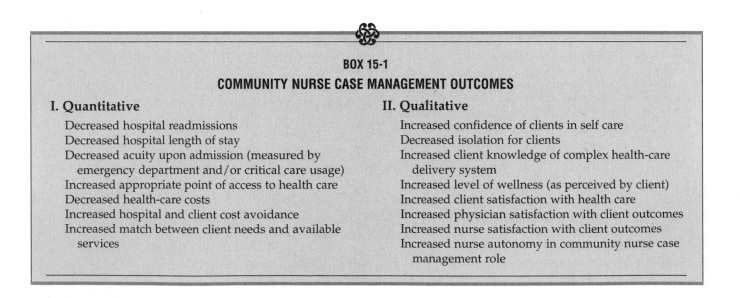

BOX 15-1
COMMUNITY NURSE CASE MANAGEMENT OUTCOMES

I. Quantitative

Decreased hospital readmissions
Decreased hospital length of stay
Decreased acuity upon admission (measured by emergency department and/or critical care usage)
Increased appropriate point of access to health care
Decreased health-care costs
Increased hospital and client cost avoidance
Increased match between client needs and available services

II. Qualitative

Increased confidence of clients in self care
Decreased isolation for clients
Increased client knowledge of complex health-care delivery system
Increased level of wellness (as perceived by client)
Increased client satisfaction with health care
Increased physician satisfaction with client outcomes
Increased nurse satisfaction with client outcomes
Increased nurse autonomy in community nurse case management role

have her check on you. I think I would be more depressed if she didn't come to help me. Some people don't have families, and they need help and don't have a way of getting it here in the Valley."

2. "She has helped my wife's and my situation 100%. I know if we didn't have her we would have been back in the hospital a dozen times. She knows how to help us and she knows how to talk to us. She has helped us get our medicine and our sugar supplies real cheap, where before it was costing us almost everything we made. We have nine children and grandchildren living with us and we need our money to help feed, clothe, and send them to school. We don't have to pay for her (the c-NCMr) visits, whereas before when the home care nurse was seeing us, we worried about how we could pay the $100 per visit. A guess it was fortunate that we don't qualify for home care anymore."

3. "I know she has kept me out of the hospital at least twice. She comes to check on me when I need her and she calls my doctor when I need help, so that I don't have to go to the emergency room. When I got bad before she came to see me, I usually had to go to the hospital where they put this machine on me and I had to stay for several days."

Based on satisfied client and staff responses and the overwhelmingly supportive quantitative outcomes identified, the medical center will further measure and validate the value and applicability of C-NCM not only in rural settings, but in other settings as well.

CONCLUSION

In this time of change in health-care delivery, this rural medical center has taken the first steps in the transformation from episodic care to a focus on wellness promotion. It is evident that future decisions to provide care across the continuum will not be based solely upon reimbursement concerns: a client's ability to pay for care; or a desire to fill hospital beds. Winchester Medical Center will continue to support the provision of care at the most appropriate level, with the least amount of cost, and certainly where the most positive client outcomes can be achieved.

REFERENCES

Ethridge, P. (1991). A nursing HMO: Carondelet St. Mary's experience. *Nursing Management, 22* (7), p. 22-27.

Joint Commission on Accreditation on Accreditation of Hospitals Organization. (1992). *The 1993 joint commission accreditation manual for home care* (Vol. 1-2). Oakbrook Terrace, IL: Author.

Martin, K. S., & Scheet, N. J. (1992). The Omaha system: applications for community health nursing. Philadelphia: W. B. Saunders Co.

Rogers, M., Riordan, J., & Swindle, D. (1991). Community-based nursing case management pays off. *Nursing Management, 22* (3), 30-34.

Chapter 16

Parish Nursing

Anne Marie Djupe, MA, RNC

OVERVIEW

*Parish nurses provide nurse case management services
to faith communities, especially those
that are poor and underserved.*

Parish nursing is an emerging community-based nursing role in which the population served is the faith community. The services provided by the parish nurses include health education, personal health counseling, resource and referral, organizing and supporting volunteers, and interpreting the relationship between faith and health. These services are provided in the church, in homes, nursing homes, on the telephone, and in the community. Faith communities are being recognized as an important health resource, particularly in our poor and underserved communities. The parish nurse, working in the faith community, is positioned to integrate the resources of individuals, the community, and related health-care institutions.

Working with different client populations requires all the resources and creativity of an entire community. One of the often overlooked community-based resources is the local congregation. The church is the one social institution uniquely structured to affect intellectual, spiritual, and physical dimensions of human behavior. More than 60% of this nation's citizens belong to a faith community, and more than 40% attend a worship service at least once a week (Drucker, 1993).

"Worship places are health places by virtue of the wellness they promote. Every faith tradition gives its adherents hope, a sense of meaning and purpose, a core set of values that shape personal and communal identity, a commitment to social justice and equity and a desire to serve others" (Droege, 1994). Churches have traditionally been havens to the underserved, the outcasts, the marginalized. Religious traditions underscore the imperative to protect and defend the poor and vulnerable and to work for peace and justice.

The congregation as a microcosm of the surrounding community must respond to the needs of those individuals it serves. This becomes even more critical as neighborhoods go through transitions with more poor and underserved moving in. These outreach activities include soup kitchens, food pantries, hot lunch programs, overnight shelters, clothing outlets, day care for children and adults, and teen programs. Churches are also used for self-help groups such as

Alcoholics Anonymous, support groups, and after-school programs. According to a recent survey of Protestant congregations, more than three quarters responded that they are addressing at least one health concern, whereas over half responded that they are addressing three or more. The three most commonly reported were nutrition, substance abuse, and mental health (NCC Survey report, 1991).

Former president Jimmy Carter stated, "Fully two-thirds of the years of life that are lost before the age of 65 could be saved by using current technology, convincing individuals to make better lifestyle choices and drawing on the available resources already present in most communities" (Carter, 1994a). For this to happen, education that is culturally sensitive and understandable must be available, resources must be accessible, and technology must be used appropriately. An emerging nursing role serving in this community setting is the parish nurse. The parish nurse is a community-based nurse whose population is a faith community and who clearly embraces the spiritual dimension of those she serves (Djupe, Olson, & Ryan, 1994). The services provided by parish nurses include health education, personal health counseling, resource and referral, organizing and supporting volunteers, and interpreting the relationship between faith and health. These services are provided in the church, in homes, and nursing homes, on the telephone, and in the community. The parish nurse functions as a member of the pastoral team which includes participation in worship and the total life of the congregation. The parish nurse while distinct from, works in collaboration with, the home health nurse, school nurse, or nurse in Medicare care settings. The parish nurse is not engaged in invasive nursing procedures or delegated medical functions and is able to maintain long-term relationships with clients.

PARISH NURSE PROGRAM

In 1984, Lutheran General Health System (LGHS) initiated the first institutionally-based paid parish nurse program in the United States by partnering with six local congregations, four Protestant and two Roman Catholic (Figure 16-1). Lutheran General funded the parish nurse faculty and continuing education program, the congregations provided facilities, and the institution and congregation shared salary costs. Professional liability for the parish nurse and the congregation were provided by the institution. Usually, parish nurses provide these services while working part-time. Most of the LGHS parish nurses work in one congregation but several serve multiple congregations. In 1988, United Medical Center (now Trinity Medical Center [TMC]), a hospital system in the Quad Cities area of western Illinois, initiated a sister program. Over the past 10 years, the two programs have grown to include 53 parish nurses who serve 59 rural,

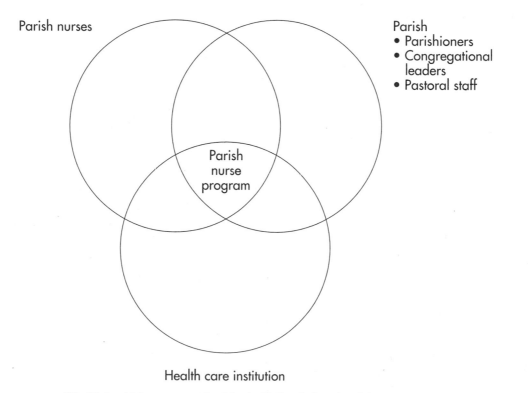

FIG. 16-1   Major components of the institutionally based parish nurse program

inner city, urban, and suburban congregations with a population of more than 80,000 congregational members. These programs are in congregations of 13 different denominations. LGHS and TMC continue to partner with these congregations by sharing salary costs and providing education, supervision, and support (Lloyd & Djupe, 1994). Surveys by the National Parish Nurse Resource Center (NPNRC) suggest that parish nurse programs are developing nationwide and that there are now more than 2,500 practicing parish nurses (Lloyd & Solari-Twadell, 1994).

Roles of the Parish Nurse

Health educator. The parish nurse seeks to raise the health awareness of the parish community and to foster an understanding of the relationship between lifestyle, personal habits, attitudes, faith, and well-being. This is accomplished through a variety of formats from seminars and classes to newsletters and bulletin boards. In addition, the parish nurse encourages parishioners to take their actions seriously in relation to the environment and the society in which they live. In 1993, 419 educational programs were presented or coordinated by 32 parish nurses. A total of 11,263 individuals participated in these sessions. Support groups addressing such issues as parenting, caregiving, and weight loss were attended by 1,788 individuals (Box 16-1).

Parish nurses have been instrumental in enhancing the worship facility to accommodate persons with disabilities by having ramps built, improving lighting in stairways, having large print bulletins and hymnals available, providing hearing devices, and even keeping lap blankets available for the elderly in the winter.

Personal health counselor. Parish nurses are available to all parishioners to discuss personal problems, to recommend medical intervention when necessary, and to make hospital, nursing home, and home visits. Frequently, these concerns include topics such as par-

enting of children, dealing with teens, aging parents, and relationships with a spouse or other family member. As the elderly and their families face decisions regarding safety and living arrangements, they frequently turn to the parish nurse for advice and counsel. For example, questions may be directed toward evaluating various housing options available to them and the pros and cons of choosing one option over another. One family member wrote:

> As a daughter who lives far away from aged parents who are church members, I have found the parish nurse program to be invaluable. My father whose health was deteriorating, was able to remain in his home largely because of the support provided by this program. My mother, residing in a nursing home, is visited weekly by the parish nurse. I call the parish nurse to get an update on my mother's condition regularly. From her, I learn about my mother's overall well-being and take comfort in knowing her care is being overseen by a knowledgeable and compassionate advocate (Lloyd & Djupe, 1994).

Parish nurses also facilitate conversations with individuals and family members regarding end of life decisions. These have occurred in formal classes, in homes, and even in crisis situations in hospitals. The pastor and parish nurse can help address this difficult issue in the context of one's faith and values. The parish nurse also helps to translate the medical information so that the family can make more informed decisions.

Resource and referral. The parish nurse draws on health-related resources from families, the congregation, and the community and often advocates on behalf of the parishioner with these agencies or groups. These include physicians, self-help groups, federal, state or community agencies, food pantries, shelters and housing, nursing homes, retirement facilities, hospitals, legal and financial counselors, psychotherapists, and home care and elder care specialists (Figure 16-2). For example, Elizabeth is the parish nurse in a low-income Hispanic neighborhood. The parish is located on the border of a major dividing line between two large gangs. The closest medical clinic is located across this dividing street that does not have a convenient stop sign or light. It is not enough to recommend that individuals go to the clinic for needed medical care. Elizabeth is also working as a member of the board of the clinic with the city to put in a stop sign. She is also working with the city to provide more security measures for individuals and families in the neighborhood.

The parish nurse collaborates with other health-care professionals and assesses ways in which she and the congregation can support individuals and families. For example, the parish nurse may visit parishioners in the hospital and discuss with the staff what the needs will be for that individual upon discharge. This may involve meals, transportation, visits, bringing

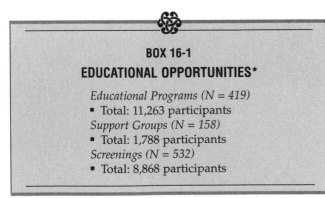

BOX 16-1

EDUCATIONAL OPPORTUNITIES*

Educational Programs (N = 419)
- Total: 11,263 participants

Support Groups (N = 158)
- Total: 1,788 participants

Screenings (N = 532)
- Total: 8,868 participants

*Source: Monthly Utilization Reports submitted by LGHS & TMC Parish Nurses, January 1993 to December 1993.

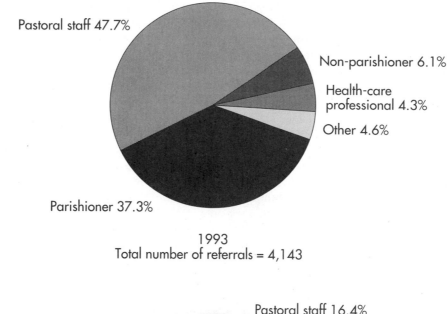

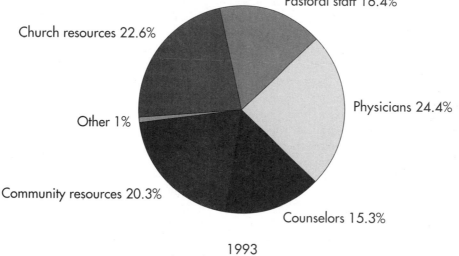

FIG. 16-2   Above, referrals from selected sources to the parish nurse. Below, referrals made by the parish nurse to various resources (Source: Monthly utilization reports submitted by LGHS and TMS Parish nurses, January 1993 to December 1993.)

communion, and helping individuals and families understand or reinforcing their treatment plan.

Working with volunteers. The parish nurse collaborates with congregational volunteer structures which might be in place. The parish nurse serves as a clinical resource and support to volunteers to broaden and extend the sources of help within the parish. As of December, 1993, the parish nurses representing 40 sites reported that a total of 1,519 individuals served with them in a volunteer capacity by either assisting with planning and implementing programs or participating in delivery of support services to members of the congregation. The parish nurse may guide volunteers to reach out, for example, to individuals who have

recently sustained a loss or to families attempting to care for an ill or dependent family member at home. The parish nurse will often conduct follow-up assessments and make referrals for individuals being visited by a volunteer.

Interpreter of relationship between faith and health. In all of these functions, the parish nurse, in conjunction with the pastoral team, lay leaders, and health committees, seeks to help congregations rediscover their historic role in the area of health and well-being. Parish nurses have chosen this specialized work because of the unique opportunity to speak with individuals and families about the deeper values and beliefs that affect their health. Although the parish nurses have not been specifically identified as case managers, much of their time centers on care management activities, as defined by Cohen and Cesta (1993). The parish nurses complete monthly reports to log their activities. On these reports, they identify the category of intervention by using the Omaha Documentation System (Martin & Scheet, 1992). In 1993, the parish nurses reported their interventions in the following manner: Health Teaching/Guidance (35%), Case Management (35%), and Surveillance (30%). These responses begin to verify our assumptions regarding the role, recognizing the emphasis varies in different churches and communities. This offers an opportunity for further inquiry. During 1993, the parish nurses documented 24,501 contacts with individuals of all ages. In our experience, 55% of the contacts are with individuals over 65 with increasing numbers each year in the over-80 category (Figure 16-3). Individuals bring to the parish nurse a wide variety of concerns. Over the past three years, the primary concerns have revolved around issues of access to services, loneliness, isolation, relationships, grief and loss, hospitalization, and questions related to specific diseases.

Working in the Inner City

Urban crime and poverty are national issues that are a reality in Chicago. This reality hits the young and the elderly the hardest. Already vulnerable by either youth or age, when in an environment characterized by scarce resources, violence and drugs, they are at particular risk for death, injury, poor health, and social isolation. It is in these neighborhoods that the congregations and parish nurses of the inner-city parish nurse programs are working.

"Society, community, and family have to deal with whatever problem arises" (Drucker, 1993). This statement certainly reflects the experience of the parish nurses. As one parish nurse wrote, "A frequent entry point into the lives of families is assisting them to resolve problems of inadequate housing, food, clothing and heat." When one addresses the needs of the inner city, one must think of medical issues within a social context. Teen pregnancy must be understood within the context of the culture, the environment, the setting in which the teen lives. Tuberculosis is a growing concern and must be addressed in terms of the social issues related to homelessness and lack of medical care.

Issues of the inner city. An increasingly difficult issue in our inner cities is the large number of immigrants and refugees. When these individuals come to this country, they are profoundly impacted by our culture. One of the most difficult losses is the community network they had in their home country. Many of these individuals are alienated from their families and their support systems. The language barrier is itself a problem, but more complicated is the cultural interpretation and meaning of words. Individuals without documentation are afraid to seek medical care for fear of being discovered and returned to their native country. Consequently, they wait until the situation becomes severe or at crisis stage before seeking help.

We are losing children at an incredible rate because of violence in our cities. "Violence was the top worry of parents and children alike in 1993 according to a *Newsweek* poll" (Edelman, 1994). Children are losing hope of growing to adulthood. This violence occurs in the home as well as on the streets. Parish nurses report the increasing amount of domestic violence occurring in the homes of their parishioners. It takes time and a very trusting relationship for a spouse to admit this and seek help. Much of this violence is related to drug use.

There is generalized fear in the neighborhoods. Individuals may not feel free to ask neighbors for

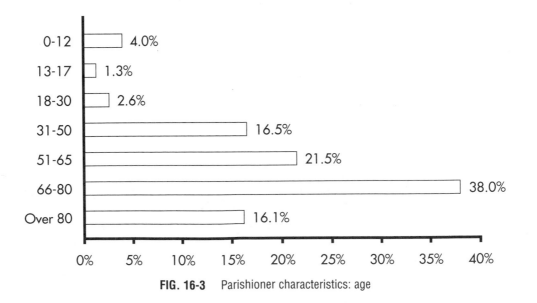

FIG. 16-3 Parishioner characteristics: age

help and so feel like prisoners in their own homes. They are often fearful of going beyond the boundaries of their ethnic neighborhood into other communities. All of these factors lead to increased feelings of isolation and loneliness.

Homelessness is a growing problem in the city and is spreading into the suburbs. The most rapid growth is among women and children. More and more churches are participating in programs to open their churches as shelter or provide resources to others.

A major issue for persons in the inner city is just the largeness of the city and its bureaucratic systems. It may take hours to travel across town to get to a social service agency and then many more hours waiting for service. Along with the cost of transportation, there is the cost of time lost from work. People feel frustrated and overwhelmed by trying to access these complicated systems. It is not surprising that individuals will not seek preventive care such as screenings when it is so difficult just to receive basic or even emergency care.

How do we respond? Individuals look to the church as a place of help, a place where someone will take time to listen to them, and a place for direction or resources as needed. One of the unique aspects of the local church is that it involves persons of all ages, individuals, and families. When individuals move into a community, they often seek out a church and may turn to the pastor for assistance in locating health-care resources. People turn to the church at special times of life—birth, death, marriage, confirmation, baptism. Individuals turn to the church when they have felt abandoned by other segments of society and often trust the church when they do not trust other community organizations.

Zander identifies consistency of provider as a key characteristic of case management (Cohen & Cesta, 1993). This clearly relates to the parish nurse role because she is the person who becomes the anchor for individuals and families as they relate to a wide variety of community resources. The parish nurse becomes the one who supports the individual and family through many challenging life events such as marriage, birth, illness, disability, and death.

Some of these activities occur in formal settings such as classes or office visits and many others occur informally, on the street, drop in at the church, or in one's home. One of the parish nurses began regular visits to an elderly woman of the parish to check her blood pressure. The woman began to invite neighbors to be at her home when the parish nurse came. It has become a regular event. The women now gather for their regular blood pressure check while they talk about their families, share their experiences of life, grief and loss, and informally support each other.

The parish nurse often must begin by sorting out the issues and prioritizing them. This can be a very challenging task with the complex nature of the physical, social, and emotional problems that are presented.

One of the most effective efforts, though time consuming, is to accompany individuals to the doctor, to the clinic, to the public aid office. Individuals do not seek appropriate medical care because of inaccessible transportation, (several busses), fear for their safety, lack of knowledge about the system, and inadequate finances. For individuals who cannot speak English, navigating through the complicated health-care system can be an especially overwhelming task. Fortunately, more agencies are providing translators to assist these individuals. Even those who have insurance may not receive appropriate care because they cannot communicate their needs effectively. The parish nurse not only assists in the translation but advocates on behalf of the individual so that they receive appropriate care and understand the treatment plan which the parish nurse can reinforce in the days to come.

When one considers providing health programs, one must consider the opportunity to reach a wide variety of individuals beyond parishioners who may come in contact with the church during the week. This includes children in day care, seniors, and the homeless as well as many who attend self-help groups. Many opportunities arise in the congregation for the parish nurse to impact children as well as adults. A program was given for young children, "Your Body, God's Gift," which coincided with events of the calendar year. For example, a discussion of the skeletal system occurred during Halloween and the cardiovascular system was discussed during the Valentine season. When the organist in a congregation died of AIDS, the parish nurse organized support activities and provided education for all age groups about the disease as well as facilitating a discussion of the ethical and spiritual issues related to dealing with this disease.

The parish nurses write newsletters and bulletin articles emphasizing health topics with a whole person perspective. From a survey of over 1,000 parishioners, 90% reported that they read the newsletter or bulletin article written by the parish nurse (Lloyd & Djupe, 1994). Parish nurses have also promoted national health observances such as those published by the U.S. Department of Health and Human Services, World Health Day, and the National Observance of Children's Sabbaths.

It is well understood that the parish nurse cannot work in isolation and needs the resources of many volunteers to carry out this type of ministry. Working with volunteers can be very challenging, however. First of all, individuals have very little time or energy to give to the church. Secondly, they need education and support related to the task. Individuals cannot be asked to visit the homebound without specific directions given and boundaries explained. One of the parish nurses working at Chicago Uptown Ministries, in collaboration with the Chicago Department of Health, Providence of God Parish, and the St. Luke Society developed a training program for lay health promoters. The first group of participants consisted of an average 20 to 25 people per week and attended classes on communication, hypertension, diabetes, lead poisoning, cancer, drugs and alcohol, AIDS, family planning, well-baby care, and self defense. The parish nurse provides ongoing support and resources for these health promoters who are working out in their communities. These individuals represent a wide range of ethnic groups and their primary responsibility is to serve as a link between the community and the health delivery system. They also provide some basic education to their families and neighbors related to these health issues (Tazelaar, 1993). Because they are members of the community themselves, they are more likely to be trusted by other community members.

Clients as partners. There has been much written in recent health reform literature about partnerships between the various levels of health-care providers. As resources become more scarce, this becomes even more critical. With parish nursing, we have taken this a step further in two directions. First, we have developed partnerships between local congregations and a large health-care system. This has taken a great deal of commitment, flexibility, and sponsorship on both sides. Second, we have moved toward a philosophy of working with clients as partners. Helping individuals and families to become active participants in decisions about their health care and management of their health-care resources means a shift in approach from "knowing what is best for the client" to mutually agreeing on a plan and then empowering the individual and family to carry out the plan. This becomes even more of a challenge when we are working with underserved and mentally ill clients. Sometimes, the most profound assistance is in the "journeying" with people instead of the "doing for." This can be particularly challenging for nurses who tend to be "doers." There is now only a beginning appreciation of the power of presence and caring. To involve the client as partner, it is imperative to respect the individual and truly listen to their needs. This means putting aside on a daily basis one's prejudices, dealing with one's own frustrations, and tuning in to the stories and needs of the client.

What have parish nurses learned? Parish nurses have learned many things from people considered the "underserved." Taking the time to listen results in the clients becoming teachers and sharing their stories. Among the lessons learned are:

- That all individuals, including the homeless and mentally ill, search for God, for meaning in life. All search for direction and clarity in a world of ambiguity and confusion.
- That "one does not give up on people because they do not do what you tell them to." This means committing to a long-term relationship and supporting individuals through many challenges of life even when they take turns or make decisions that seem inappropriate or detrimental at the time. It means holding the belief that each person is sacred and must be treated with respect and dignity.
- That one must be cognizant of each person's ability to be responsible. This means taking the word responsibility apart to "response-ability" and addressing each client according to individual abilities and challenges posed by their environment (Walker, 1994). One must explain and translate complex information so that it is understood. It is very easy to become frustrated with individuals when they do not take responsibility for themselves, when in reality, they do not have the ability or support to do so. Parish nursing services are designed to build on and strengthen capacities, limited though they may be, of individuals, families, and congregations to understand and care for one another.
- That one must build relationships with individuals—a process that may take a very long time for those who have very little trust. This means being in tune with the needs of the client and moving at a pace that they can tolerate. We live in such a hurried world and have expectations of immediate response. Many of these individuals with whom one works do not have that same sense of urgency or capability of response. One learns to look for very small incremental victories and celebrate them whenever possible.
- That we must be sensitive to what clients believe they need and not act on one's own prejudices and suppositions. For example, Harold is a 62-year-old man who has been homeless for about three years. He is edentulous and has a severe skin condition. One part of his life that is very important to him is that he reads scripture at masses in his Catholic church. It is very important for him to see his name in the bulletin as lector. The parish nurse meets Harold for lunch once a month. She says that his prayer before the meal is very moving and always is a blessing to her. For Christmas, she gave him a portable radio. He loves the radio, particularly a classical music

station and has become quite knowledgeable about classical music. He also enjoys bird-watching and reports to her about the birds he has observed. Recently, the pastor came to the parish nurse with a question. Several parishioners offered to buy Harold new dentures, believing this was what Harold needed most. It was believed that this would improve his appearance. The pastor sought out the parish nurse's counsel as to the best way to present this to Harold in the most sensitive manner. In discussion with the parish nurse, she suggested that perhaps what he needed more was new shoes and foot care because he made his living by collecting cans and copper wire. The pastor and parish nurse decided to approach Harold to determine what he felt he needed and how they might assist him. This needed to be done out of mutual respect for Harold. What Harold wanted and was willing to accept was an eye exam and a new pair of bifocals to replace the pair he had found in the dumpster. One of the important lessons from such individuals as Harold is the importance of "being called by name," that each of those individuals in the crowd has a name. Harold also reminds nurses of their own frantic pace when he tells about the birds that he sees and the music he hears. People like Harold help the parish nurse to stop and assess her own priorities and needs.

- That one must recognize the need to let go. At times when one feels failure and loss, one must look critically at one's own limits and recognize when to say no and determine boundaries. This means a great deal of insight for the nurse and support in looking at one's own feelings. As one parish nurse said, "As we are privileged to listen to the stories, struggles, and suffering of others, we are changed."

Parish nurses struggle with their own limitations and ability to make things better. This means assessing when one is therapeutic and when one is not. One of the benefits of having the parish nurses work as employees of LGHS is that they come to LGHS twice a month for a day of education and support. Several hours of this time is spent in a small group format where individual cases are presented. The group provides feedback and direction to the parish nurse. The focus is more on how the experience impacted the parish nurse professionally and personally rather than the impact on the client. A frequent focus of these sessions is on limit-setting. It is through these activities that the parish nurses receive support and direction which sustains them in this challenging work. Parish nurses also call upon the LGHS faculty, which consists of a physician, a nurse, and two chaplains, for individual support, direction, and consultation.

Sr. Elizabeth Gillis, an inner-city LGHS parish nurse, recently wrote in her annual report:

Increasing the well-being of individuals and families, a goal of parish nursing, is often attainable. Satisfying basic human needs of food, clothing, shelter, and safety helps people move along the health-illness continuum toward well-being and enables them to discover their own inner resources—emotional, intellectual, and spiritual. With the collaboration and support of sharing parishes, concerned parishioners, neighborhood resources, and the parish staff, a more wholesome and healthy environment has been assured for some vulnerable families who have come with hope and trust to our parish. Such encounters strengthen our faith in God and the human spirit, and validate the reasons for staying in the struggle with others and for being a parish nurse in the inner city (Parish Nurse Annual Report, Columbus-Cabrini Medical Center, 1993).

CONCLUSION

Former president Carter has said:

Wouldn't it be wonderful if faith groups adopted one close-by geographical area and made sure . . . that every single child was immunized against the basic diseases? that there was no hungry person in that area? that every person had a basic medical exam? that every woman who became pregnant would get prenatal care? that every elderly person was contacted daily? Suppose these congregations convinced parents and children to fight the presence of guns. Suppose they made a commitment to provide the kinds of alternatives needed to reduce the violence that afflicts the poorest among us. These are very exciting and redemptive options for the faith groups of our nation (Carter, 1994b).

Certainly faith groups cannot address these issues alone but represent an important partner in impacting the health of this nation. Parish nursing is one model that presents a unique opportunity for health-care institutions to align themselves with community-based congregations to provide preventive health services. The parish nurse is clearly emerging as a trusted provider of health promotion and prevention services. In this capacity, the parish nurse, working in the faith community, is positioned to integrate the resources of individuals, the community, and related institutions.

REFERENCES

Carter, J. (1994a). *Faith & health: newsletter of interfaith health program.* (Available from the Carter Center of Emory University, One Copenhill, Atlanta, GA 30307).

Carter, J. (1994b). *The challenges of faith and health: the report of the national conference of the interfaith health program.* Atlanta: The Interfaith Health Program of The Carter Center of Emory University.

Cohen, E. L. & Cesta, T. G. (1993). *Nursing case management: from concept to evaluation.* St Louis: Mosby.

Columbus-Cabrini Medical Center Parish Nurse Program. (1993). *Annual Report.* Chicago, IL: Author.

Djupe, A. M., Olson, H., & Ryan, J. A. (1994). *Reaching out: parish nursing services—an institutional/congregational partnership* (2nd ed.). Park Ridge, IL: National Parish Nurse Resource Center.

Droege, T. (1994). *Faith & health: newsletter of interfaith health program.* (Available from the Carter Center of Emory University, One Copenhill, Atlanta, GA 30307).

Drucker, P. (1993). *Post-capitalist society.* New York: Harper Business.

Edelman, M. W. (1994, August). *Newsletter of national observance of children's sabbaths.* (Available from Children's Defense Fund, (202) 628 8787).

Lloyd, R. C., & Djupe, A. M. (1994). *Expanding our understanding of health and well-being: the parish nurse program.* Park Ridge, IL: National Parish Nurse Resource Center.

Lloyd, R. C., & Solari-Twadell, P. A. (1994). Organizational framework, functions, and educational preparation of parish nurses: national survey, 1991 and 1994. *Proceedings of the 8th Annual Granger Westberg Parish Nurse Symposium,* Northbrook, IL.

Martin, K. S., & Scheet, N. J. (1992). *The Omaha system: applications for community health nursing.* Philadelphia: W. B. Saunders.

NCC Ecumenical Child Health Project. (1991). *Results church health survey.* Washington: Author.

Tazelaar, G. (1993). Increasing access to health care with lay health personnel. *Health and Development, 4,* 3-9.

Walker, S. N. (1994). Health promotion and prevention of disease and disability among older adults: Who is responsible? *Generations: Journal of the American Society of Aging, 18* (1), 45-50.

The author acknowledges the Trinity Medical Center and Lutheran General HealthSystem parish nurses, and Bethany Johnson, Office Coordinator for Parish Nursing Services at LGHS, for their contributions to this chapter.

Chapter 17

Nurse Case Management and Long-Term Care

Sunny R. Howe, MS, RN, CNAA

OVERVIEW

Use of a nontraditional case management process in a long-term care facility with scarce nursing resources has produced positive outcomes for both clients and staff.

Lack of registered nursing staff and traditionally task-oriented practice in the long-term care arena have generally precluded use of case management. Nevertheless, one nursing home had success by developing and implementing use of special data collection tools, permanent assignments for all staff, and continuing quality improvement (CQI) leadership talents of nurse managers. This nontraditional case management model has resulted in significant cost savings, decreased staff turnover, and improved resident and staff satisfaction.

The case management model of care exemplifies the core values of nursing as a profession. This care delivery model creates a method to meet regulatory requirements, provides optimal efficiency and productivity, and addresses the expectations of health-care consumers.

Many directors of nursing in the long-term care practice arena have been aware of the benefits of case management but have been reluctant to implement such a model. There seemed to be good reasons for this:

- Long-term care facilities have a limited number of registered nurses (RNs) on their staffs; that is, 15% of direct care staff by 1990 State of Wisconsin statistics (Department of Health and Social Services [DHSS], 1991).

- Traditionally, care models in nursing homes have been "task oriented" in nature (Deckard, Hicks, & Roundtree, 1986).
- The majority of direct care provided to nursing home residents is by unlicensed assistive personnel (70%) (DHSS, 1991).
- State and federal regulations require that comprehensive resident assessments, care plans, and extensive documentation for each resident be done by an RN.
- Historically, there has been a high turnover of staff; that is, 46%, by State of Wisconsin statistics of nursing homes (DHSS 1990).
- The limited reimbursement to long-term care institutions by Medicaid or Medicare funding sources has precluded the hiring of larger numbers of RNs.

When facing any challenges, the implementation of any change in the current system can seem overwhelming. Case management models implemented in acute care settings have, however, had a favorable impact on many elements chronically plaguing long-term care nursing, such as staff turnover, staff satisfaction, patient satisfaction, cost effectiveness, and quality of care (Cohen, 1991; Ethridge, 1989).

PREPARATION FOR IMPLEMENTATION OF THE MODEL

The first step in the establishment of case management is to present the concept to senior administration. Articulating what implementation of the model could accomplish must be described in sufficient detail. This step cannot be taken lightly since, in many instances, a case for the model will need to be made to nonnursing personnel. The overall cost savings expected with implementation should be highlighted because there will be some increased costs for education.

Once approval for the implementation has been received, discussion of the vision with the management team can occur. If the plan involves changing job roles or the elimination of a specific job description, the persons involved should be assessed as to their skills, abilities, and willingness to be a partner in the upcoming change. They should be approached individually before any group discussions are held. Having a committed team is crucial to the project's success. Continually reassessing that commitment of all members is the ongoing challenge of the director of nursing. A member of the staff or the director who is knowledgeable in case management should do the presentations and be involved in the teaching. Having a consultant take this part is an option but not necessary. Whatever the method chosen, the discussions should be facilitated using a *continuous quality improvement* (CQI) process (Marszalek-Gaucher & Coffey, 1990). The following elements should be considered for inclusion:

- Problems with the current system and model of care
- Identification of need for change
- Identification of goals to be achieved by a change to case management
- Description of various styles of case management
- Identification of how each style would or would not meet the needs of the facility
- Identification of possible adjustments in the styles to fit the unique needs of the facility
- Plans for making those adjustments
- Plans for inclusion of all staff in both the change process and in determining the specifics of the implementation plan along with time lines

- Plans for evaluation of the implementation process
- Educational and assistance resources available
- Education of staff in the case management process and the management team in transformational leadership skills of teaching, mentoring, and coaching (MacGregor-Burns, 1978)

From these discussions the goals of case management in the long-term care setting were identified (Box 17-1).

Depending on the size of the facility, it may not be practical to consider changing to a case management care delivery model on all units; however, the benefits of having the entire management team "buy in" to the concept at the same time are significant. When defining the vision it is appropriate to inculcate the understanding that, while the concept may be static, the implementation on individual units can be quite different (Cohen & Cesta, 1993, p. 6). The director of nursing must reiterate this fact and express support of individual management styles and recognize the existence of unique resident population's needs. Taking frequent opportunities to do this can greatly contribute to acceptance of the vision by the management team.

The major issue in the implementation of case management in a nursing home revolves around the number and expertise of the RNs available to perform the components of the model. Since this limited resource is probably not going to change and may further decrease, a more efficient way to utilize the talents of the available RNs must be explored. To this end, some nursing homes have used the unit's nurse manager or care coordinator as the case manager for as many as 48 residents in a unit that has no other or only part-time RNs (Smith, 1991). Although this has been successful and has met many of the individual resident's goals, in general it has proved to be an overwhelming task for one person and can easily contribute to burnout and turnover.

At Alexian Village of Milwaukee (a continuing care retirement community for 400 residents with an 87-bed skilled nursing facility), a decision was made by the management team to modify the traditional case man-

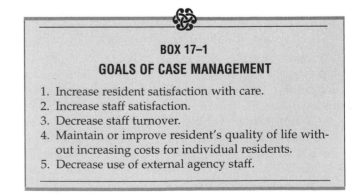

BOX 17–1
GOALS OF CASE MANAGEMENT

1. Increase resident satisfaction with care.
2. Increase staff satisfaction.
3. Decrease staff turnover.
4. Maintain or improve resident's quality of life without increasing costs for individual residents.
5. Decrease use of external agency staff.

agement model, in which all case managers were RNs, in favor of using LPNs in this role for selected residents. Considering the educational preparation and regulatory practice requirements of the LPN, such a decision seemed radical. Nevertheless, it was well recognized that LPNs have been the backbone of nursing homes' resident care delivery system for many years. They have had intimate knowledge of resident's needs and expectations and have appropriately met those needs. Not to capitalize on the strengths of the LPNs and their close and beneficial relationship with residents seemed to be both devastating and nonproductive. In making the decision to use LPNs as case managers the following premises were considered:

- Based on CQI principles, decision making needs to occur as close to the customer as possible to have the most beneficial results.
- The assessment and evaluation pieces of the nursing process that are exclusively the domain of the RN are based on data. If the data were collected by an LPN that had a vested interest in the resident and that data proved to be both of sufficient quantity and quality, the RNs' time could be minimal in collaborating with the LPN to complete these sections of the process.
- To accomplish the foregoing, a high degree of consistency in practice assignments by all staff nurses would be required.
- An RN taking responsibility for the actual assessment and evaluation would need to be able to trust that the data collected by the LPN were accurate.
- A thorough educational process in use of the data collection instruments would be required for both LPNs and RNs. Use of the Health Care Financing Administration (HCFA) mandated forms would be an appropriate starting point because training guides exist for their use.
- The development of and training in additional data collection tools that would act as adjuncts to the HCFA forms would be necessary for a more complete data base.
- LPNs and RNs unfamiliar with the Minimum Data Set (MDS) and Resident Assessment Protocols (RAPs) would need to receive specific education in the paper compliance activities of the case manager role before taking on the more creative and collaborative parts of the role. Management would need to provide assurance that nurses would not be expected to increase their individual involvement in case management until they felt prepared to do so.
- The nurse manager of the unit would retain case management accountability while the learning process for staff was accomplished.

INITIAL PHASE: UNIT NURSE MANAGER SERVES AS CASE MANAGER

Taking advantage of the nurse manager's skills, education, and managerial expertise can serve as the basis for case management implementation. In many settings, this person has already been responsible for completion of many of the federal, state, and facility paper compliance requirements (i.e., MDS, RAPs, care plans). Because the nurse manager will ultimately become a pivotal person when implementing the model with staff nurses, it seemed logical to have that person serve as case manager during this phase. This allowed time necessary for the structuring of the model for staff "buy-in" and to provide the necessary education for all staff.

Functioning in this role for all residents during the primary implementation phase allows the nurse manager to:

1. Gain an indepth familiarity with residents and their families.
2. Gain an understanding of the case management concept.
3. Be in a position to identify potential case management system problems.
4. Discover opportunities to find solutions to those problems by using trial and error approaches.
5. Become recognized as an expert so that teaching staff the concept and details of the model will take place with greater ease.

During the implementation phase the opportunity is present for management team building to occur as both case management skills and transformational leadership qualities are discussed with the director of nursing and other members of the management group.

The period of time for this phase may take between six months and one year. During this time the nurse manager requires more than the usual amount of support by administration. Methods must be sought to relieve or assist managers with as many of their other duties as possible. The burdens may need to be absorbed by the director of nursing, assistant director, administrator, education coordinator, and other nondirect care staff. Because the ultimate benefits of the model will not be experienced for a while, all of the nondirect care staff along with the nurse managers must be a party to and share in the ultimate vision of the case management model. It is the responsibility of the director of nursing to maintain the flame of excitement concerning the model for both the management team as a group and for the nurse managers in particular. All must understand the ultimate vision and believe that they will not have to serve in dual roles indefinitely.

DURING THE INITIAL PHASE

Depending on the number and type of residents living on the individual units, the nurse manager may select several residents to case manage and then add to that number after gaining expertise. As this learning curve progresses, education sessions are necessary for the managers. The content should include case management principles and practices and can be provided by a consultant, seminars, or texts on the subject. As the group's knowledge base expands, they will be able to offer valuable input as to the creation of the policies, procedures, and assessment tools necessary for full implementation of the model. It should be noted that how the finished model will ultimately function is still not known; only the concept is a solid vision. This is an important point to reinforce. At this time, informational and educational sessions that outline the case management model and its goals will need to occur with all licensed staff. Skilled facilitation techniques will be required at these sessions to elicit ideas and engender healthy discussion while still maintaining the goals defined by the management team. In particular, the LPNs' attitudes toward accepting an expanded role should become clear. Individual LPNs may have difficulty understanding how the differentiation in nursing practice between RNs and LPNs and their role as a case manager under the direction of the nurse manager can be reconciled. The director of nursing and nurse managers will need to meet individually with these LPNs.

Another of the director of nursing's challenges during this time period is to manage the level of discontent some staff will feel with this nebulous situation while encouraging progress and enthusiasm. Incorporating case management wording in memos, speech, and discussions with staff and other disciplines at every opportunity will validate the manager's efforts. Individual conversations will need to be held with members of other disciplines that have "managed" segments of the resident's care.

During change, it is normal that departments or individuals within a department feel threatened. To avoid "turf wars" the director of nursing needs to meet proactively with other disciplines and individuals that are concerned. These discussions should clearly identify that the goals of quality resident care are paramount in this endeavor and that the value of their partnership in providing personal services and expertise are recognized as integral to any model of care. Depending on the degree of involvement various disciplines have had in resident care issues, it may be appropriate to include them earlier, rather than later, in decision making that affects many of the details of the model. From the time the nurse manager begins to function as a case manager to the time when individual resident's care management is transitioned to a staff nurse, the highest regard must be placed on the value of partnership to achieve the best results for the resident. The director of nursing will need to continue to facilitate the collaborative process between the nursing department and all other disciplines.

MIDPHASE OF IMPLEMENTATION

While the unit nurse managers are acting as case managers, discussions with all staff concerning the ultimate vision of the case management model must continue in earnest. The director of nursing, along with the nurse manager, can serve as facilitators of such discussions conducted with each unit's staff. The individual issues of staff mix, working schedules, resident population types, and similar issues for each unit will be highlighted. Adjustments in the case management process for any particular area will be made. This makes the model each unit's own. As individual staff nurses take an increasing proprietary interest, the nurse manager can begin one-to-one education and coaching in the case management role. The nurse manager than can relinquish selected cases to specific nurses. Depending on the skills and abilities demonstrated by the staff nurse, she can choose to retain some or none of the decision making connected with the resident's care. At Alexian Village, our experience at this stage proved to be very exciting. Staff nurses, RNs, and LPNs eagerly accepted the challenge of learning case management. Many had "favorite" residents for whom they wished to be more responsible. They gained greater autonomy and satisfaction as they were empowered to have a greater influence over their nursing practice and their collaboration with other disciplines. The nurse managers gained great satisfaction as they watched their staff's growth and development. As the nurse manager coached staff for success, positive reinforcement for their use of transformational leadership qualities was achieved.

In the Alexian Village model, each staff nurse who worked a minimum of five shifts in a two-week period were designated to be case managers. When scheduled, they were assigned to complete the daily tasks of medication and treatment administration, documentation and directing execution of the care plans for 22 residents. The resident's daily personal needs were addressed by nursing assistants assigned to perform the personal care for the residents. In addition to this "daily work," each nurse was eventually assigned between three and seven residents as a case load, depending on the amount of hours they were scheduled to work in a two-week period. These residents were part of the 22 for whom they had responsibility on any given day. They knew these residents and their families well and served as the liaison between the resident and members of the interdisciplinary team. They were responsible for the following related to their case residents:

- Completion of the MDS, RAPs, and care plan on a quarterly and annual basis.
- Review of the residents' charts and care plans on a regular basis to ensure appropriateness of all medications, treatments, orders, and other interventions.
- Regular discussions concerning the achievement and progress toward care plan goals with other caregivers and in particular the nursing assistant assigned to the resident.
- Serving as liaison with other disciplines, the family, and physician regarding care issues for the resident.
- Reviewing notes from other nurses who have provided care for the resident in the absence of the case manager.
- Assuming accountability for having residents' care goals achieved or goal adjustments made.

While this transitional period was occurring, the data collection tools were developed to help the novice case manager in the new role. As with any change, a large degree of staff involvement in the development of forms and tools helped ensure acceptance by the staff as a whole. As the tools were developed, educational sessions were held to explain not only the tool itself but how it was to be integrated in the case management process. One example of a tool is in Appendix 17-A. This addresses the complex issue of behavior monitoring and the appropriateness of psychotropic drug use. This data collection form calls for the case manager to collaborate with the resident, his family, the pharmacist, and the physician before making a decision in this area of care. Notice that this form indicates that the nurse manager would still need to approve the recommendation made by the case manager. This provides a coaching mechanism for the nurse manager. In the final phase of the model's implementation the RN case manager would have decision-making autonomy; the LPN would still require the nurse manager's review.

There were some casualties encountered as it became accepted that case management was to be the model of care practiced at the facility. This presented the challenge of recruiting staff to be a part of the model from the beginning of their employment. During this time there was some attrition of nondirect care staff as discontent with changing roles was unable to be satisfied. On a positive note, there was relatively little difficulty in finding staff who were eager to be empowered and learn the case management model.

The nursing staff recognized that nursing assistants needed to be an integral part of the case management system. To this end, the team wanted nursing assistants to be identified as practice partners for specific residents under the direction of the RN or LPN case manager. To effect such a change, the nursing assistants had to have more consistent resident assignments; however, permanent assignments for this group had been tried before and met with little enthusiasm. Even though there was some trepidation at trying again, a concerted effort was made to include the nursing assistants in the decision process by allowing them a choice of which assignment they wanted. They were also assigned a case load of three to four residents on their regular assignment. They knew these residents well and were responsible to give frequent feedback to the case manager regarding care specifics. When at all possible, the assigned nursing assistant attended care conferences for those residents. A mechanism was put in place to allow the nursing assistant to have a respite from the permanent assignment should they request it. Numerous care seminars were held for nursing assistants. The goals of these seminars were to explain case management and their part in the process, increase their knowledge base, and affirm their value to the organization and the case manager of the residents to which they were assigned. It's interesting to note that 15 months after following the institution of the permanent assignments, no one wanted to return to rotating assignments! Having a consistent direct caregiver had obvious positive outcomes for the residents. It also had a further positive impact on the case management process because the nursing assistant was able and willing to give more comprehensive input to the case manager. The nursing assistant felt valued and encouraged to participate in not only the care planning process but the evaluation of that care. Because the mechanism was now in place for more productive discussions to occur between the licensed and unlicensed staff, educational seminars were held in the use of communication and delegation techniques.

END PHASE AND EVALUATION

This phase begins when all residents have a staff nurse case manager. The unit manager can now devote efforts toward coaching and evaluating the progress and goal achievement of the case management process. At this point, in the Alexian Village experience, some changes were instituted on individual units. The staff of one unit decided that, because of their working schedules, night shift nurses could not be effective as case managers. Nevertheless, their input to case managers working other shifts was crucial. It was agreed that the entire night shift staff would act as a "case team." Communication methods and tools were instituted to provide the case manager with data concerning their resident's behaviors and concerns arising during the night shift hours. Although this resulted in other nurses taking larger case loads, this process has proved to be a successful and rewarding.

On another unit, a majority of the night staff worked 12-hour shifts and felt that they could maintain case management responsibilities for stable, longer term residents. They felt there were adequate opportunities to interact with families, residents, and others during the evening hours. This system has worked equally well; however, at times the unit's nurse manager has had to assume some coordination tasks for these nurses.

As issues with the case management process were encountered (i.e., the need for more extensive data collection tools, better delineation of accountabilities, assistance with complex resident care or involved family dynamics), they were individually addressed. Trial solutions were proposed, implemented, and evaluated by the unit's staff. The nurse manager facilitated this process, one that frequently involved members of other disciplines. The director of nursing's role becomes that of mentor for the nurse managers and the development of their coaching skills.

This style of case management—using the talents of both staff LPNs and RNs—has been very successful in practice at Alexian Village of Milwaukee.

Staff turnover rate for the year 1989 was 42% for licensed staff and 78% for nursing assistants. In 1994 the licensed staff rate was 20%, a decline of 117%, and the nursing assistant turnover rate fell to 44%, a 229% decrease. These statistics reflect both voluntary and nonvoluntary causes. All those resigning did so for reasons other than dissatisfaction with the case management model. Exit interviews conducted with nurses indicated a high degree of satisfaction with the case management process. Nationally, costs associated with turnover of staff have been estimated at $7,911 per nurse and $2,558 per nursing assistant (Caudill, & Patrick, 1990). The cost savings to the institution are obviously significant. Residents and families repeatedly voice their ongoing satisfaction with having greater consistency of caregivers and knowing that they have a specific nurse that is coordinating their care. A negative effect that we noted and continue to see is evidenced when changes in caregivers or case managers for residents is necessary. These changes occur on occasion as a result of changes in working schedules, room changes by residents, resignations, or significant increase in acuity of a resident. It seems to be very distressing for both the staff and the residents during these times. The reason for this may be the normal fear associated with relinquishing such a comfortable and rewarding relationship. In many instances,

residents and staff had never experienced such a close relationship until case management became a reality; therefore, were reluctant to face a change. Staff satisfaction is evidenced through the decrease in turnover; however, satisfaction with their increase in autonomy, status, and value to the residents is evident.

There are indicators that illustrate improvement in quality of life: decrease in incontinence, decrease in use of restraints, and increase in ability of specific residents to perform activities of daily living. Although improvement in these and some other areas in the nursing home's population was and continue to be noted, quality remains a difficult task to evaluate. Two reasons for this are (1) the expected decline in the health of the majority of residents at this time in their life, and (2) the increase in the acuity of residents being admitted to long-term care facilities, secondary to decrease length of stay in acute care setting.

CONCLUSION

An example of the effectiveness of case management for a specific resident is the best way to illustrate the model's effectiveness (see Case Study).

It would be difficult to quantify the joy that E. B. felt when she tasted chocolate again (this was her greatest food desire) or could breathe normally again or communicate her wishes easily, but it was clearly written on her face. It would be equally difficult to quantify the joy that the case manager, the unit's nurse manager, and her caregivers felt as each step in her progress was made; however, one look at any of them demonstrated the pride and satisfaction felt by this team.

There were monetary cost savings as well. The cost of tracheostomy supplies and equipment, gastrostomy tubes, and tube feedings averaged $150 per day above

---

CASE STUDY

E.B. was 76 years old and had resided in a nursing home for almost five years after a stroke that resulted in hemiplegia. She had a tracheostomy and gastrostomy tubes in place. She had come to the nursing home after being weaned from a ventilator; however, she still required a significant amount of airway management. Her nutritional intake was totally via the gastrostomy tube. She had not eaten anything or talked in almost five years.

This former dental assistant, wife, and beauty pageant winner was transferred to Alexian Village in 1991 and assigned a case manager. Within seven months the tracheostomy tube was removed; within nine months the gastrostomy tube was discontinued. Her depression was reversed, and she became a dynamic, vocal resident.

the daily room rate. The annual cost savings to the resident and Medicare was estimated at over $54,000.

This success story exemplifies the core values of nursing as a profession and the achievements that could be experienced from case management in particular.

REFERENCES

Caudill, M., & Patrick, M. (1990). Costing nurse turnover in nursing homes. *Nursing Management, 20* (11), 61-64.

Cohen, E. (1991). Nursing case management: does it pay? *Journal of Nursing Administration, 21* (4), 20-25.

Cohen, E. L., & Cesta, T. G. (1993). *Nursing case management: from concept to evaluation.* St Louis: Mosby.

Deckard, G. J., Hicks, L. L., & Roundtree, B. H. (1986). Long-term care nursing: how satisfying is it? *Nursing Economics, 4* (4), 194-200.

Del Togno-Armanasco, V., Olivas, G., & Harter, S. (1989). Developing an integrated nursing case management model. *Nursing Management, 20* (5), 26-29.

Department of Health & Social Services (DHSS), Division of Health. (1991). *1990 nursing home report.* Madison, WI: State of Wisconsin.

Department of Health & Social Services, Division of Health, Center for Health Statistics. (1990). *Use and analysis of health data.* Madison, WI: State of Wisconsin.

Ethridge, P. (1989). Professional nursing case management improves quality, access and costs. *Nursing Management, 20* (3), 30-35.

Goodwin, D. R. Nursing case management activities, how they differ between employment settings. *Journal of Nursing Administration, 24* (2), 29-34.

MacGregor-Burns, J. (1978). *Leadership.* New York: Harper & Row.

Marszalek-Gaucher, E., & Coffey, R. J. (1990). *Transforming healthcare organizations.* San Francisco: Jossey-Bass.

McCloskey, J. C. (1990). Two requirements for job contentment: autonomy and social integration. *Image 22* (3), 140-143.

Smith, J. (1991). Changing traditional nursing home roles to nursing case management. *Journal of Gerontological Nursing 17* (5), 32-39.

Resident Behavior and Psychotropic Drug Use Monitoring Review

TO: _____ _____
     Case Manager   Date

FOR: _____

     Resident

Current Psychotropic Medication(s) in use _____

_____ OR

Assessment for Initiating Medication Use

_____

Purpose/Rationale

1. To identify the most specific behavior of a resident who needs observation to determine course of treatment (i.e., nondrug vs. drug intervention or a combination of the two).
2. To identify how and for whom the behavior is a problem.
3. To analyze the behaviors and determine the possible causes or patterns of behavior.
4. To analyze documentation of behaviors, interventions and effectiveness. (If possible, monitor for at least one week before a psychotropic drug is started or changed.)
5. To determine what nondrug interventions may be or are the most helpful. (Nondrug interventions must be tried before psychotropic drug is given.)
6. To assess if the medication(s) prescribed is/are appropriate for the behaviors that you have identified.
7. To modify the resident's case plan.
8. To modify the CNA assignment sheet and the interdisciplinary monitoring sheet.
9. Provide information for appropriate follow-up and reevaluation.

I. IDENTIFICATION OF THE MOST SPECIFIC PROBLEMATIC BEHAVIOR FOR THIS RESIDENT

What exactly does the resident do/not do that affects one of these five things?
A) Safety of the resident
B) Threatening to resident him/her self
C) Potential or actual threat to other resident(s)
D) Interferes with staff's ability to deliver necessary care to the resident
E) Reduces or fails to maintain the resident's functional status, either physical or mental

IDENTIFY A, B, C, D, OR E THEN EXPLAIN

_____

_____

II. ANALYSIS OF BEHAVIOR

1) How long has this behavior been an issue?

_____

_____

2) Discussion with the family and/or past caregivers as well as review of the past history to determine "normal" pattern(s) of behavior.

_____

_____

3) Who is present during the behavior? Is there a pattern?

_____

4) Where and when does the behavior usually occur? Review of the Interdisciplinary Behavior Monitoring Sheet and discussion with other disciplines will be helpful. DEFINITELY DISCUSS WITH CNAs ASSIGNED TO RESIDENT.

_____

_____

5) List nondrug interventions to be tried (added to the Behavior Monitoring Record) and/or those attempted along with the effectiveness of the approaches.

_____

_____

_____

6) Review all current medications for possible side effects that may result in the type of behavior seen.

_____

_____

_____

Date/results of last Tardive Dyskinesia Monitoring _____

_____

Discuss review with pharmacist. _____

_____

_____

_____

7) Assess if/how the psychotropic medication(s) prescribed is/are appropriate for the behaviors that you have identified.
     Consult with pharmacist regarding:

Class of drug _____

Dosage _____

Length of continuous use _____

_____

8) Have all medical reasons for the behavior been ruled out or a coinciding diagnosis for the behaviors identified?
Discuss your review done thus far with the physician AND/OR
Discuss your intent to monitor current behavior before use of psychotropic drugs.
If appropriate, consider Psychiatric consult and/or option to be seen by the psychologist.

_____

_____

_____

_____

III. PLANS FOR FOLLOW-UP

1. Add to or change care plan or place Temporary Problem (Two-week duration or less).
2. Add to or change CNA assignment sheet.
3. Add to or change the Interdisciplinary Behavior Monitoring Sheet.
4. Evaluate behaviors and interventions after one week of monitoring using Section II questions/cues.
5. If nondrug interventions are unsuccessful redo Section II with new action plan and evaluation.
6. Should an antipsychotic drug be chosen as one of the approaches to be used for this resident an Informed Consent Form must be signed by the resident or the resident's family/DPOA (at this time only antipsychotics require an informed consent; however it is appropriate to discuss the review and your plans with the family/resident).
7. Reevaluate quarterly or sooner, if needed.

PLAN OF ACTION: (WITH NEW INTERVENTIONS OR MEDICATIONS AND DIAGNOSIS)

_____

_____

_____

_____

Case Manager _____ Date _____

FORWARD TO NURSE MANAGER FOR REVIEW

Nurse Manager _____ Date _____

COMMENTS: _____

_____

_____

_____

RETURN TO CASE MANAGER

EVALUATION _____

_____

_____

_____

Part Four

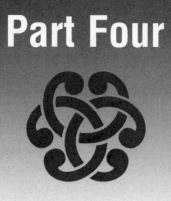

THE NURSE CASE MANAGEMENT PROCESS

Perhaps the central difference that distinguishes the professional nurse case management approach . . . lies in the context of the professional relationship between the client and the nurse case manager.

Judith Papenhausen

Part Four offers data on outcomes that have resulted from implementing nurse case management in various environments. Chapters 18 through 26 describe the cost savings to the organizations and the benefits of nurse case management to clients. These chapters identify data-collection processes, raise issues of design of new systems, and discuss problem-solving techniques that have been successful as well as those that have presented challenges.

Chapter 18

Case Management as a Response to Quality, Cost, and Access Imperatives

Kathleen A. Bower, DNSc, RN
Carol D. Falk, MS, RN

OVERVIEW

As case managers, nurses contribute to care coordination and significantly influence access, quality, and cost of health care.

• Maximum quality, appropriate access, and managed costs are three desired outcomes of today's health-care systems. When used in conjunction with care coordination strategies such as managed care, resource management, program management, and critical paths, case management can be an effective and efficient client care strategy that positively affects quality, access, and costs. Case management simplifies the care processes and comprehensively identifies clients' needs for resources and services, locating institutions within established networks that can provide the necessary services. This chapter explores the framework for case management and shows how this care strategy can be used to direct, coordinate, and provide care effectively over an episode of illness or across the continuum of care.

LINKS TO CARE COORDINATION

Case management is a means not the goal. It is one of several strategies for the effective and efficient coordination of client care. As a goal, care coordination ensures that the care of all clients is managed with minimal overlapping of and no gaps in roles and processes. Care coordination is a means for achieving better quality, cost, and access. Care coordination is also a framework for organizing multiple approaches including case management, care management, critical paths, program management, and resource management.

Although case management is an important strategy in coordinating client care, it cannot be used in isolation. To be effective, case management must be used in conjunction with other strategies such as the ones outlined above. In this way, case management becomes a focused, cost-effective approach to managing quality, cost, and access issues.

QUALITY, COST, AND ACCESS

To meet the needs of multiple constituencies, health-care systems must demonstrate maximal quality, managed costs, and accessibility.

Quality

Interest in quality has escalated in recent years with an emphasis on issues of definition and measurement.

A number of definitions of quality have emerged. One frequently used definition suggests that quality is meeting or exceeding customer expectations. Within the context of health care, however, "customer" may mean the patient or client, the family, or significant others, providers, payors (insurers and employers), and the community within which care takes place. In addition to the definition, the expectation or standard against which quality is measured is also complex and multidimensional and includes client satisfaction and clinical outcomes.

Various approaches to quality improvement have arisen within the past several years. Despite the apparent diversity, there are core principles common within each of the approaches. Those core quality improvement principles are:

1. Consumer orientation
2. Scientific, data-based approach
3. Teams and team work
4. Understanding and refining processes
   ▪ Simplifying processes
   ▪ Eliminating nonvalue added activities
5. Reducing variation
6. Managing the organization as a system (Bower & Falk, 1993).

In the current environment, there is a shift toward more intensively examining *outcomes* of care rather than the earlier emphasis on care processes. *Outcomes* can be defined as *"the anticipated, desired condition of the patient at discharge or at specified points along the episode/continuum"* (Bower, 1991). In conjunction with the concept of continuum, the outcomes movement dramatically affects approaches to defining and measuring quality. Specifically, these concepts mandate that quality measures be reoriented in terms of focus, time, and location.

Changing the focus of quality measures means that the traditional markers of quality (such as morbidity, mortality, readmissions, infection rates, complaints, unanticipated incidents, medication errors, length of stay, and charges) are no longer sufficient. Rather, the focus must be expanded to include such issues as health status, functionality (activities of daily living, family role, and job), pain management, symptom management, and mobility and activity. It also suggests that measurement must encompass client perception as well as objective findings.

Continuum- and episode-focused care also create the need to assess quality at points other than the traditional timeframe of acute care. Specifically, within finite, episode-based health issues, quality must be examined at various points along the episode and at the end of the episode. Likewise, for ongoing health issues, measurement is needed at defined points throughout the continuum, but there is no end point as there is with episode-focused care. To measure quality for both requires moving from the conventional, acute care foundation into the community, including the client's home, physicians' offices, clinic settings, and extended-care facilities.

In summarizing quality, it can be said that *quality* is *"the right care, at the right time, in the right place, by the right provider, and at the right cost"* (Falk, 1992). As such, it incorporates the concepts of appropriateness (Should it have been done?), effectiveness (Did it reach the desired results?), and efficiency (Was it done at the most appropriate cost?). Case management is one strategy supporting the achievement of quality outcomes.

Cost

Cost is a significant concern and, in the current environment, is often directly related to survival. Cost measurement depends upon the perspective of the audience. Clients look at cost from multiple dimensions, such as money (direct and indirect), time, and convenience. Clients also tend to relate perceived value and cost.

Providers also look at costs from many perspectives. Key perspectives are the relationship between costs and reimbursement and the contributions of individual components to the overall cost.

The relationship between cost and reimbursement is increasingly essential as the reimbursement system moves from a charge-based or discounted charge-based methodology toward per-case and capitated approaches. The latter methodologies provide a financial incentive to establish continuum-focused care by reducing the emphasis on costs of the fragmented components of care and focusing on the whole. Case-based and capitated reimbursement methodologies give providers more control and freedom over how the health-care dollars are spent for individual clients as well as populations of clients. Simultaneously, these reimbursement approaches incur more risk for the providers, increasing their accountability for the total dollars and for the associated outcomes of care.

Payor perspectives of cost are changing in the current environment. The definition of payor has shifted radically within the three decades. Initially, payors were either individual clients or a limited number of commercial insurance plans, such as Blue Cross/Blue Shield. The onset of Medicare immediately and dramatically introduced the federal and state governments into the payor world. Driven by the need to manage costs more effectively, multiple players have entered the payor arena, including health maintenance organizations and preferred provider organizations. Recently, employers again shifted the concept of payor by negotiating directly with providers for health care for their employees. Payors are seeking managed costs yet demand that quality parameters be met as well. Increasingly, the payors are examining total costs, including the entire episode and continuum of care. They are also demanding that satisfactory outcomes be demonstrated in addition to cost effectiveness, again demonstrating the consistent interaction between cost and quality.

Access

Access, defined as *availability of resources and services,* can be viewed from both a quality and a cost standpoint. From a quality perspective, access means that the resources and services are appropriate to client and family need. The cost standpoint indicates that the needed resources and services are readily accessible and are not inadequate nor excessive but sufficient to meet client and family need.

Case management has emerged in this complicated environment as one approach to quality, cost, and access imperatives. The discussion will now turn to a description of case management.

CASE MANAGEMENT

A strategy for care coordination, *case management* is ultimately an approach to managing quality, access, and cost. It can be defined as *"a role and process that focuses on procuring, negotiating, and coordinating the care, services, and resources needed by individuals with complex issues throughout an episode or continuum"* (Bower & Falk, 1993). There are many goals served by case management, including:

- Enhancing the health status and functionality of clients;
- Maximizing client access to health-care services;
- Cost-effective resource use; and
- The integration and coordination of service delivery activities provided by multiple disciplines (Falk, 1994).

Conceptually, case management can be summarized in five principles. Those principles suggest that case management:

1. Focuses on clients and families with complex issues;
2. Involves negotiating, coordinating, and procuring services and resources needed by the focus clients and families;
3. Entails using a clinical reasoning process;
4. Involves developing a network based on multiple, interdisciplinary relationships; and
5. Is episode- or continuum-focused (Bower & Falk, 1993).

CLIENT POPULATIONS

As the first principle indicates, case management focuses on clients and families with complex issues. Case management is a resource because it involves the creation of distinct positions; therefore, it is best focused on individuals most in need of an additional, intensive resource. This tends to be people with complex issues.

In designing case management systems, acuity is less an issue than is complexity. Complexity is related to the interaction of multiple concerns, including health, social, economic, spiritual, psychological, emotional, and environmental. It is common for individuals with complex issues to receive their care from multiple providers and in multiple sites, increasing the likelihood of fragmentation, overlaps, or gaps in care. As a result, these individuals are at risk for increased use of resources, for difficulties in self-management of disease processes, and for less than optimal clinical and cost outcomes. They also are typically the individuals who require above average amounts of staff time and effort.

One useful approach is reflected in the idea that "all patients need their care managed; not every patient needs a case manager" (Bower & Falk, 1992). This means that a system for care coordination encompasses various strategies. Some of those strategies are outlined in Box 18-1. A well-integrated system for care coordination of all clients includes the roles and processes of case management, care management, program management, and resource management. In addition, a plan of care is needed for all clients to promote continuity and consistency of plan. For patternable and predictable client populations, an multidisciplinary team can prospectively prepare a standardized plan that is used as a template to address the usual needs of a defined client population. The standardized plan is then modified to meet the needs of individual clients. *Critical paths* are an example of this approach. The remainder of the clients who are not appropriate for critical paths require the concurrent development of an individualized plan to reflect their complex, changing, or unpredictable needs. Within this framework, case management is a supplemental strategy applied in approximately 20% or less of the total client population, whereas the other four strategies (care management, program management, resource management, and critical paths) are used in much larger proportions of the client population.

The Episode and Continuum Nature of Case Management

The episode and continuum nature of case management is important because it distinguishes case management

BOX 18-1
STRATEGIES FOR CARE COORDINATION

Care management (or patient care coordination) is the process and system developed to organize and orchestrate the care of all patients within a specific geographic area or discipline in such a way that it is directed toward meeting desired or anticipated outcomes within an appropriate length of stay and resource utilization.

Resource management is the process of identifying, confirming, coordinating and negotiating benefits and resources for the patient. This includes screening for benefits eligibility; communicating with the patient and the health-care team, especially when benefits and the plan of care are out of alignment; communicating and negotiating with payers regarding the anticipated plan of care; identifying postdischarge needs and benefits; and arranging for postdischarge care and community resources.

Program management is the process of developing a formal system of care, including services and resources, for an identified population of patients with similar needs, often over an episode or continuum. Within program management, consistent availability of services is developed and a means of patient access to the program is established.

Case management is a clinical system that focuses on the accountability of an individual or group for coordinating a patient's care (or group of patients) across an *episode or continuum* of care; ensuring and facilitating the achievement of quality, clinical and financial outcomes; *negotiating, procuring, and coordinating services and resources needed by the patient and family;* intervening at key points (or significant variances from the anticipated plan of care) for individual patients; addressing and resolving consistent issues that have negative quality or cost impact; and creating opportunities and systems to enhance outcomes.

Critical paths are a grid that outlines categories of interventions on one axis (usually the vertical) and time (or other indicators of clinical progression) on the other. They are developed for defined, homogeneous patient populations by a multidisciplinary team that represents as much of the episode or continuum as possible. They are used to coordinate, plan, deliver, monitor, and review care concurrently by individuals from all disciplines. By comparing the patient's actual status with that anticipated on the critical path, variance can be identified, addressed, and resolved at the individual and aggregate levels. Aggregate variance is used retrospectively for continuous quality improvement (CQI).

Copyright 1994, The Center for Case Management. Developed in conjunction with C. Falk, Carondelet Health Care.

from other strategies for coordinating care and, in many respects, defines the focus of the case manager's role.

An episode is finite; it has a defined timeframe. Alternatively, continuum-related health-care issues may have a defined beginning but may continue into infinity. For example, a client undergoing a total hip replacement experiences an *episode* of care. Most chronically ill individuals (for example individuals with chronic obstructive pulmonary disease [COPD]) have health issues that extend over the continuum. It is also possible to have episodes within a continuum. Returning to the example involving clients with COPD, it is suggested that, although the trajectory of their underlying illness extends throughout the remainder of their lives, they may experience exacerbations or episodic acute problems such as pneumonia or acute respiratory failure. The continuum nature of chronic illness implies that case management design must facilitate supporting selective clients and their families for extended periods of time, perhaps even years. The distinction between episode and continuum is an important design consideration for case management, specifically when planning for the duration of the case manager-client relationship. In continuum-based practices, that relationship may extend over several months or years. In episode-based case management, the relationship with the client is likely to extend over the course of days to a few months.

Describing case management as episode- or continuum-based prevents it from being confined to a given geographical area and positions the case manager to work with individual clients and their families when and where they most need support. As such, case management *is not* a unit-based system for care but an approach that links various settings and geographic areas where care is provided. This has major implications for enabling the case manager to coordinate care and influence quality, access, and cost.

The Case Management Network

Within case management, the need to develop a network moves the process away from an isolated, solo practitioner perspective and toward an integrated, interdisciplinary process. Case managers are only as successful as the networks and relationships they build. The network can best be visualized as a wheel, with the case manager and the client in the hub connected via spokes to the needed services and resources. An example of such a network is provided in Figure 18-1.

The network may be established on a more fixed basis in situations where the case manager's practice focuses on a specific care issue or client population. It is then modified by including disciplines and resources within or external to the organization to meet the needs of the individual client. In this situation, the case manager and the network constituents have a relationship at both the formal and informal levels which allows client needs to be met rapidly. When the case manager's practice is of a more general nature, the network will be established for individual clients. Although it is equally effective, the process of developing the network in this situation is likely to take more time and effort. In both situations, the network enables case managers to access services and resources needed by the individuals in their caseloads with maximal efficiency and effectiveness.

Case Management and a Clinical Reasoning Process

The last principle listed involves the use of a clinical reasoning process. That process includes:
- Referral and screening;
- Assessment of needs, issues, resources and goals;
- Definition and integration of goals;
- Coordination and implementation of a plan through direct or indirect interventions;
- Evaluating the effectiveness and efficiency of the plan; and
- Revising the plan based on changing needs and assessments (Bower & Falk, 1993).

This clinical reasoning process continually focuses the case management strategy on clients and their needs, creating a highly individualized response. In effect, case management is a needs-response approach to addressing the complex needs of individuals at risk. All clinicians use most, if not all, of the process outlined above; the exception may be the referral and screening phase. What makes case management different from other approaches to care is (1) the focus on highly complex individuals, and (2) its episode and continuum nature.

THE INFLUENCE OF CASE MANAGEMENT ON QUALITY, COST, AND ACCESS

Case management affects each of the dimensions of quality, access, and cost through the process of care coordination. The influence of case management on those dimensions will be described in this section.

Contribution to Quality

Case management enhances the likelihood that quality outcomes will be attained. It is an intense process that focuses on the client as an individual, as a customer. In effect, case management provides a partner for the client and the client's family to problem solve issues as they arise and to smooth the course of care. A process-oriented strategy, case management supports eliminating or at least minimizing nonvalue

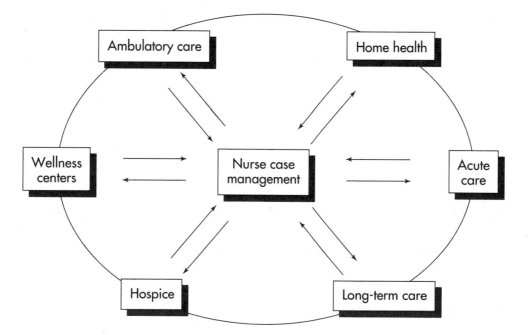

FIG. 18-1   The nursing network (Courtesy of Carondelet St. Mary's Hospital and Health Center, Tucson, AZ)

added activities and assists in simplifying the care processes for the focus clients. Although managed costs are a desired outcome of case management, the primary focus is on clinical outcomes, including functionality and enhanced self-management of diseases and symptoms.

Because it is an episode and continuum-based process, case management facilitates assessing and measuring outcomes along the entire trajectory of care. Case managers have the opportunity to evaluate client status at various points of the care process, often extending over a long period and within the multiple sites in which clients receive care.

In case management, quality management is both a concurrent and retrospective process. Concurrently, case managers use the clinical reasoning process to evaluate the effects of care in view of established goals. Retrospectively, issues experienced by clients within the case-managed population are examined for patterns and trends and addressed at a system level. Essentially, case management operationalizes quality management processes.

Contribution to Access

Case management also creates opportunities for managing appropriate *access* to care. Using the clinical reasoning process, case managers comprehensively identify client needs for services and resources within the context of established goals and desired outcomes. The network component of case management creates and facilitates the link to needed resources and services. In some situations, case managers advocate earlier access to care when the needs are less acute and intense and, therefore, less expensive. By working with clients and their families over time (i.e., either an episode or throughout the continuum), case managers can identify patterns in illness and client responses to interventions and situations. Through the resulting relationship, they then have the opportunity to identify in a timely manner those changes in patterns that indicate a deterioration in the client's condition or an ineffective response to treatment.

In addition, case managers can reflect back to clients an example-based description of their patterns to support positive changes in them. This process enhances client knowledge about the disease process, symptom management, wellness promotion, and health-care system use. In this way, clients acquire the skills they need to identify appropriate points and time for accessing the health-care system.

The case management network also facilitates appropriate and timely access. Specifically, case managers go directly to the resource or service needed. This frequently involves negotiating with the payor. In many situations, the case manager knows exactly who to contact within the service agency to effect the desired results. This enhances access to services and resources to the clients at the most opportune point in their care trajectory. The relationship that evolves between the case manager, the network members, and the client fosters creative solutions to the unique issues that case-managed clients present. Those creative solutions can often be beyond the usual scope of response by the providers or the payors.

Contribution to Managing Costs

Cost is influenced by case management through all of the processes outlined earlier. In addition, because case managers procure, negotiate, and coordinate needed services and resources, costs are managed more effectively. By focusing on clients who typically incur high costs, case managers have the effect of reducing the costs of care, especially at the more expensive end of the range. Rather than cost shifting (for example, from acute care to ambulatory care), case managers work within an episode or continuum. This enables them to identify when care will be most effectively provided, what care is needed, and to link the care to the client efficiently at the time of need.

Crisis management is expensive. Individuals in crisis often need more and intensive resources than at other times. There are fewer options available to resolve the situation. Resources and services must be brought to bear on the situation in an unplanned manner. Case management seeks to avoid or prevent crisis when possible. In essence, "case managers seek to keep individuals out of crisis and, when in crisis, to manage it" (Falk, 1994).

By having a long-term perspective of clients and their issues, case managers can negotiate having resources available at nontraditional times and in nontraditional places. They have the opportunity, time and mandate to craft new and different approaches to the complex issues presented by clients.

By negotiating with payor sources, they can create options that might not otherwise have been feasible. Case managers often create options and possibilities that are not activated in the usual course of care. Case managers smooth transitions from one care site to another and from one provider to another. Transitions are periods when care can become fragmented and disjointed, creating the possibility of increased costs. Case managers coordinate the client's progression throughout the episode or continuum, from one care site to another, from one provider to another.

Although various client populations can benefit from case management services, perhaps the most responsive populations are the chronically ill. These individuals are the most susceptible to the negative results of fragmented care and who are the most fragile in terms of need for coordination of care. They are also the individuals who experience repeated admissions to acute care and who frequently present for care in physicians' offices, clinics, and other care sites. This results in higher costs over time, even when hospitalizations do not always result.

Many of the issues within a case management practice are related to clients' ability to manage their own care and the associated symptoms. When clients experience difficulty in or barriers to managing their own care, they need the support of a clinician, often in the role of a case manager, who can support them through those situations.

CONCLUSION

Case management is emerging as a popular approach to coordinating the care of clients. It is not a stand-alone strategy but one that complements the other approaches to care coordination including care management, program management, resource management, and critical paths. The ideal design incorporates each strategy and focuses it on the most appropriate client population.

Rather than use case management for all clients, it is best focused on those most in need and at risk for experiencing negative consequences when care is not coordinated. Clients selected for case management have needs that extend beyond those of the usual clients within a population. They are the most vulnerable to issues arising from inadequate or poorly timed access to care and services, and they are most likely to be outliers when quality and cost are measured. In these situations, case management becomes a resource and a strategy to more effectively manage access to quality and cost of care.

REFERENCES

Bower, K. (1991). Unpublished case management seminar material.* South Natick, MA: The Center for Case Management.
Bower, K., & Falk, C. (1992). Unpublished case management seminar material.* Tucson, AZ: Carondelet Health Care System.
Bower, K., & Falk, C. (1993). Unpublished case management seminar material.* Tucson, AZ: Carondelet Health Care System.
Falk, C. (1992). Unpublished case management seminar material.* Tucson, AZ: Carondelet Health Care System.
Falk, C. (1994). Unpublished case management seminar material.* Tucson, AZ: Carondelet Health Care System.

---

*These references to works by Kathleen Bower and/or Carol Falk are excerpts from copyrighted materials and require authors' permission for use.

Chapter 19

Risk Identification: Management versus Avoidance

Joann Clough, MAOM, RN

OVERVIEW

Nurses play a key role in the risk-identification process, which aims to manage risk rather than avoid it.

Risk identification is a process of discerning relevant risk groups and targeting programs and services. This process is especially beneficial in managing the health care of those with chronic illness. The need for risk identification is increased as health-care organizations enter into financial risk arrangements with payors and other health-care providers. This chapter will assist the reader to understand the indicators for high risk and the various components of the risk-identification process. This will be accomplished partially via a thorough review of the literature on indicators of risk for high-service utilizations. In addition, a case study will highlight the experience of a health-care organization in the Southwest that used risk identification as a method of managing the health care of enrollees in a capitated health plan.

Risk identification is a process of identifying and intervening with individuals who are at risk for high service utilization. This chapter will explore various facets of risk identification, including a literature review of the indicators of high risk, risk identification methods, the steps involved in the risk identification process, a health-care organization's experience with risk identification, and considerations for health-care organizations implementing a risk-identification system.

INDICATORS OF HIGH RISK

Research studies have demonstrated that the primary indicators of risk for high utilization of health resources are in the following areas:

- Previous service utilization
- Perceived health
- Type and number of conditions/pathologies related to functional ability
- Number and type of medications
- Age

Previous service utilization was one of the most common findings among researchers.

Previous Service Utilization

In 1985, Levkoff et al. conducted an extensive study that looked at health-care utilization among 863 elderly HMO enrollees for whom there was at least one full year of utilization data. The distribution of inpatient admissions showed that the majority of members

(86%) were not admitted to an acute care hospital. At the other end of the spectrum, 3.5% of members accounted for 45.4% of all inpatient admissions.

Hospitalizations accounted for the largest proportion of health-care expenditures. A similar pattern of utilization was found among hospital outpatient visits. Over three quarters of the sample did not make any hospital outpatient visits, whereas 3.8% of the sample made almost 40% of all outpatient visits. A disproportionate percentage of all physician visits was also found, with 13.4% of the sample making almost one-third of visits. The number of years since the last hospitalization was the second most important predictor of expenditures, with individuals who were hospitalized most recently at higher risk for increased expenditures.

Two other researchers found previous utilization to be an important predictor of future service use. According to Wasson et al. (1987), those clients averaging 19.2 hospital days per year would be called the high-use group, and all others the not-high group. In a study done by Boult et al. in 1993, a hospital admission or more than six physician visits in the previous year indicated a risk for future hospitalization.

Perceived Health

Individual's health perceptions also influence utilization of health-care services as found by Connelly et al. in 1989. The analysis revealed that clients with low health perceptions make more office visits, more telephone calls to the physician, and had more office charges than clients with higher scores. The study concluded that health perceptions are an important factor contributing to the use of health care by clients, regardless of the client's actual physical health. In a separate study, Boult et al. (1993) also found poor self-rated health to be an indicator for repeated hospital admissions.

Type and Number of Conditions and Pathologies

Type of diagnosis and the presence of multiple conditions or pathologies have been closely linked to functional disability as indicators for risk. Wasson et al. (1987) found that a greater number of diagnoses or major mobility and dependency limitations were generally associated with a greater likelihood for using medical care. The most common diagnoses in the high-use group were degenerative arthritis (54%), hypertension (49%), atherosclerosis (47%), and chronic respiratory disease (28%).

Further definition of groups of individuals who had inappropriately high health-care utilization was attempted by Smith et al. in 1986. The authors studied a group of chronically ill clients to determine their characteristics, symptoms, functional health status, and amount of health-care utilization. They found this group to have multiple complaints and a history of multiple medical examinations. The group was functionally disabled, spending an average of seven days ill in bed each month, and perceived themselves as severely ill. They were willing to undergo multiple hospitalizations, diagnostic studies, and operations. Their health-care charges were extraordinary, averaging $4,700 annually. The average hospital care expenditure per year was $2,382 as compared with the U.S. per capita hospital care expenditure of $385 in 1980.

Another study that supports multiple chronic conditions along with functional limitations was done by Rice in 1986. Rice found the number of hospital days per 1,000 persons rises from 314, for those with one chronic condition causing limitation of activity, to 441 for those with two causes, and 570 for those with three or more causes. Forty-six percent of the elderly who were limited in activity because of a chronic condition accounted for 63% of physician contacts, 71% of hospitalizations, and 83% of all the days that older people spent in bed because of a health condition.

Number and Type of Medications

Levkoff et al. found in their 1985 study that the number of reported medical conditions was not statistically related to expenditure rate, whereas the number of drugs taken for those conditions was a significant predictor. In fact, these researchers found that the total number of drugs taken by an individual was by far the most significant predictor of average annual per capita expenditures. Their research demonstrated that the number of drugs a person reports taking is a more precise indicator of utilization than the individual's self-reported number of conditions. This could be related to more accurate reporting of the number of medications they are taking versus the medical conditions that require medication use. Alternatively, medication use may serve a a proxy for severity of illness. Some sufferers of heart disease may, for example, require medication, whereas others are able to control their condition through exercise and diet. Individuals whose illness warrants medication usually have more severe illness than those not requiring medication. Levkoff et al. found that the three classes of medications most highly associated with average annual per capita expenditures are cardiac, diuretic, and antiinflammatory drugs, those most often prescribed for heart disease and arthritis.

Age

Age was found to be the only social demographic variable statistically associated with average annual per capita expenditure in the 1985 study by Levkoff et al. The average annual per capita expenditure increased from $1,031 for individuals 60 to 64 years of age to $2,656 for persons 80 to 84 years old—an increase of 158%. Research indicated that the prevalence of chronic conditions increases with age, and therefore the use associated with these conditions also increases with age. Age was also an indicator of repeated hospitalizations in the research done by Boult et al. in 1993.

RISK IDENTIFICATION METHODS

Research has demonstrated that there are certain health measures that can predict high utilization of health services. How then, can these risk indicators most efficiently and accurately be determined? Researchers have studied this question and have found self-report methods to have been successful.

Ferrano (1980) found self-assessments of health to be good measures of health status. Weinberger et al. (1986) found them to be an economical means of gathering data on the health of older people and useful in predicting hospital admission and nursing home placement in older persons. Siu et al. (1993) concluded that brief measures of health and self-reported physical functioning in persons over 85 years of age have acceptable validity and may be appropriate to use as a substitute for the costly collection of observed performance measures.

Levkoff et al. also strongly recommended the adoption of a self-report health questionnaire among prepaid plans that provide care to the elderly. They found the questionnaire they used in their study to be relatively easy to administer and an inexpensive method of identifying individuals who were likely to incur high health-care expenditures.

RISK IDENTIFICATION PROCESS

The National Chronic Care Consortium (NCCC), an alliance of 24 leading health networks representing 16 states was formulated in 1991. Members of the NCCC are dedicated to the efforts required to transform the delivery of chronic care services. Risk identification has been identified by the NCCC as an essential component of chronic care services. A task force was implemented in 1994 to work on risk identification. In an interim report compiled by the NCCC (1995), the task force defines *risk identification* as a *three-step process that results in specific interventions*. The three steps include risk appraisal, risk screening, and risk evaluation (Figure 19-1).

The risk identification process needs to be initiated when a person or enrollee enters into a relationship with a health plan or a health-care provider network. Enrollees bring their health, knowledge, skill, and abilities to the relationship. It is imperative to the success of the health plan that those enrollees who are at risk for poor outcomes be identified and linked with appropriate interventions.

Risk Appraisal

The first step of the risk-identification process is *risk appraisal*. The risk appraisal questionnaire should be given to all enrollees and should separate the well group from the chronic disease or functional limitation group. Interventions targeted at the well group would consist of those related to primary prevention and health promotion, (e.g., diet, exercise, immunizations).

Risk Screening

The chronic disease and functional limitation groups then enter into the second phase of the risk-identification process, *risk screening*. Risk screening separates those individuals who had the presence of high-risk indicators from those who did not. Interventions directed toward the chronic functionally impaired group not considered to be high risk include secondary prevention activities, (e.g., early detection, education, and aggressive treatment). Primary prevention and health promotion interventions can also be applicable to this group.

Risk Evaluation

The third step of the risk-identification process is *risk evaluation*. This step is usually performed by a health professional for the purpose of targeting specific tertiary interventions. Tertiary interventions are aimed at maintenance and decreasing the modifiable risk. These interventions could be as simple as referring to a home-delivered meals program or as complex as providing comprehensive case management.

This author has found that risk identification is often confused with comprehensive assessment, e.g., geriatric assessment. Geriatric assessment can be an intervention related to risk identification but is not the starting point of the process. Risk identification can be interwoven into existing interdisciplinary services and programs as an ongoing process that needs to be repeated as an individual's health status is likely to decline.

A CASE STUDY IN RISK IDENTIFICATION: THE LUTHERAN HEALTHCARE NETWORK EXPERIENCE

In 1989, Lutheran Healthcare Network (LHN) implemented case management as their client care delivery system—a comprehensive approach to the management of client care across the continuum. Components of the LHN model include critical pathways, total care pathways, coordination of care across the continuum, case management beyond the walls, and wellness centers.

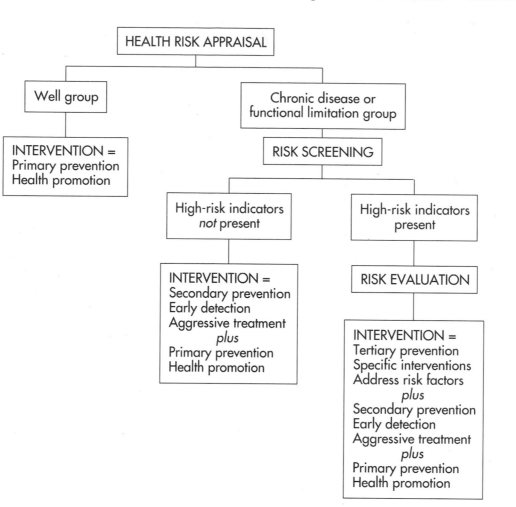

FIG. 19-1   Risk identification process

Case management beyond the walls was implemented in 1990 to work with high-risk Medicare beneficiaries to reduce health-care costs. High-risk clients were generally identified through hospital discharge planning based on the following criteria: frequent admissions, certain types of chronic illness (e.g., CHF, COPD), lack of support systems, and history of inability to comply with medical plan of care.

Periodic financial studies were done to determine the success of LHN case management. One such study was done in May of 1993 (Table 19-1). The analysis included 336 clients. These clients were compared against themselves, looking at equal time frames of utilization before and after case management was initiated. The before-case-management time period started with the date of client enrollment and ended May 6, 1993. The before-case-management time period equaled the after-case-management time period. For example, if a client had been on case management for six months before May 6, 1993, the before-time period would have started November 5, 1992.

The study showed positive changes in admission patterns for the clients who were enrolled in case management including a 28% reduction in emergency room visits, a 40% reduction in inpatient visits, and a 20% increase in utilization of outpatient services. Length of stay was reduced 0.26 days as a result of case management which equalled a total savings of 78 days. The study also showed that case management intervention reduced costs to LHN by $824,942. The cost comparison time period was for the number of months that the client was on service. If the client had been on case management for six months, then the cost of care for the six months before case management was compared with the cost of care after case management. The cost of providing the care was $160,000.

In January of 1993, LHN entered into a Medicare risk contract whereby the payor, selected physicians, and LHN became partners in assuming financial risk for meeting the health-care needs of the enrolled population. Case management was a key to success with this contract due to the positive financial impact that had

TABLE 19-1   Financial outcomes of LHN case management

	Before case management		After case management		Results of case management
	NUMBER OF ADMISSIONS	AVERAGE COST	NUMBER OF ADMISSIONS	AVERAGE COST	COST SAVINGS
ER	219	193	158	256	1,819
Inpatient	496 (LOS 7.38)	4,070	299 (LOS 7.12)	3,950	837,670
Outpatient	283	339	341	324	−14,547
				Totals	824,942

already been demonstrated. The case management team identified an opportunity to implement a more proactive approach to identifying high-risk individuals, whereby enrollees would be screened to determine "risks."

The Health Needs Assessment tool (see Appendix 19-A) was developed by nurses in the case management department based on their experience with high-risk individuals. The nurses knew from experience which health indicators could be intervened upon by them to prevent or reduce hospitalizations. These indicators were in areas of health that included chronic illnesses and conditions, patterns of hospital usage, numbers of prescriptions and non-prescription drugs, support systems, self-rated health, and instrumental activities of daily living (IADLs).

Implementing the Risk-Identification Process

The risk-identification process began in January 1993 with the screening tool being mailed to all new enrollees of the health plan. The enrollee completes the questionnaire and sends it back for the case manager to score (see scoring guidelines in Appendix 19-B). A combined score of greater than 10, or a positive response to questions concerning the enrollee's need for information regarding their chronic condition and medication usage will result in further risk evaluation via a phone call from a case manager.

A variety of interventions may result from the risk evaluation. The case manager will gather additional information from the enrollee to determine the most appropriate action. Frequently, the enrollee needs questions answered regarding the chronic disease, condition, or medications. Other times, the case manager provides information regarding the health plan, (e.g., drug formulary, importance of primary care physician, and appropriate use of the emergency department). Many of the enrollees contacted receive information related to the community resources that are available to them. Some of the individuals need more intensive follow-up and an ongoing plan of care.

Depending on the extent of the need and the functional ability of the enrollee, the case manager will refer the individual to the wellness center. Wellness centers are used as much as possible for follow-up because they are less resource intensive. The enrollee comes to the wellness center for an appointment with a nurse practitioner and a plan of care for education related to self-care management is implemented. A case manager is indicated when the enrollee cannot get to a wellness center or when more extensive education and self-management needs are apparent.

The return rate of the risk screening questionnaire continues to be 70%. A study done in June of 1994 demonstrated that 35% of those that returned the risk screening tool received risk evaluation and intervention, with 3% to 5% being assigned to a case manager.

LHN is concerned with the 30% of the population who do not return the form. Are high-risk individuals being missed? What are the cost and benefit of determining who the 30% are and attempting other methods of screening them? Krmpotic (1994) studied enrollees who had completed the Health Needs Assessment and found that there was a direct correlation between an enrollee's risk score and the overall cost of the enrollee to the plan. Based on these findings LHN is developing a plan for a second mailing to the enrollees who did not respond.

Risk Identification in Maternal and Child Populations

Most of the work completed to date has been in the area of risk identification in the elderly. Lutheran Healthcare Network (LHN) has broadened its focus to include the maternal-child population when it entered into a shared-risk contract with Arizona's Health Care Cost Containment System (AHCCCS), Arizona's Medicaid system. Eighty five percent of the population for whom LHN is responsible in this contract is composed of mothers and children.

A "High Risk Maternal Case Management Referral Form" (see Appendix 19-C) was developed and implemented in 1994. This form is generally initiated by physicians or the managed care office when a high-risk pregnancy enrollee presents. Any one item checked on the form warrants a high-risk referral. The maternal case manager makes contact with the high-risk mother for further assessment and implementation of a plan of care.

The maternal and child case management program has developed a second form to identify mothers at risk. This questionnaire, called a "Prenatal Health Assessment" (see Appendix 19-D), will be completed via a phone call to all women on the plan who are pregnant and who may not be referred by the physician. The goal of the form is to identify women who could benefit from education and follow-up from the maternal case manager.

A pediatric form called the "Pediatric Case Management Referral Form" has also been developed to be used by physicians, emergency rooms, and managed-care staff in identifying high-risk children who could benefit from case management. This tool (see Appendix 19-E) is currently being implemented.

Considerations for Risk Identification and Assessment

Risk identification is a fairly new concept. Health-care providers involved in the process have learned effective strategies to aid in the development of risk identification. The last segment of this chapter will discuss several important aspects of risk identification that need to be considered when implementing the process.

Type of risk. Each health-care provider needs to determine the type of risk needing to be modified. The LHN example demonstrated the desire to minimize the risk of costly utilization of hospital resources. Other health-care providers may want to identify risk of nursing home placement or risk of increased disability. The questions asked will be directed at the type of risk to be identified.

Linking risk with interventions. It is important to be aware of the types of interventions that are available as a result of risk identification. The intent of the risk tool is to identify relevant risk groups for targeting specific interventions in order to reduce modifiable risk. Interventions can be at the service or program level. The LHN example demonstrated case management as a programmatic intervention for a person at risk for hospitalization. Establishing and communicating advanced directives is an example of a service intervention that could enhance quality of life and reduce health-care costs.

Screening process. When determining the screening process, it is essential to look at the cost-benefit of each proposed method. The method must be designed so that the yield of people at risk is high. For this rea-

son, mailing the tool is a commonly chosen method; however, when the tool is mailed there is always the issue of nonreturn. Each health-care organization must decide for itself which method is the most resource-conserving to reach the greatest number of individuals.

The length of time between initiating the risk questionnaire and interventions based on the response also needs to be considered. For example, in the early stages of the LHN risk-identification process, the time frame between mailing the questionnaire and the case manager interventions was as high as six months after the health plan enrollment date. This time frame is not acceptable when trying to identify and intervene proactively with high-risk individuals, because excess expenditures have already taken place. The system was refined to complete the process within six to eight weeks, which was still longer than desired. An alternate method to mailing the questionnaires would be calling all enrollees on the phone, which is resource intensive. Even though there is not an established benchmark for turnaround time, each health-care provider needs to find the system for them that identifies individuals as quickly as possible while using the least resources.

Tool presentation. The development of a risk screening tool must include consideration of both content and format. The content will be those risk factors or indicators known to be related to adverse events. Format characteristics contribute positively or negatively to a tool's performance and effectiveness. It is important to ask the following questions when developing the tool.

1. What is the layout and appearance of the tool? Large block letters with legible typeface is preferable. Wide margins with large amounts of white space make the tool less intimidating. Directions and key phrases need to be in bold type. The tool should be single sided or stapled to open like a book.

2. What is the estimated time to complete the tool? The questionnaire should be as short as possible to separate out the high-risk group. Remember, there will be further evaluation for those determined to be at high risk.

3. Is the rationale clear? The reason for why the information is being collected and how the information will be used needs to be clearly explained on the questionnaire or in the cover letter.

4. Is the tool easy to read and complete? The responses should require minimal writing either by checking or circling. The sentences should be short and crisp. Jargon and clinical terms should be avoided with language that is sensitive to client perceptions.

5. What is the flow of the questions? There should be a friendly tone to the questions. The questionnaire

should start with questions that make most sense to the enrollee and deal with sensitive or controversial questions later.

Rescreening. There is currently much discussion among providers related to the issue of rescreening. Should it be done on a yearly basis, after hospitalization, or does the cost of rescreening outweigh the benefits? No studies have been published to date that demonstrate the cost-benefit relationship of rescreening. Health-care organizations embarking on risk identification will need to determine for themselves the point at which resources expended for rescreening outweigh the dollars saved.

Integrating risk information into the health record. It is essential that the information discovered in the risk identification and assessment process be included in the health record so that other providers within the system have access to the information. At LHN, the Health Needs Assessment questionnaire is copied and mailed to the primary care physician, along with notes from the case manager. Ideally, the information would be entered into an automated system whereby it could be linked to other demographic and clinical information related to the enrollee.

CONCLUSION

Case management has been born in an era when there is impetus to implement strategies that increase the quality of health care and at the same time reduce the costs. Case management effectiveness is dependent on early identification of those people who are at high risk for declining health and high utilization of health-care resources. A managed approach to care whereby there is an enrolled population provides an opportunity for case managers to screen the entire population for those at risk for hospitalization.

Risk identification in this context is a new concept of risk—not one to avoid but one to acknowledge and manage. The goal of risk identification is to modify or eliminate risk through interventions that foster independence and self-care, enhances quality of life, prevent

or reduce functional decline, and reduce hospitalization, nursing home placement, and death. Risk identification is a three-tiered process consisting of health risk appraisal, risk screening, and risk evaluation. Each step of the process results in the assignment of the enrollee to a risk category with corresponding interventions.

Health-care organizations interested in managing risk need to consider several components of the process: (1) the type of risk they want to manage, (2) interventions that will decrease the modifiable risk, (3) the type of screening process that will be used, (4) tool layout, (5) if and when rescreening will be done, and (6) integrating risk information with demographic and clinical information.

REFERENCES

Boult, C., Thereat, B., McCaffery, D., Could, L., Hernandez, R., & Krulewitch, H. (1993). *Journal of the American Geriatric Society, 41,* 811-817.

Connelly, J., Philbrick, J., Smith, R., Kaiser, D., & Wymer, A. (1989). Health perceptions of primary care patients and the influence of health care utilization. *Medical Care, 27* (3), 99-108.

Ferrano, K. (1980). Self-ratings of health among the old and the old-old. *Journal of Health and Social Behavior, 21,* 377-383.

Krmpotic, D. (1994). [Health needs assessment and cost outcomes]. Unpublished raw data.

Levkoff, S., Wettle, T., Coakley, E., Jordon, H., Hartline, D., & Szmusszkovicz, D. (1985). Predictors of service utilization by Medicare HMO enrollees. *HMO Practice Research, 2* (2), 58-65.

National Chronic Care Consortium (NCCC). (1995). *Risk identification: exploring a conceptual framework and identifying implementation issues.* Author. Bloomington: Minn.

Rice, E. (1986). The medical care system: past trends and future predictions. *New York Medical Quarterly, 6,* 39-70.

Siu, A., Hays, R., Ouslander, J., Osterwell, D., Valdez, R., Krynski, M. E., & Gross, A. (1993). Measuring functioning and health in the very old. *Journal of Gerontology, 48,* 10-14.

Smith, R., Monson, R., & Ray, D. (1986). Patients with multiple unexplained symptoms. *Archives of Internal Medicine, 146,* 69-72.

Wasson, J., Sawigne, A., Balestia, D., Mogielnicki, P., Nelson, E., Frey, W., & Webster, S. (1987). Capitation for medical care. *Medical Care, 25* (10), 1002-1005.

Weinberger, M., Darrell, J., Tierney, W., Martz, B., Hiner, S., & Barker, J. (1986). Self-related health as a predictor of hospital admission and nursing home placement in elderly housing tenants. *American Journal of Public Health, 76,* 457-459.

Lutheran Healthcare Network
Health Needs Assessment

Name _____

Street Address _____

City _____ Zip Code _____

Telephone _____

Primary Care or Family Physician's Name _____

1. Has a doctor ever told you that you have any of the following conditions? Circle all that apply.
   A. High blood pressure/Hypertension
   B. Stroke
   C. High blood sugar/Diabetes
   D. Cancer
   E. Heart problems/Congestive heart failure
   F. Heart attack/Angina/Chest Pain
   G. Lung problems/Emphysema/Asthma
   H. Kidney failure
   I. Alzheimer's disease/Dementia
   J. Psychiatric disorder
   K. Disabling arthritis
   L. Hip fracture

2. If you circled any of the above, do you feel that you have all the information you need in order to take care of yourself effectively? ❑ Yes ❑ No

3. Have you been hospitalized in the past 2 years? Check the correct response.
   A. ❑ Not hospitalized in last 2 years
   B. ❑ 1-2 times
   C. ❑ 3-4 times
   D. ❑ 5 or more times in last 2 years

4. List the reasons for the above hospitalizations.

   A. _____

   B. _____

   C. _____

   D. _____

5. How many prescription medicines are you taking now? _____

6. How many over-the-counter medications are you taking now (i.e. aspirin, vitamins, etc.)? _____

7. Do you have questions you need answered regarding any of your medications?
   ❑ Yes ❑ No

8. Do you live alone? ❑ Yes ❑ No
   If no, is anyone who lives with you in ill health or disabled? ❑ Yes ❑ No

9. How would you rate your health? Circle the correct response.
   A. Excellent
   B. Good
   C. Fair
   D. Poor

10. Do you need assistance with any of the following areas? Circle any of the tasks that apply to you.
    A. Shopping
    B. Meal preparation
    C. Housekeeping
    D. Laundry
    E. Transportation
    F. Medications
    G. Bathing
    H. Dressing
    I. Walking
    J. Telephone access/Making appointments

Thank You! Please return this survey in the postage-paid envelope we've provided.

Lutheran Healthcare Network
Health Needs Assessment Scoring

1. Each disease circled or written in = 1 point
2. Y = 0 points
   N = 2 points
3. A = 0 points
   B = 1 point
   C = 2 points
   D = 3 points
4. Not scored
5. 0-3 = 0 points
   4-6 = 1 point
   7+ = 2 points
6. 0-3 = 0 points
   3+ = 1 point
7. Y = 2 points
   N = 0 points
8. Y = 1 point
   N = 0 points
9. A = 0 points
   B = 1 point
   C = 2 points
   D = 3 points
10. Each circled or written in item = 1 point

Lutheran Healthcare Network
High Risk Maternal Case Management
Referral Form

Date Referred _____

Choice Plus _____

AHCCCS Select _____

FHP _____

Referred By _____

Other _____

MEDICAL RISK FACTORS

____ History of Premature Labor/Delivery

____ Chronic Diseases _____

____ Diabetes

____ STDs _____

____ Multiple Births

____ Anemias

____ History of Previous C-Section

____ Placenta Previa

____ Preeclampsia, PTH

____ >2 Second Trimester Miscarriages

____ Polyhydramnios

____ Other _____

PSYCHOSOCIAL RISK FACTORS

____ Age < 17 years

____ Age > 35 years

____ African American

____ Hispanic nonEnglish Speaking

____ All CPS Referrals

____ Any Psychological Problems

____ Abuse/Violence

____ Chronic Appointment Failures
(2 or more)

____ Unmarried/Limited Support
Systems

____ Other _____

NUTRITIONAL RISK FACTORS

____ < 100# Prepregnant Weight

____ Failure to Gain Weight (<2# per month)

____ Excessive Weight Loss in the 1st
Trimester (6 or more #)

____ History of Anorexia/Bulimia

____ Other _____

SUBSTANCE ABUSE FACTORS

____ ETOH

____ Cocaine

____ Heroin

____ Marijuana

____ Tobacco

____ Amphetamines

____ Other _____

COMMENTS: _____

_____

_____

_____

Lutheran Healthcare Network Prenatal Health Assessment

1. Is this your first pregnancy?   ❑ Yes ❑ No
   G ___ P ___ AB ___
2. Have you seen an obstetrician yet?   ❑ Yes ❑ No
   Date _____ Dr. _____
3. Has your prenatal blood work been done?   ❑ Yes ❑ No
   Date _____
4. Are you on any medications?   ❑ Yes ❑ No

   List: _____

   _____

5. Do you have any health problems?   ❑ Yes ❑ No

   List: _____

   _____

6. Do you have any questions about prenatal care needed? ❑ Yes ❑ No
   Explain:
7. Do you have any questions about your pregnancy? ❑ Yes ❑ No

   Explain: _____

   _____

8. How is your support system? Do you have
   family or friends to help you?   ❑ Yes ❑ No

   _____

   _____

9. Are you on WIC or AFDC?   ❑ Yes ❑ No
10. Are you aware of the prepared childbirth classes
    at Mesa Lutheran Hospital? Give Info.   ❑ Yes ❑ No

    _____

    _____

11. Are you aware of covered benefits under your
    health plan and how the plan works?   ❑ Yes ❑ No

    _____

    _____

Lutheran Healthcare Network
Pediatric Case Management Referral Form

Name _____ ·   Id# _____

Address _____

Phone # _____

Date Referred _____   Choice Plus _____

    AHCCCS Select _____

Referred By _____   Other _____

MEDICAL RISK FACTORS

____ Congenital Anomalies _____

____ RDS

____ Failure to Thrive

____ Prematurity

____ IUGR

____ Seizure Disorder

____ Hyperbilirubinemia

____ Chronic Diseases _____

____ Other _____

PSYCHO-SOCIAL FACTORS

____ Abuse/Violence

____ Limited Support System

____ All CPS Referrals

____ Any Psychosocial Problems

____ Parent < age 17

____ Other _____

NUTRITIONAL RISK FACTORS

____ SGA

____ Failure to Gain Weight

____ Diarrhea/Dehydration

____ Poor Nippling/Sucking Habits

____ Anorexia/Bulimia

____ Obesity

____ Other _____

SUBSTANCE ABUSE FACTORS

____ History of Maternal Use

____ S/S of Drug Withdrawal

____ ETOH

____ Cocaine

____ Heroin

____ Marijuana

____ Tobacco

____ Amphetamines

____ Other _____

COMMENTS: _____

_____

_____

Chapter 20

Issues of Design and Implementation from Acute Care, Long-Term Care, and Community-Based Settings

Marilyn J. Rantz, PhD, RN
Kenneth D. Bopp, PhD

OVERVIEW

Nurse leaders are well positioned to identify barriers to and strategies for implementing nurse case management services.

Sixteen nurse leaders across the United States who have successfully implemented case management were interviewed to explore the obstacles they had encountered while bringing about this model of care delivery. The nurse leaders had experiences implementing case management programs that bridged the continuum of care. Common themes across the settings of acute, long-term, and community-based care were financial barriers, lack of administrative support for case management, human resource management inequities, turf battles, and the lack of information system support. Strategies to overcome these obstacles include communication and education, relationship building, and demonstration and documentation of benefits and costs.

What are the obstacles to case management design and implementation? To gain a current national perspective about that question, we interviewed 16 nurse leaders across the United States who have successfully implemented case management and asked, from their point of view, what obstacles they had encountered. Although most had implemented case management in acute care settings, there were several who had experienced implementing programs that bridged the continuum of care. There were common themes across the settings of acute care, long-term, and community-based care. These themes were financial barriers, lack of administrative support for case management, human resource management inequities, turf battles, and the lack of information

system support. In this chapter, we will explore these common obstacles, discuss the perspectives of the 16 people interviewed, discuss current literature related to implementation of nurse case management, and suggest strategies to overcome obstacles to implementation. Fundamental to the obstacles are differences in perspectives of the key players involved in case management: administrators and chief financial officers, nurses, physicians, and other health-care professionals. We will explore the points of view of key players and how they relate to the obstacles across all settings.

With few exceptions, we conducted these interviews with nurse executives whose health-care systems were not totally operating within a managed care environment, nor reimbursed totally by capitated payment. Being capitated or preparing for capitation is a strong fiscal incentive for offering preventive services, especially tertiary prevention. Hence, administrators and payors are more likely to consider nurse case management service for people at high risk in a different light, and the barriers identified in a nonmanaged care, fee-for-service environment may no longer be as large an issue.

PERSPECTIVES OF KEY PLAYERS
Administrators and Chief Financial Officers

Administrators and chief financial officers of acute, long-term, or community-based health-care delivery organizations are educated and function in their administrative jobs from a fiduciary perspective. Although they are concerned about cost and quality, their primary focus is on maintaining the financial viability of their organization. They are heavily invested in ensuring that their organization survives and has adequate revenues to carry out its mission. This preoccupation with revenues, however, does not commonly take into account a clear understanding of expenses and subsequent losses that can be involved in delivering care to resource-intensive clients. Focusing on revenues is further reinforced by third-party payment reimbursement systems. Case management is not usually a revenue-generating program in the direct sense of the word "generating"; it is a revenue-"protecting" program that minimizes losses related to cases that are resource intensive. For administrators and chief financial officers to buy into the concept of case management, they must be shifted from their revenue-generating perspective by compelling financial data that nurse case management reduces losses and protects the organization's bottom line.

Nurses

Although administrators are preoccupied with financial issues, nurses as health-care providers are concerned about quality of care and the needs of clients. They view case management as an opportunity to ensure that clients are getting the care they need. Nurses value enhancing self-care capacities and maximizing independence of clients. They can see the value in investing in improving clients' capabilities to manage their chronic illnesses better, avoiding acute episodes requiring expensive health-care interventions. Obviously, the perspectives of nurses are not all the same. Some nurses do not have a good understanding of care delivery in a variety of settings; they tend to focus on their particular setting to the exclusion and understanding of other settings. Although nurse

administrators have learned to focus on the financial implications of care delivery within their setting, in general, the nursing perspective has not been focused on maximizing revenues to assure the financial viability of their health-care organization. Traditionally, it has been focused on care needs of clients and how those needs could be addressed.

Physicians

The physicians' point of view is consistent across all care delivery settings. They see themselves as "*the* case manager." Their perspective is reinforced by historical health-care reimbursement systems, by their traditional perspective of "I'm the captain of the team," and by managed care contracts that designate primary-care physicians as gatekeepers. As physicians work with nurse case managers, however, they begin to understand that the nurse case manager's role is different from the physician's role as a case manager. Like nurses, physicians are concerned about quality of care and meeting the medical needs of clients. Typically, they are often frustrated when dealing with the management of chronically ill clients whose conditions are unresponsive to treatment or are long term. After working with nurse case managers in the community, they are more than willing to refer chronically ill clients with multiple health problems for case management by nurses. Historically, the physician's perspective has not been focused on assuring financial viability of health-care organizations. For them to buy into the concept of nurse case management, they must be convinced it will improve the quality of care and benefit clients.

Social Workers

Social workers are the other prominent group of health-care team involved in case management. The roots of the term "case management" are grounded in the field of social work. In many settings, turf battles are common between nurses and social workers and may be related to the perspective that social workers hold that *they* should be the case manager. In settings where case management has been successfully implemented, social workers tend to focus on social and financial issues, whereas the nurses tend to focus on client care needs and providing, or assuring services are provided, to meet those needs. Typically, the social workers' perspective has focused on the social and financial impact of illness on clients and their families. Historically, just like nurses and physicians, they have not focused on assuring the financial viability of their health-care organization.

Blending Perspectives

In settings where case management has been successfully implemented, a key seems to be that physicians, nurses, social workers, and other health-care providers have been able to work collaboratively and appreciate each person's role in care delivery for clients. In these settings, each professional's perspective and contributions are valued. Systems are in place that differentiate each role and avoid duplication of effort and competition between providers. From the client's point of view, they need services from a variety of health-care providers. At times, they need services from the physician (and from the physician's medical management perspective), at times they need services from the nurse (and from the nurse's nursing perspective), and at times they need services from the social worker (and from the social worker's perspective) to assist with medical, nursing, social, and financial problems that they are facing as a result of their chronic condition. A key to successful implementation of case management is to develop an appreciation of each provider's role and blend the philosophical perspectives so that each provider focuses on the client's well-being rather than their discipline's point of view.

OBSTACLE: FINANCIAL BARRIERS

Because most third-party payers do not directly reimburse health-care organizations for case management, administrators do not view nurse case management as a valuable revenue-generating activity. They view case management as an expense. They see salaries of nurses who work as case managers that must be paid without corresponding revenues to offset salary costs. Under current fee-for-service or DRG-based reimbursement, case management has to be presented to administrators as a cost-saving activity. When presented in this way, the burden is on nurse case managers to demonstrate *intially* and *continually* how case management impacts cost by reducing resource utilization to within limits of reimbursement or by reducing institutional losses related to high-cost clients.

In general, nurses have not focused on financial issues; many nurses lack knowledge or awareness of how costs relate to the care clients receive and how reimbursement systems work in health care. In settings where implementation of nurse case management has been successful, however, nurse case managers are very attuned to capturing data that can substantiate the impact of their efforts on reduction in resource utilization and subsequent cost savings to the agency (Cohen, 1991; Ethridge & Lamb, 1989; McKenzie, Torkelson, & Holt, 1989).

Within current reimbursement systems, physicians and agencies are primarily paid on a "piece-work" basis (Reinertsen, 1994). Physicians under fee-for-service reimbursement are oriented toward activities for which they can bill third-party payors and that generate revenue for their practices. Like administrators, initially, they do not view case management as a necessary or valued activity. When nursing administrators decide to pursue implementation of nurse case management, the onus is placed on them to justify the cost of implementing nurse case management and clearly demonstrate that nurse case management can free the physician from time-consuming care coordination activities in order to use that time to perform activities that are reimbursed. This is a subtle, important point of view and a major obstacle to implementation. Ferreting out costs of high-cost clients is difficult or nearly impossible with many computer systems and hard-copy medical record systems. The nurses we interviewed have been creative in pursuing ways to obtain information to overcome the financial barriers to obtain data to justify nurse case management implementation financially.

OBSTACLE: LACK OF ADMINISTRATIVE SUPPORT FOR CASE MANAGEMENT

With financial barriers clouding the issue of cost, the stage is set for a lack of administrative support when nurse administrators decide to implement case management. If the nurse administrator is successful in convincing administrators and chief financial officers to implement case management and yet does not obtain their full administrative support, the lack of commitment and support for case management can be manifested in a number of ways. Some of the people that we interviewed discussed problems with inadequate resources for funding case managers, adding the case management function to preexisting job responsibilities of some nurses, a myriad of difficulties obtaining medical records and cost data to establish baseline costs and costs after implementation, postimplementation criticism of the validity of evaluation data elements selected, and a lack of administrative support to help overcome resistance to change inherent to the introduction of case management.

It is imperative that there be administrative support to remove organizational barriers as case management is implemented. These barriers may include interdepartmental communication barriers, overlapping job responsibilities, policies and procedures that may impinge upon the various departments, as well as the major issue of handling resistance and opposition by other stakeholders in the organization who resist change. There is always resistance to change. Those people who have a stake in the change to nurse case management must be identified and their concerns about case management and its implications for them must be addressed. There must be administrative support to assist case managers in resolving concerns and overcoming resistance.

Lack of resource commitment to case management often results in case management being added to nurses' existing responsibilities. In a dual role, responsibilities are usually too great for the nurse to perform both jobs well. Often the case management role gets slighted as the urgency of line management nursing activities or in-hospital activities take precedence. Even when case managers are hired for the case management function across the continuum, many of them are frequently pulled out of their case management role to fulfill urgent staffing needs in traditional nursing functions.

Lack of administrative support for case management can be manifested in failing to assist the nurse administrator to obtain cost and medical record data necessary for evaluation and criticism of the relevance or validity of evaluation criteria selected to measure effectiveness. One nurse leader explained how she overcame this obstacle by forming an administrative support team that included the chief financial officer, information specialist, and other key stakeholders to gain their commitment and support before implementation regarding the data elements targeted as outcome criteria. By participating in the decision-making process, they were unlikely to dismiss the relevancy of the evaluation data and withdraw their support at a later date.

OBSTACLE: HUMAN RESOURCE MANAGEMENT INEQUITIES

As the nurse administrator implements nurse case management, there are several human resource management issues that can become inequities and, therefore, obstacles. These include the case manager role, nursing preparation for the case manager role, and monitoring the performance and activities of case managers.

Typically, the case manager's role does not fit traditional health-care human resource management policies and procedures. Because case managers manage cases rather than supervise other employees, they wreak havoc on traditional human resource management systems (Davenport & Nohria, 1994). The skills, compensation schedules, job classification criteria, performance evaluation criteria, and career paths of nurse case managers are incongruent with traditional health-care human resource management systems. Several of the nurse case management leaders we interviewed pointed out problems of fitting nurse case managers into current salary schedules and problems relating nurse case managers to the clinical ladder systems commonly in place in hospitals. Pay inequities can sabotage even the most carefully planned case management implementation.

In most human resource management systems, nurse case managers with greater knowledge, skill requirements, and decision-making responsibilities would be classified at lower job classification and therefore lower salary levels than nursing supervisors working on hospital nursing units. Traditional human resource management systems recognize and compensate line management responsibilities to a greater degree than nonline responsibilities. Although the case manager is actually "managing" multiple cases, they are not considered line management and are penalized in many traditional human resource management systems. Furthermore, most human resource management systems do not have a career path for case managers as they do for traditional nursing job classifications.

Another major obstacle is that most nurses are inadequately prepared for the case management role. Nurse case managers need to have strong problem-solving skills; they must be able to make independent judgments and have knowledge of care processes and practices across the broad continuum of behavioral, health, and social services. Not only must they be able to problem-solve these issues, but they must be able to integrate the multidisciplinary and interdisciplinary care approaches for individual clients. Experts we interviewed and some literature (Bower, 1992; Cronin & Maklebust, 1989; Gibson et al., 1994) indicate a growing realization that advanced practice nurses may be best prepared to assume the case management role.

Nursing education has traditionally prepared nurses to function in highly structured institutional settings. The case management role demands flexibility and the ability to work independently within each client's changing environment. That may require the case manager be able to work within a hospital system while the client is hospitalized, with home health services when the client is discharged from the acute care setting, or with nursing home staff as the client receives long-term care services after hospitalization. It is important that nurses who are selected for case manager roles be able to function within a variety of health-care settings. Many nurses are uncomfortable playing the boundary-spanning role of coordinating care across professions and across organizational boundaries that is required of the nurse case manager.

Most nurses have experienced and consequently view health care from a narrow, segmented, acute care nursing unit perspective. They lack knowledge of multiple-care delivery settings and the continuum-of-care perspective. Consequently, most nurses are codependent in the hierarchial structure and support of a hospital or nursing home environment and few are prepared to make the independent decisions required of case managers. A fundamental question that must be addressed is how to educate and orient nurses to prepare them adequately for the case management role.

Another human resource management obstacle to implementation is monitoring and evaluating the case manager's activities and performance. When case managers function across the health-care continuum, they work independently. Traditional methods of productivity analysis and management performance review become difficult.

Typically, case managers are not observed as they interact with clients within their homes or in the various care delivery settings across the continuum. How can the case manager's supervisor identify performance problems and appropriately guide those in the case management role to improve? Other issues surrounding the evaluation of the case manager's performance are important. Should the case manager be held accountable for client outcomes? Should the case manager be held accountable for financial outcomes? Determining appropriate outcome criteria and performance criteria for case managers must be resolved for successful implementation.

Nurse administrators and individual nurse case managers we interviewed who have successfully implemented case management were carefully tracking not only financial outcome data but also client outcome data to evaluate the overall performance of their case management program. These data, however, were not translated to the individual employee level for performance criteria. Evaluation of individual employees's performance and productivity is an issue that needs further exploration.

OBSTACLE: TURF BATTLES

As discussed, there are philosophical differences in perspectives of the key players providing direct services in case management: physicians, nurses, and social workers. These philosophical differences can become an enormous source of stress and conflict as case management is implemented. The primary strategy in dealing with these philosophical differences is to focus on what the *client* needs. Turf battles disappear if professionals are able to focus on the needs of the client and how best to go about helping the client meet those needs. In almost every interview we conducted, case managers or nursing administrators who had implemented case management explained that primary-care physicians view themselves as *the* case manager. This is usually an initial perspective that must be overcome if nurse case management is going to be successfully implemented. Once physicians understand, however, that nothing is being taken away from them as the client's physician, and that the

focus is on the care of the client and how to meet the client's priority needs, physicians become cooperative. Once physicians actually experience the model in practice, they actively refer clients for case management and become supportive of efforts of the nurse case manager.

There is confusion about the definition and role of case management. Because there is a lack of industry standards, people seem to be reinventing the wheel rather than learning from each other's experience. Carondolet St. Mary's educational efforts through its courses, consultation, and multiple publications has gone far to assist other settings in the implementation of the model and clarify much of the confusion (Ethridge & Lamb, 1989: Michaels, 1992). American Nurses' Association (ANA) publications defining and describing case management by nurses have also assisted in clarifying the role, activities, and use of case management (ANA, 1988; Bower, 1992). Nevertheless, there remains a basic lack of understanding and controversy about what case management is and who is qualified to do it (Gibson et al., 1994; Rogers, Riordan, & Swindle, 1991). Some experts we interviewed required master's-prepared, advanced-practice nurses in community case manager roles. Others said they would like to use advanced-practice nurses, but that they had been unable to do so because of supply in their geographic region. Subsequently, these programs required bachelor's-prepared nurses. Some hospitals have clearly differentiated practice within their hospital and community-based programs. These places have delineated how nurse case manager roles relate to staff nurses prepared at various educational levels. These limited locations aside, there is no clear consensus about who is best prepared and best qualified to perform the nurse case management functions. Consensus may be moving toward the advanced practice nurse as the best prepared and best qualified. The ANA recommends that the *minimal* preparation for a nurse case manager be a baccalaureate in nursing with three years of appropriate clinical experience (Bower, 1992).

There is confusion about how utilization review and case management discharge planning differ. Sometimes staff interpret the case manager role as one of utilization review. In some settings, the terms utilization review and case management are interpreted as having the same negative meaning. In settings where this is the case, the negative connotations of case management terminology have led some nurse administrators to rename case management so that financial watchdog connotations of utilization review are clearly separated from the coordinated care functions of case management.

Additionally, there is confusion surrounding defining case management in terms of tools of case management such as critical pathways. There is a misperception that if one implements critical pathways, case management is automatically implemented. There is also confusion regarding the case manager coordinating and caregiving role versus other caregiving roles of other providers. The case manager must be able to articulate the differences between job functions as a nurse case manager versus the job functions of home health nurses or other providers such as social services or physical therapy.

Turf barriers can inadvertently be constructed from policies and procedures that are directed at maximizing performance within individual disciplines, departments, and care settings. Although policies and procedures are established to optimize components of the continuum of care, barriers can result that inhibit case management efforts for coordination and performance across the entire system. The case manager must be able to withstand the pressures from individual disciplines, departments, and care settings to maintain his point of view. The case manager must be able to bridge components of care across the continuum and actively tear down barriers between disciplines, departments, and care settings.

Because the case manager role is a professional role, there is professional autonomy in clinical decision making. However, there are problems related to professional autonomy that must be overcome. A major problem is trust. Trusting each other as assessments are made and conclusions drawn from those assessments is rare between disciplines as well as individual providers within the same discipline. A functional distrust among professionals has been promoted. It is commonly believed that you cannot trust someone else's judgment. There is a belief that each professional should reassess each situation to verify that the other professional assessed the situation correctly. Because the case manager role is an autonomous role that demands independent decision making, other members of the health-care team must learn to trust the judgment of the case manager and respond to the needs of the client as interpreted by the case manager. If this fundamental problem is not overcome, the effectiveness of the case manager is seriously impaired.

OBSTACLE: INFORMATION SYSTEM SUPPORT

The need for information systems that can support case management was universally discussed by all of the experts interviewed. Most health-care information systems have been built along functional or departmental lines, even within the hospital, and few health-care organizations have information systems that interface across the broad array of health, behavioral health, and social service programs and sites

with which community case managers must interact. Most of the experts interviewed were concerned about the lack of integrated databases that can deliver relevant information from across the institution or continuum to the case manager's work station in a timely manner.

The information that needs to support case management includes:

1. Client demographics such as name, address, birth date, education, occupation, family structure/support.
2. Assessment data such as medical and social history, nursing assessment, health and medical care goals and preferences, biopsychological status, and care needs.
3. Care plan protocols such as critical pathways that organize, sequence, time, and coordinate the major interventions of health-care providers. (The information system should allow case managers to access treatment protocols developed by various health-care disciplines and care settings to assist them in compiling care plans for a client's particular case type or illness that involves multiple disciplines, multiple parts or departments of an organization, and multiple parts of the continuum of care.)
4. A resource database that allows case managers to determine capability and capacity. (The capability component of the database provides case managers with an inventory of health, behavioral health, and social services—skilled health care professionals, equipment, facilities—that are available in the organization or community to serve client needs. The capacity component of the database provides the case manager with information regarding the times the resources are available to be scheduled to serve the client.)
5. Information that allows case managers to monitor and track not only service delivery, but also changes in service delivery.

Developing an information system to deliver these types of information to the case manager's desk will be difficult for most health-care organizations because most systems in the past were built along functional lines. Building such a customer-focused system often involves building the system from the ground up. Because the cost and the time required to build integrated information systems is frequently high, most case managers are patching together databases to support case management. To get the data that they need to carry out their case management responsibilities and to document the benefit-cost of case management, case managers often have to compile data manually. The experts interviewed agreed that having an information system that provides the information described above, transmits it across the continuum of care, and integrates it at the case manager's work station is an important infrastructure need of case management.

OVERCOMING OBSTACLES

Although some strategies have been alluded to in the previous discussion of specific obstacles, there are a select group of strategies used by the experts we interviewed to assure the successful implementation of nurse case management. These strategies include communication and education, relationship building, and demonstration and documentation of benefits and costs.

Communication and Education

The introduction of nurse case management requires administrators and health professionals to understand, accept, and sometimes adjust their patterns of practice to accommodate case management. Consequently, the initiation of case management must be accompanied with communication and education from the outset.

The overlay of nurse case management on the traditional relationship patterns among health professionals often causes confusion of roles and turf issues. Communication with physicians, staff nurses, social workers, and other health-related professionals that identifies and clarifies the role of case managers is essential. The experts interviewed indicated that one-on-one, face-to-face communication was most effective in clarifying roles and eliminating the threats for these stakeholders. Because other professionals often have preconceived ideas regarding what case management is (utilization review, discharge planning, home health), nurse case managers have to educate other professionals about what case management is *not* as well as what it is. One expert indicated that her organization defined the role of the case manager as an advocate, a broker of services, a coordinator of services, and a caregiver. Using this definition, physicians can understand that they are not case managers because they do not have the time to do all the functions. Other health professionals were then able to see that the case manager's role is much broader, and they could focus on discussions with case managers to reconcile the role issues in the one area of overlap—caregiving.

Another educational issue that was raised by the panel of experts is the preparation of nurses to function in the case management role. Nurse case managers need to have strong problem-solving skills, knowledge of care processes and practices across the continuum of care, and the ability to make independent judgments.

The experts indicated that the minimum preparation for the case manager role is a BSN with five years of diverse clinical experience. The ideal candidate for the case manager role is the advanced-practice nurse. Further, the experts suggested that most nurses, including advanced-practice nurses, need additional training to maximize their performance as case managers. They suggested that the enhancement of nurse competencies should include basic negotiation skills, conflict resolution techniques, critical thinking, delegation, and financial issues.

Relationship Building

Nurse case managers function where the organization interfaces with clients and family caregivers and health providers across the continuum of care. Not only are they liaisons between different health-care professionals and clients, but they also may actually provide some services previously done by other professionals. Introducing nurse case management requires negotiation and mutual adjustments to fit case management into the organization's structure and caregiving processes.

The experts interviewed identified several relationship-building activities that facilitated the integration of case management into the organization's structure and care processes. In some organizations, the implementation of case management has been facilitated by establishing an advisory group made up of the chief of medical staff, administrative vice presidents, the chief financial officer, information systems representatives, and other interested physicians, nurse administrators, and nurse case managers. The group meets regularly to clarify the nurse case manager's role and relationship to the other health-care professionals, to develop goals, to identify critical paths that need to be developed, to decide which cases are high cost or complex and need to be case managed, and to approve the data elements to be used for the evaluation of the effectiveness of the nurse case management program. The group is a mechanism for internal marketing and enhances the probability that nurse case managers get the cooperation they need from administration, finance, information systems, and other nursing and non-nursing departments across the continuum of care. The group also can help manage the normal organizational resistance to change.

The experts also suggested that the selection of nurses to begin a case management program is a critical factor in the success of the program. They indicated that the people chosen to be the first case managers should be known and have already established rapport, credibility, and relationships with physicians, nurses, and other health professionals across the continuum. Trust is essential to the case manager's effectiveness. Case managers known and respected for their management and clinical skills already have achieved a level of trust with the professionals with whom they can build the trust necessary to achieve the full potential of case management. As they work with other professionals on a daily basis, they must continue to build credibility and trust.

Finally, the experts suggested that the approach to implementing case management should be low key. The program should be piloted and its effectiveness should be demonstrated before it is broadly implemented throughout the organization and across the continuum. Easing the program into place and demonstrating its effectiveness reduces stakeholder uncertainty and increases their acceptance of case management.

Demonstration and Documentation of Benefits and Costs

Effectively executed nurse case management is a win-win situation for clients and their informal caregivers, organizations, physicians, and nurses. The burden of proof, however, is on nurse case managers. The key stakeholders who must be persuaded of the value of nurse case management are physicians and administrators.

Physicians see themselves as "case managers" and must be convinced, and case managers must clarify the complementary nature of the nurse case manager's role to the role of the physician and demonstrate how these case managers can be supportive of the physician's practice. Moreover, nurse case managers must demonstrate that case management is good for clients. If case managers can demonstrate that clients benefit, physicians will buy into nurse case management.

As indicated earlier in this chapter, administrators do not view nurse case management as a valuable, revenue-generating activity. They view case management as a cost. Consequently, the burden is on case managers to demonstrate that case management has a positive impact on the organization's financial bottom line.

The experts interviewed suggest that case managers start with a client population on which case management can have a significant impact. Most of the leaders interviewed started with the frail elderly with multiple chronic illnesses and high utilization of the hospital's emergency room and acute inpatient facilities. By breaking the cycle of frequent ER visits and hospital readmissions, these leaders were able to justify the use of case managers quickly because cost savings were clear in service utilization. Demonstrating that case management more than pays for itself in reducing hospital utilization for persons with complex illnesses gets the program off the ground and establishes credibility for the service.

CONCLUSION

The key to successful implementation of case management is measuring and documenting outcomes in terms of benefits to clients and dollars. In measuring the benefits and costs of case management, leading case management efforts have focused on quantifying the impact of case management in terms of reduced emergency room visits, admissions and readmissions to inpatient units, length of stay, increased client and family caregiver satisfaction, and health-care provider satisfaction (Cohen, 1991; Ethridge & Lamb, 1989; Rogers, Riordan, & Swindle, 1991). Successful case management programs have been able to demonstrate that clients win, family caregivers win, the organization wins, physicians win, and staff nurses win as a result of case management. Overcoming obstacles to implementation of case management is well worth the effort. Careful analysis of the obstacles, stakeholders perspectives, and implementation strategies can assist the nurse to plan and implement nurse case management successfully.

REFERENCES

American Nurses Association. (1988). *Nursing case management.* Kansas City, Mo: American Nurses Association.

Bower, K. A. (1992). *Case Management by Nurses.* Washington, DC: American Nurses Association.

Cohen, E. L. (1991). Nursing case management: does it pay? *Journal of Nursing Administration, 21* (4), 20-25.

Cronin, & Maklebust, (1989). Case-managed care: capitalizing on the CNF. *Nursing Management, 20* (3), 38-47.

Davenport, T. H., & Nohria, N. (1994). Case management and the integration of labor. *Sloan Management Review, 35* (2), 11-23.

Ethridge, P., & Lamb, G. S. (1989). Professional nursing case management improves quality, access, and costs. *Nursing Management, 20* (3), 30-35.

Gibson, S. J., Martin, S. M., Johnson, M. B., Blue, R., & Miller, D. S. (1994). CNS-directed case management: cost and quality in harmony. *Journal of Nursing Administration, 24* (6), 45-51.

McKenzie, C. B., Torkelson, N. G., & Holt, M. A. (1989). Care and cost: nursing case management improves both. *Nursing Management, 20* (10), 30-34.

Michaels, C. (1992). Carondelet St. Mary's nursing enterprise. *Nursing Clinics of North America, 27* (1), 77-85.

Reinertsen, J. L. (1994). The tyranny of piecework. *Health-Care Forum Journal, 37* (4), 19-24.

Rogers, M., Riorgan, J., & Swindle, R. D. (1991). Community-based nursing case management pays off. *Nursing Management, 22* (3), 30-134.

Chapter 21

Staff Development for Nurse Case Management

Virginia Davis, MSN, RN

OVERVIEW

Nurses can develop the competencies needed by nurse case managers through staff development efforts that focus on education, practice, and peer review.

Developing case managers is a process that supports accountability of the case managers first to the population served and then to the employing organization. Given the various methods, settings, and objectives used in nurse case management, this chapter provides a framework for developing case managers to meet the identified needs. Development of case managers builds sound professional nursing practice by further defining the four roles that differentiate nurse case managers: caregiver, advocate, broker, and coordinator. Role definition and required competencies can be defined by population needs. Competency development depends on the particular required knowledge, skill, and ability to apply both knowledge and skill when needed for each role. Processes for ongoing competency validation and role development are vital in effective nurse case manager (NCM) development.

This chapter provides a framework for identifying the needed NCM competencies. It also discusses methods for developing those competencies through education, practice, and peer review. The competencies and development process are woven around the four roles of caregiver, coordinator, advocate, and broker.

ORIENTATION AND ROLE DEVELOPMENT

Registered nurses, assuming the responsibility and accountability for case management, will require orientation to the role and ongoing development in the role. The orientation process for case managers should be built upon the foundation of a theoretical framework, philosophy, and standards designed to meet the needs of the population served. The four major roles of case managers—caregiver, coordinator, advocate, and broker—provide a framework for standard competencies and education. This chapter not only describes an orientation and development program that verifies the required competencies for those roles but also identifies methodologies for ongoing development for case managers.

NEEDS, MISSION, PHILOSOPHY, VISION, AND STRATEGY

The orientation and development of case managers must be designed to meet the identified needs of the populations served and to support the goals and strategic direction of the agency (Figure 21-1). When considering the implementation of a case management program, certain questions are pertinent. The answers to these questions will help shape the orientation, development, and evaluation of case managers. Some of these questions include:

- *What are the characteristics (e.g., age, culture, language)?* The characteristics of the population are key elements in determining the knowledge required by the case manager. If the population to be served is primarily a geriatric one, a thorough knowledge of geriatric assessments and intervention is imperative. The culture(s) of the populations served is an important variable in the acceptance of case management interventions. Various cultural groups will be better served if the family is highly involved as opposed to working primarily with the individual.

- *What are the population needs (e.g., common nursing or medical diagnoses, health-care access, support services available)?* The common nursing and medical diagnoses of the population shape the required knowledge base and competencies of the case manager. The pathophysiology, the emotional toll, the end-beginning, or quality-of-life dilemmas faced by the population are all key components in developing competencies of the case manager.

- *What is the agency's stated, implied, or lived mission in relationship to the population to be served (e.g., improved health status, improved quality of life, disease prevention)?* The agency's mission should help shape a case management program. The case manager may be working with a group of teens at risk for pregnancy, with a focus on prevention of low-birth-weight infants. To extend the mission to one of improving the quality of life, mothers and infants identified as at risk for abuse or neglect may be followed by a case manager for two to three years. The case manager's interventions should support appropriate use of health-care resources and reinforce effective parenting skills.

- *What is the theoretical framework used as the basis for nursing care?* A theoretical or conceptual framework will help guide the case manager's practice. The foundation for nursing, the nurse-client relationship, is fundamental in nurse case management. This framework provides an organized structure for identifying client strengths, problems, and interventions required (Figure 21-1).

- *What is the vision of the agency and other providers (e.g., collaborative team to make **health** everyone's experience, or low-cost, high-quality provider)?* Implementation of a case management program will be supported if the agency's vision is supported. The *collaborative* approach to make *health* a reality demands a highly developed set of case-manager competencies related to collaboration, health assessments, and interventions that support lifestyle changes. The vision of being the preferred low-cost, high-quality provider demands full knowledge and application of costs of care, correlation between cost and reimbursement, and quantification of outcomes.

- *What are the agency's major strategic initiatives and the assumptions upon which those initiatives are developed?* Agency strategic initiatives supported by case management influence the required orientation and development of case managers (see Figure 21-1). Physician hospital integration will require systems that will appropriately use physicians' and other health professionals' talents. For example, the case manager who is supporting a physician's practice must understand the operation of the physician's office and clinic and how to improve the clients' health status while making the office more efficient. Participation with managed care companies in capitated arrangements necessitates low-cost, highly effective delivery systems. Reducing hospital costs of care and making desired outcomes more consistent requires a case manager to be expert in the utilization and variance analysis of critical pathways. This expertise can be further developed through the agency's orientation and development process. Short- and long-term health goals for a population require effective, therapeutic, and continuous relationships focusing on healthy lifestyles and self-responsibility. A case management service which is supporting long-term health for a population will require that case managers be competent in health assessments, health education, and lifestyle change methodologies.

IDENTIFICATION OF COMPETENCIES

Once the objectives of the case management services are clarified, competencies can then be identified. A competency program should be used during the orientation of case managers and on a regular basis, at least annually, to identify needs for ongoing development of

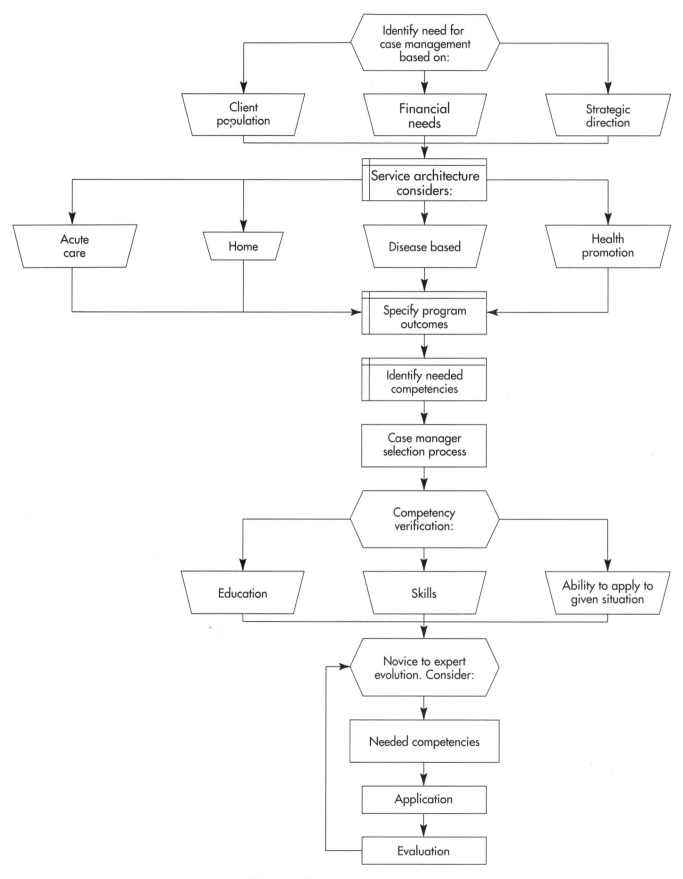

FIG. 21-1   Case manager development

the case managers. The competency-based orientation and evaluation program (CBO&E) can verify knowledge and skills required for case management and the ability to apply both knowledge and skill when needed. Competency programs have received much deserved attention in the last several years. Regulatory and licensing agencies have clearly and specifically identified the need for such a program.

As seen in Figure 21-1, the case manager's competencies should be based on needs identified and outcomes desired. The standards of care and practice, based upon the needs of the population served, will provide additional resources for identifying competencies. Clearly, the case manager role encompasses the use of the nursing process as well as several major roles such as caregiver, coordinator, advocate, and broker.

The *caregiver's* role in nurse case management is founded upon the nurse-client relationship and the use of nursing art and science. The caregiver's role depends on the use of nursing process and fosters the client's self-reliance. When considering the competencies needed for the caregiver's role, attention required by the client, application of applicable principles, intervention, and use of critical thinking are required. Below are some of the competencies related to the *caregiver* component of case management.

- Assesses all clients and identifies priorities with client and family using agency's theoretical or conceptual framework.
- Establishes priorities and intervention based on need for care, teaching needs, multidisciplinary needs and referrals, nursing and medical diagnoses.
- Identifies desired outcomes and establishes time frames for accomplishment with client.
- Evaluates client's progress toward identified outcomes, evaluates, and revises plan or critical pathway.
- Initiates activities to resolve lack of progress toward outcomes, critical path trajectory.
- Ensures that the relationship and accountability are established and maintained with the client, family, and other team members.
- Uses applicable standards and practices to guide intervention choices.
- Uses interventions that foster prevention or restoration.
- Identifies trends in exacerbation of illness and fosters use of identified trends by client to develop preventive strategies.

The *coordinator* role in nurse case management requires an understanding and use of clinical pathways, the queuing of activities, and integration of information for use by clinicians and clients. Coordination as part of case management requires arrangement, in due order, of needed services and activities, and combining these in a harmonious relation. Below are competencies related to the *coordinator* role.

- Selects and applies appropriate critical pathway.
- Provides continuity through care provision, communication and assurance of plan implementation with other team members, agencies.
- Collaborates to ensure desired client outcomes with client, family, physicians, other disciplines, agencies.
- Demonstrates overall accountability for achievement of outcomes with appropriate resource utilization.
- Uses knowledge of available resources and services and coordinates utilization of such to meet client needs.

The case manager, as *advocate*, supports the client in meeting goals, defends and espouses the client's cause, and generally acts on behalf of the client as needed. Rushton (1994) defines *advocacy* as *safeguarding and advancing the interests of another*. These are competencies related to the *advocate* role.

- Identifies cases for case management.
- Actively pursues desired outcomes.
- Fosters independence of client.
- Considers and respects cultural and generational factors in procurement and delivery of services.
- Educates client to use resources and services.
- Encourages client's appropriate decision-making methodology.

The *broker* role used in nurse case management fosters the procurement of needed resources and services for the client. Traditionally, a broker serves as a middleman or agent in bringing resources or services to the client. Competencies that relate to the *broker* role include:

- Maintains needed communication with payors and uses eligibility requirements to procure appropriate services.
- Negotiates for simple or complex services to meet client needs.
- Advocates for scarce resources that may not be covered by traditional reimbursement mechanisms.
- Establishes services that are not available to meet client needs.
- Monitors and manages resource utilization.

Each of the competencies can be supported with more detailed expectations or modular objectives (Appendix 21-A).

EDUCATIONAL DEVELOPMENT

During the process of developing case managers, education of case managers and those with whom they will work is vital and fundamental to the success of the program.

The educational process is an evolutionary one and should continue to be based on identified role expectations, identified learning needs, changes in client population, and changes in payors. Clear understanding of case management and differentiating the case manager's role as it will be implemented in the particular agency should be an overriding theme in any educational session. Integrating the case manager role with the values and philosophy of the organization is a key component of the educational process. Many authors have identified the various components of case management educational programs (Bower, 1988; Cohen & Cesta, 1993; Etheredge, 1989).

During the development of the education content, concepts or threads related to the organization's philosophy and values can be incorporated. *Concepts* relate to the needed components of practice such as accountability, development of nurse-client relationships, and collaboration. The *threads* relate to the organizations values and weave those values into the role concepts (Table 21-1). After integrating the identified roles and needed competencies with the threads and philosophical concepts, the content of educational offerings can be developed. Box 21-1 outlines content for didactic presentation to provide the framework and knowledge base for educating case managers.

In addition to didactic lectures and group discussions, other learning options can reinforce educational sessions and should be available for self-teaching or reinforcement. Such options include review of articles and other professional publications, self-guided case studies, and case reviews.

TABLE 21-1   St. Mary-Corwin Regional Medical Center, case manager curriculum threads

Role/*Thread*	Definition	Application concepts description
MEMBER OF THE NURSING PROFESSION *Attitude of Collaboration*	The nurse is accountable for the ethical, legal, and professional responsibilities related to all other roles.	Accountability Critical thinking skills Use of nursing process Promotion and recognition of nurse's optimal contribution Incorporating nursing research into practice
CAREGIVER *Respect for Persons*	The nurse, using accepted standards of practice based on the nursing process, helps the individual/family/group to identify and meet basic health needs in a wide variety of settings and with appropriate interventions.	Gordon's functional health patterns Lifespan implication Use of nursing process Standards of practice Collaboration/teamwork/interdisciplinary
ADVOCATE *Value-Oriented Management*	The nurse promotes a climate in which individual/family/group may act in their own interest. The nurse intervenes when they are unable to do so by taking on their cause as her/his own.	Client: nurse relationship Client outcomes Collaboration/teamwork/interdisciplinary
BROKER *Stewardship*	The nurse acts as the negotiator and procurer for client need management by connecting the client/family/group with the necessary service and/or product.	Client-nurse relationship Client outcomes Collaboration/teamwork/interdisciplinary Financial implications (for client and organization)
COORDINATOR *Value-Oriented Management/Stewardship*	The nurse coordinates care of the individual/family/group by using a multidisciplinary, holistic approach. The nurse as manager works to achieve desired outcomes through coordination of individual and family care with effective use of personnel, equipment, supplies, and work systems.	Collaboration/teamwork/interdisciplinary Resource use Client-nurse relationship

Developed by Zschokke, D. (1994). St. Mary-Corwin Regional Medical Center, Pueblo, Colo.

BOX 21-1
OUTLINE FOR EDUCATING CASE MANAGERS

Lecture I: Case Manager Roles: Caregiver, Coordinator, Broker, Advocate

A. Define case management and response to identified needs.
B. Describe roles in correlation with values.
C. Apply concept of accountability and nurse-client relationship to case managers.

Lecture II: Delegation and Inclusion

A. Determine appropriate delegation.
B. Prioritize client needs, interventions requires, other work.
C. Application to the coordinator role.
D. Determination of what to delegate and to whom.

Lecture III: Collaboration, Teamwork, and Negotiation

A. Review effect on communication techniques.
B. Define collaboration and application to the coordinator role.
C. Apply to concept of continuity and seamless care.

Lecture IV: Client Education

A. Review adult learning principles.
B. Identify various teaching methodologies and appropriate application.
C. Describe application of client education to self-care and independence.
D. Review application of client education to caregiver and advocate role.

Lecture V: Discharge Planning

A. Assess needs for post acute care services.
B. Review community and agency resources and referral process.
C. Apply to caregiver, coordinator, and broker roles.

Lecture VI: Critical Pathways: Development and Use

A. Review purposes and uses of critical pathway.
B. Describe agency's process for critical pathway development.
C. Define variances and mechanisms for tracking and analyzing variances.
D. Quantification of critical pathway use.
E. Describe use of critical pathways as tool for case managers.
F. Apply critical pathway use to caregiver and coordinator roles.

Lecture VII: Financial Aspects of Case Management

A. Identify financial impact of case management; *cost savings*.
B. Describe reimbursement mechanisms and payor trends impacting organization and service available.
C. Correlate costs of intervention and supplies as identified on critical pathways to reimbursement and to outcomes.

CASE MANAGER EVOLUTION

Establishing mechanisms for reinforcement and continually expanding the development of case managers early in the case management program will help solidify the implementation (Figure 21-2). Suggested methodologies include regular case review with peers by using an established format (Box 21-2). Presentation of case managers' own exemplars will use the process of reflection and self-learning.

ORGANIZATIONAL SUPPORT

The support of the case managers must be evident. The development of nurse case management, in congruence with the organizations vision, goals, and strategies, strengthens the acceptance of the program.

Other supporting mechanisms include scheduled reports at department head meetings, by case managers regarding the impact of the process, articles in medical staff publications, reports to the board of trustees, and integration of program results at identified committee meetings.

CONCLUSION

Identification of needs, developing the case manager role in relationship to those needs, and evaluating the impact of interventions solidifies the case management program. Initial and ongoing development of proficient case managers is one of the vital elements to client outcomes and successful case management programs.

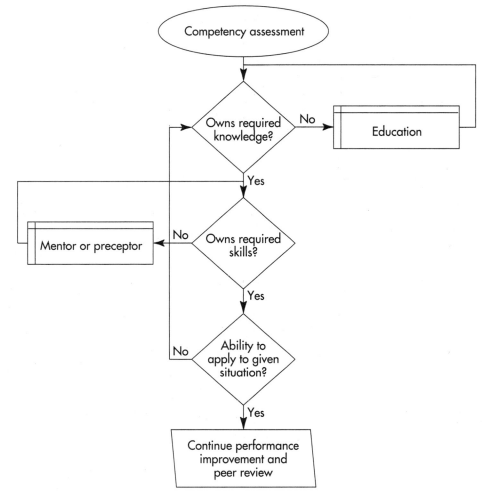

FIG. 21-2   Case manager evolution

BOX 21-2
CASE REVIEW FORMAT

I. Case Summary

A. Medical and nursing diagnoses
B. Stated goals of client
C. History and pattern of exacerbations of illness: dependency and resource utilization

II. Decision Points for Client

III. Short-Term Goals

IV. Analysis and Conclusions

PEER REVIEW

	OUTCOMES IDENTIFIED	ASSESSMENT	DONE (Y/N)	ACTION	OUTCOMES ACHIEVED
Dx 1	1. 2. 3. 4. 5.	1. 2. 3. 4. 5.			
Dx 2	1. 2. 3. 4. 5.	1. 2. 3. 4. 5.			
Dx 3	1. 2. 3. 4. 5.	1. 2. 3. 4. 5.			

Comments:

St. Mary-Corwin Regional Medical Center. Pueblo, Colo.

REFERENCES

Bower, K. (1988). *Case management by nurses.* Washington, DC: American Nurses Publishing.

Cohen, E., & Cesta, T. (1993). *Nursing case management: from concept to evaluation.* St Louis: Mosby, pg. 90-100.

Etheredge, M. (1989). *Collaborative care: nursing case management.* Chicago: American Hospital Publishing, pg. 39-51.

Fawcett, J., & Carino, C. (1989). Hallmarks of success in nursing practice. *Advances Nursing Science 11* (4), 1-8.

Rushton, C. (1994). The critical care nurse as a client advocate. *Critical Care Nursing 6,* 102-106.

St. Mary-Corwin Regional Medical Center
Division of Nursing
Competency Based Orientation
and Evaluation Program

Nursing Generic Competencies

This competency-based orientation and evaluation (CBO-E) program is designed to enable you to base your nursing practice upon the St. Mary-Corwin Regional Medical Center philosophy of nursing and standards of care. You will use the nursing process to provide care for clients in a dynamic client and family environment while developing your potential as a professional nurse.

Upon completion of orientation, the nurse will demonstrate the listed generic competencies. These competencies are expected of all RNs in any area of the hospital.

DIRECTIONS

Each orientee and preceptor is responsible for maintenance of the program. At the beginning of the orientation the orientee will review the program and indicate the criteria the orientee is already capable of meeting. At the first meeting, orientee and preceptor will review each criteria and plan the orientation based on the agreed upon learning needs. The Clinical Manager and the nurse educator will serve as resources to the orientee and preceptor.

Orientees will choose learning options and document on the competency list.

Preceptors will choose evaluation options for determining competent performance and document in the evaluation column on the competency list.

The preceptor will indicate the date the criteria is competently performed and initial.

The orientation is completed when all performance criteria are met. In the event that clinical experiences are not available to meed all competencies, and adequate experience cannot be obtained in a lab-like situation, the orientee will contract with the preceptor to enlist assistance when performing the competency for the first time.

During the orientation process, weekly meetings will be held with the orientee, preceptors and nurse educator to evaluate progress with the program.

At the completion of orientation, the entire program is reviewed by the orientee, preceptor, nurse educator and department director. Goals are then planned for the next

three months. The tool is retained as a permanent part of the orientee's record of employment.

DEFINITION

The preceptor is an experienced and competent staff nurse who serves as a clinical role model and resource person to newly employed staff nurses. The preceptor performs the following functions:

- Executes the case manager role as defined by the job description
- Facilitates the orientee's socialization in the work group
- Assists the orientee in identifying critical learning needs
- Works with the orientee in mutually planning learning experiences
- Bases teaching and learning content on nursing standards, professional publications and care texts and journals
- Implements the learning plan
- Evaluates the orientee's learning performance

The preceptor is guided by the nurse educator and works within the competency based orientation program. An individual's performance on the preceptor role is evaluated by the department director with input from the nurse educator, staff nurse, peers and the orientee.

Self-assessment: In the column marked "self-assessment," please indicate the number that corresponds to your present ability in relation to each competency:

0 = not presently able to perform   1 = able to perform with assistance   2 = able to perform independently

Perceptor I have observed and validated _____ perform the signed-off competencies. I have confidence she/he can independently perform them safely and competently.

Initials   Signatures

_____   _____

_____   _____

_____   _____

Orientee I feel confident that I can demonstrate and perform the signed-off competencies safely and competently. For those competencies not signed-off, I will ask a resource person to validate them when the opportunity arises.

_____   _____

Signature   Date

St. Mary-Corwin Regional Medical Center
Division of Nursing

Competency: Case Manager: Caregiver Role

PERFORMANCE CRITERIA	SELF-ASSESSMENT	LEARNING OPTIONS	EVALUATION MECHANISMS	DATE MET/ SIGNATURE	COMMENTS
▪ Assess client and identifies priorities using theoretical and conceptual framework		▪ Read nursing philosophy and framework for care delivery ▪ Use self-study module for assessment and documentation review	▪ Discussion ▪ Observations ▪ Documentation		
▪ Identifies trends in exacerbation of illness, etc., and fosters use of identified trends by client to develop preventive strategies		▪ Texts related to diagnoses ▪ Use of case study self-learning module	▪ Discussion ▪ Case study presentation		

St. Mary-Corwin Regional Medical Center
Division of Nursing

Competency: Case Manager: Coordinator Role

PERFORMANCE CRITERIA	SELF-ASSESSMENT	LEARNING OPTIONS	EVALUATION MECHANISMS	DATE MET/ SIGNATURE	COMMENTS
• Selects and applies appropriate critical pathway		• Educational session on critical pathways	• Observation • Documentation		
• Collaborates to ensure desired client outcomes with client, family, physicians, other disciplines, agencies, etc.		• Read *ANA Social Policy Statement* with focus on collaboration • Attends continuing care rounds • Spend time during orientation with other disciplines caring for client population	• Case presentation in continuing care rounds • Observation • Referrals, consultations made		

St. Mary-Corwin Regional Medical Center
Division of Nursing

Competency: Case Manager: Advocate Role

PERFORMANCE CRITERIA	SELF-ASSESSMENT	LEARNING OPTIONS	EVALUATION MECHANISMS	DATE MET/ SIGNATURE	COMMENTS
• Identifies cases for case management		• Educational session on case management	• Identifies self as case manager as seen with leaflet to client, input in computer system		
• Cultural and generational factors are considered and respected in procurement and delivery of services		• Reading materials and videos, i.e., common cultures and age groups	• Discussion • Appropriate revision of care plan/critical pathway • Client satisfaction		

St. Mary-Corwin Regional Medical Center
Division of Nursing

Competency: Case Manager: Broker Role

PERFORMANCE CRITERIA	SELF-ASSESSMENT	LEARNING OPTIONS	EVALUATION MECHANISMS	DATE MET/ SIGNATURE	COMMENTS
• Monitors and manages resource utilization		• Critical pathway educational session • Self-study module, i.e., costs of care and variance analysis	• Identifies variances from critical pathway • Discussion • Documentation		
• Negotiates for services to meet client needs		• Read *Getting to Yes* • Attend educational session on negotiation	• Observation • Discussion		

Chapter 22

Marketing Nurse Case Management Services

Donna Zazworsky, MSN, RN, CCM
Joyce A. Hospodar, BS, MPA

OVERVIEW

Nurse case managers can use marketing tools to position themselves as indispensable resources for high-quality, cost-effective health-care delivery.

Nurse case management services are an important and integral component of health care today. Independent health organizations and integrated delivery networks must understand how nurse case management helps answer the demands for increased cost consciousness and quality improvement. By knowing the steps in the marketing process, nurses can translate their contribution by preparing and implementing a marketing plan. Success will ensure that nurse case management is an indispensable resource and an essential strategy now and in the future.

THE HEALTH-CARE ENVIRONMENT

Nurses and other health-care providers are challenged to meet today's changes in a creative, proactive manner. Changes include shifting from fee-for-service to managed care and capitation. Current responses are taking the form of new alliances. The goal is to stay in business and achieve a positive margin or profit, while decreasing overall costs of health care and maintaining or improving quality. One new partnership, for example, involves hospitals joining with physicians to establish Physician-Hospital Organizations (PHOs), creating an integrated delivery network along a continuum of care. As a network, the PHO is more able to negotiate contracts with payor groups and Health Maintenance Organizations (HMOs).

Another alliance focuses on larger HMOs purchasing smaller HMOs to establish a more expansive regional network. Further, even at the federal level, Medicare continues to look for cost-effective ways to provide an array of services to the growing elderly population through Certified Medicare Provider (CMP), HMOs, and such demonstration projects as the Community Nursing Organization (CNO).

How does nurse case management fit into *health-care evolution?* How will marketing help the nurse case manager become a suitable player? By using the marketing plan approach, a systematic method lends credibility to the process (Caveen, 1992). It is the language and method that administration and corporations understand and expect.

Before exploring these questions further, a brief overview of the different types of case management services and nurse case management is needed to understand the intricacies of the competition and the implications of the marketing process.

Types of Case Management

Developing out of a social framework, case management is an accepted service today. Case management services are implemented in a variety of ways, although there is currently debate about what is case management versus care coordination.

Independent case management. Independent, profit or nonprofit case management organizations have developed out of an identified need within a community to coordinate services for the high-risk, aggregate groups, such as the elderly or the disabled. For example, in many places around the country, independent case management companies are hired to coordinate services such as in-home custodial care for the elderly parents when the adult children live in another location. These companies offer an array of services ranging from screening personnel to coordinating appropriate community resources.

Hospital-based case management. Hospitals have implemented internal or clinical case management for case-specific groups, such as orthopedics or cardiac diagnoses, which offer cost reductions as well as cost savings through multidisciplinary designed critical pathways (Mahn, 1993).

Many hospitals have also established community-based case management to mange the high-risk outliers within the different payor groups. At Carondelet Health Care in Tucson, Arizona, community nurse case managers (NCMs) follow HMO clients who have been admitted to the hospital twice within the last six months or Medicare clients who have a potential for readmission within 30 days of the client's previous admission. The focus of this work goes beyond recovery from acute illness to chronic care, specifically, helping people learn to live with chronic disease and thus avoiding or minimizing hospitalization (Ethridge & Lamb, 1989).

Physician-based case management. Physician groups have recognized the value of instituting their own case management services for their clients and offer a variety of inhospital or clinic focus, depending on the group's needs. For example, a cardiology group hired a nurse case manager to coordinate follow-up care for their high-risk senior HMO clients, ensuring follow-through of regular lab work and medication management.

Insurance-based case management. Insurance companies have long offered case management services for their enrollees. These case managers tend to focus on the long-term, high-risk persons who need intensive coordination of services, such as the head trauma client who needs extensive rehabilitation care.

These examples portray the versatility of case management in meeting the needs of clients and thus the needs of health care in a proactive manner. This versatility is key to marketing strategies. In other words, each one of these examples demonstrates that needs were identified and the product or service, nurse case management, was tailored to meet the needs. The first step, therefore, in creating nurse case management service is understanding the marketplace.

THE MARKETING PROCESS

The marketing process provides a framework to analyze the current marketplace, develop a product to meet the needs of the market and respective organization, and structure a plan of implementation and evaluation. The Marketing Plan Worksheet (Appendix 22-A) provides a working guide on how to design and implement the marketing process.

Developing a Marketing Plan

Step 1.   Develop a mission statement. When creating the mission statement, make sure that it fits within the organization's mission statement. In initiating a marketing plan, the first step is to see whether nurse case management fits into the scope of the parent organization's or system's strategies. The better the match of nurse case management to the organization's mission and strategic plan, the greater will be the support for the program.

For example, Carondelet's mission is "to provide for the health-care needs of our community; to embrace the whole person, in mind, body and spirit; and, to serve all persons without distinction" (excerpt from Carondelet Health Care–Southern Arizona Philosophy, Mission and Values Statement). To fit within the system's mission, the Carondelet nurse case managers' mission focuses on "helping people with serious or chronic health care issues meet the challenge of self-care and wellness and while striving to nurture and care for the whole person with respect for each person's dignity, independence and individuality" (excerpt from Carondelet Nurse Case Management brochure).

A second approach is to market nurse case management as a contract service beyond the parent organization to outside providers, health plans, and integrated delivery networks. Matching the nurse case management mission with the external organization mission is *vital* to the success of being awarded the contract as well as meeting the contractors' goals and expected outcomes.

Step 2.   Complete a market audit. A market audit consists of a current analysis of the target markets, local and national trends, demographic profiles, geographics, community resources, professional and community groups, targeted physicians, and businesses and industries. A market audit format is provided within the Market Plan Worksheet illustrated in Appendix 22-A. The defined steps to complete the audit are:

Target markets

Identifying and understanding the first-line "customers" or clients are key to preparing the market audit. It is essential that their needs be identified. There may be subgroups within the defined target market and their characteristics need to be identified. As an example, the customers may be predominantly Spanish-speaking or not have access to public transportation.

Although knowing the client population that is being served is crucial, the real customer from a marketing perspective may be administration, the contracting referral providers, health plans, or integrated delivery networks.

Targeting the high-risk client population influenced hospitalizations and length of stay (Michaels, 1992) but still promoted a reactive response to referrals. Today, the target client population is still the same for community NCMS; however, the referral process is changing. Referrals are now encouraged through physician offices or the HMOs on enrollment. In other words, the goal is to work with the high-risk population in a proactive manner before they enter the hospital.

Community

Demographic profile. The demographics of the population to be served was briefly addressed in the target markets section of the market audit. A demographic profile is more specific and includes a detailed profile of what the service area looks like, such as compiling pertinent data gathered by census tract, zip code, age, income, race, and so forth. There are many available sources for this type of information including Dunn and Bradstreet or your own organization's planning and marketing departments. Local government agencies (i.e., health department, planning department, and others) will provide information such as mortality, morbidity, and prevalence rates by diseases.

In many cases, the demographics are defined by the payors and their impact on the system for which the case management program is being established.

Geographics. Geographics is defined as the accessibility to the services being offered. Examples include the roadway networks, availability and types of public transportation, and the locations of your organization's service sites. An understanding of those factors

---

CASE STUDY

At Carondelet, the community nurse case management group practice performed an analysis of their current client base. As a result, the major high-risk diagnoses identified were coronary heart failure (CHF), chronic obstructive pulmonary disease (COPD), and neuromuscular diseases. The analysis also showed the breakdown in ages and payor groups, as well as identified the average number of case management visits and length of need within the case management service.

From 1992 to 1994, the payor mix shifted to include an increase in per diem and capitation payments and a decrease in commercial and Medicare reimbursements. The high-risk clients (i.e., CHF, COPD, and neuromuscular), therefore, enrolled in the HMOs (per diem and capitation) as well as Medicare became the target populations for community nurse case management within the Carondelet system.

Although these targeted high-risk clients were clearly defined, another target audience was identified—referral sources. Originally, community nurse case managers (NCMs) screened hospitalized HMO clients daily, identifying nurse case managed clients and making appropriate referrals. With the increase in HMO contracts, community NCMs began biweekly, discharge planning rounds with unit-based discharge planning teams consisting of staff nurses, social workers, home health liaisons, and HMO discharge planners. This reduced the amount of time spent within the hospital and increased the staff's knowledge of referral options. A referral form was developed and distributed to the above-mentioned members of the discharge team. So not only was there a need to identify the target clients but a need to identify and train the target referral sources as well. Today, approximately 95% of nurse case managed clients are referrals from hospitalizations.

---

will provide a clearer identification of what the organization may need to provide to get the services to those people in need of them.

Community nurse case management at Carondelet covers a two-county geographic area. Although the majority of clients live within the Tucson city limits, there are rural home visits required. In rural areas in the Southwest, directions may be "turn left at the fourth post with the big saguaro cactus, then keep on going until you get to the ostrich farm, then turn right after you pass the farm and go through the wash (a dry river bed)."

To cover this territory, the community case managers are assigned to three geographic sectors, that is, East, West, and South, respectively. These geographic sectors are divided by zip code boundaries and are reevaluated as needed (every one to two years) to decide if the boundaries need to be shifted based on workload distribution.

Another consideration for geographics is to recognize barriers. For instance, although a need for services are identified in a certain geographic location, planning and establishing the delivery of the specific services are vital before marketing services. For example, community health education programs were identified as a need and were being offered to a specific community population located in the northwest part of Tucson. The programs, however, were held at the hospital, which was out of the population's travel radius. The programs, therefore, were poorly attended. An important piece of data was not collected—travel patterns and barriers for that population. As a result of this experience, a location within the population' travel radius is being sought.

Community resources. Being aware of what community resources are available within the community will help in the planning and marketing of a program. Avoiding duplication of services should be a major goal. Learning how other case management programs work within the community, for example, their referral process and criteria, job responsibilities, available services, and financial boundaries, will help position and communicate the services more effectively.

For example, Carondelet received a demonstration grant from the National Multiple Sclerosis Society to provide case management for persons with progressive MS. As the need for exercise programs was identified within the study, the nurse case manager (NCM) determined there were no existing programs and sought outside funding from local agencies and private donors, developed the classes and obtained manpower, and donated space from local churches and neighborhood centers.

Professional organizations and community groups. Knowledge of the professional and community clubs and groups within the service area will help in marketing efforts. These types of organizations have established networks and focus on serving and meeting community needs. Having these organizations align with the marketing efforts are essential. For example, as the MS exercise program at Carondelet demonstrated positive outcomes in both functional status and community referrals, the local chapter of the MS Society and MS self-help groups were approached to communicate the program to the MS community. Today, the local chapter provides the communications and registration services, whereas the NCM continues to coordinate the programs throughout the community as well as train other health professionals (i.e., nurses, physical therapists, and volunteers and caregivers) to provide the program.

For those case management services that are independent of an institution and rely on referrals from other agencies, networking provides the lifeline for survival. Regular inservices, brochures, and open houses to hospital or commercial-based case managers or social workers as well as other targeted community agencies enhance the likelihood of referrals.

Physicians targeted

Physician groups represent one segment of professional alliances that nurse case managers seek. With the increasing number of health plans and their systems, physicians are inundated with numerous client phone calls and paperwork related to service authorization, provider referral forms, and special requests from insurances. NCMs assist the physicians by offering a "one-stop shopping" service. In other words, the physician only needs to contact the NCM to coordinate home health services, equipment, supplies, and receive current health status information. The NCM provides a more efficient and productive means of communicating client problems and facilitating appropriate authorization/referral requests.

At Carondelet, the community NCMs have worked closely with physicians on staff for more than 10 years. More and more physicians refer clients to nurse case management upon hospital discharge and some contact the NCMs directly from the office or clinic setting. Greater emphasis is now placed on NCM partnerships with physicians, especially when working to create a seamless continuum of community services. Carondelet offers an array of community services that spans health promotion-disease prevention, and primary, acute, transitional, and long-term care. The NCM facilitates movement of clients across the service continuum.

Business and industry

As business and industry continue to look for ways to increase savings, case management can serve as one means of cost containment. For example, organizations are teaming to share expertise and resources, particularly in the managed care environment where shared risk is part of a contract between the provider and the HMO. At Carondelet, HMO and physician-based case managers work with Carondelet's clinical and community case managers to manage clients who are high-risk, high-service utilizers.

Trends

National and local trends in case management need to be monitored and incorporated into the market audit. The services planned for should be "at the cutting edge" within your community. The national trends in case management illustrate the diverse changes and needs of the health-care environment and the competition that drives these changes. There are payor-based (managed-care and commercial) case management programs,

---

CASE STUDY

Carondelet NCMs work in concert with other case managers to identify the best approach to benefit the client. In the case of one contract between Carondelet and a senior HMO health plan, Carondelet's *community* NCMs work with a *clinic* NCM who is employed by the HMO for their outpatient staff physician clinics to manage the HMOs high-risk, high utilizers. The clinic NCM sees the clients at the clinic and provides follow-up by telephone but does not have the opportunity to observe how clients manage their health at home. One client was referred to the clinic NCM by the client's physician because of the client's need for frequent lab work and medication management. Because the community case manager worked with this client in the home, the clinic NCM and community NCM worked out a schedule of home lab draws which the clinic case manager coordinated within the HMO system. The community NCM maintained the direct contact with the client and the physician. When the community NCM identified a need for service, she contacted the clinic case manager who expedited the services. This method of collaboration builds on the unique features and strengths of both roles. This collaboration leads to improved client care and satisfaction and demonstrates to the HMO and the organization's administration that both roles are necessary for quality and cost effectiveness.

---

physician-based case managers, and hospital-based (both internal and external) case managers—all of which aim to promote quality and enhance cost-containment outcomes. Which entity best demonstrates and communicates these outcomes is the challenge to which nurse case management must respond.

Competition

As with any business environment, there is usually competition. Who is your competition? Are they local, state, or national competitors? How are they positioned? What are their services? How do they communicate their services? How do they contract? Who does their contracting? Who are their contractors? Who are their target markets? How might you merge efforts so competition is not a threat, but an opportunity? Learn your competition!

Step 3.   Complete an internal analysis. An internal analysis takes an inventory of the strengths, weaknesses, opportunities, and threats of the organization and the case management service. This analysis is commonly called a SWOT analysis (Strengths, Weaknesses, Opportunities, Threats).

Strengths

What are the strengths of the organization and the case management program? These strengths may be windows of opportunity.

At Carondelet, the strengths of the nurse case management program include the diverse clinical backgrounds of the nurses, ranging from experience in hospice, critical care, orthopedics, maternal/child, and diabetes. The group is made up of BSNs, MSNs and PhDs. In addition, the philosophy of the group practice supports autonomy, authority, and accountability for the professional and empowerment of the client.

Other strengths include the NCM's involvement in the development of the points of service within the community continuum of care. For example, the NCMs were instrumental in the development of family wellness centers being established within a school district and a parish wellness center in the barrio. NCMs along with nurse practitioners staff the 19 community health centers throughout four counties, as well as provide education and exercise programs to high-risk populations, enhancing health promotion and well-being.

Weaknesses

What are the weaknesses of the organization and the case management program? Are the weaknesses, for example, related to image, staffing, financial, client outcomes, or lack of knowledge of the services?

For example, with the effort of creating a *seamless* integrated delivery system, the "cracks" must be addressed. At Carondelet, the cracks still exist in the referral process between points of service, primarily those services outside of the Carondelet system. For example, approximately 90% of nurse case management referrals are generated from Carondelet services—hospitalizations and home health discharges—which are clearly a reactive rather than a proactive approach, but not within the nurse case manager's control. A mechanism needs to be developed to capture referrals to nurse case management services before the client requires emergency room visits or hospitalization.

Opportunities

What are the opportunities for an organization and for case management? And how does case management fit into the organization's opportunities?

With the increase in managed care contracts, nurse case management can support the organization by working with clients to avoid or minimize use of the ER or hospital. As the quality of life for the client increases, costs will be reduced.

Another opportunity is to have the organization study what impact nurse case management has had within the system and use the results at the negotiating table.

Threats

What are the threats to an organization and how do these affect case management? For example, if the organization is at risk of losing a managed care contract, how will this impact case management?

One threat is related to how nurse case management is understood within the corporation particularly when contracts are being established with health plans or networks. If the person contracting the nurse case management services along with the other Carondelet services does not have a clear knowledge base of how nurse case management impacts and facilitates the other services of the continuum, then nurse case management may be viewed as unnecessary. In the long run, this lack of knowledge could influence the success of the service outcomes and inevitably the financial viability of the contract.

Step 4.   Develop the plan. In the planning phase, a systematic process is implemented supported by data from the analysis. Included in this plan are projected goals and objectives with detailed actions and time frames. To assist with the planning process, a strategic foundation must be developed by addressing the four P's: product, promotions, placing, and pricing (McCarthy, 1990).

Product

In nurse case management, answering the question, "What is the product?" can be awkward. Is the service an independent, stand-alone product, such as the private case management company marketed to a specific population? Or is the service part of the continuum of care within a large health-care organization? An important factor in designing a product is to use terms that the customer will understand that specifies what the product is.

Promotion

How will you promote the product or service? This must be tied to the target market(s). Many hospital-based nurse case management services target the fixed reimbursement markets (i.e., Medicare, HMOs). In these cases, promotions focus on the referral mechanisms, such as physicians, discharge planners, social workers, staff nurses, and home health. For example, at Carondelet, nurse case management referral sheets and client information brochures are provided to social workers, discharge planners, rehabilitation services, and home health services.

Another important component of promotion is the six states of buyer readiness (Kotler & Clarke, 1987). These states are broken into three categories:

- Cognitive (awareness, knowledge)
- Affective (liking, preference, conviction)
- Behavior (action)

The promotion plans must take into consideration the readiness states of the target audience and incorporate a number of different methods to inform, persuade, or remind (Kotler & Clarke, 1987). For example, continu-

ing with Carondelet's example of their target audiences, community NCMs provide regular orientation and education sessions to the above-mentioned staff as well as attend discharge planning rounds twice a week on the units to maintain awareness, knowledge, and referrals (action). Also, strategically placing referral sheets in all departments enhances the likelihood of referrals. General client information brochures are available for all staff when informing clients of the nurse case management referral.

Work with the public relations department within your organization in developing promotion plans. They are the experts in communication methods for target audiences. If the organization does not have a PR department, then an outside PR consultant is recommended.

Placing

Where to place or position services depends on the organization's positioning (Reddy, 1993). For example, if the organization is an independent mental health center, then the case management program will focus specifically on mental health issues. Whereas, if the organization is an integrated delivery system with hospitals, physicians, and multiple services across the continuum of care, case management services may focus on specific (i.e., cardiac/CABG) and general concerns (high-risk seniors) both in the hospital and community.

Pricing

Knowing how to price services requires a financial analysis of what it costs to deliver the services (i.e., manpower, supportive resources, material costs, and travel). In today's health-care market, capitation is becoming more and more prevalent. Therefore, a fee-for-service payment method may be appropriate in some contracts, but identifying services and costs under a capitated contract requires a different perspective. Again, depending on the organization's direction, case management services may be contracted separately or clumped with other services or as a part of the entire organization's capitation package. At Carondelet, an Activity Tracking Form was developed to track the type and time of services by payor to provide data for negotiating future contracts.

Step 5.   Resource needs. An estimation of what resource needs your case management practice requires is essential. Providing administration with estimates for program needs will help in budgeting and future negotiations for contracts. Categories to include are staffing, travel, supplies, space, and marketing needs (brochure development, production, distribution).

Step 6.   Service goal. As part of planning, defined goals must be outlined. These goals should focus on how the service is described and how these goals fit into the overall direction of the organization. Specific objectives and action plans are developed for each goal. For example, the Carondelet's nurse case management group practice establishes yearly goals for practice, research, and outreach.

Once the plan is developed, implementation follows. This is the *doing* part; however, implementing in phases is recommended with evaluations at each phase.

Step 7. Service outcomes. Evaluating the marketing plan determines the success of the plan and thus the program. Depending on the goals and how the goals were incorporated into the organization's goals, the evaluation methods must reflect the services outcomes toward those goals.

In other words, if the organization is geared to reduce emergency room (ER) visits, then case management may direct their services and focus their marketing plan on the ER, identifying high utilizers and outcome indicators and developing referral markers/forms for the ER staff and pertinent primary care providers for case management.

CONCLUSION

Nurse case management plays a pivotal role in today's evolving health-care system. The versatility of this approach in meeting client's needs proactively while containing costs is a key area to highlight when designing marketing strategies. Understanding the marketplace, utilizing the marketing plan approach, and presenting the plan in the language and format that administration and corporations expect are means to help ensure the marketing plan's greatest chances of success. With careful analysis and planning, nurse case managers can use marketing tools to position themselves as indispensable resources for high-quality, cost-effective health-care delivery.

REFERENCES

Caveen, W., Cheshire, L., Power, B., & Wooley, D. (1992). Following a course to improve standards: a professional development course for nurse practitioners in stoma care. *Professional Nurse, 7* (9), 580-585.

Ethridge, P. E., & Lamb, G. S. (1989). Professional nurse case management improves quality, access and costs. *Nursing Management, 20,* 30-35.

Kotler, P., & Clark, R. N. (1987). *Marketing for health care organizations.* Englewood Cliffs, NJ: Prentice-Hall.

Mahn, V. A. (1993). Clinical nurse case management: a service line approach, *Nursing Management, 24* (9), 48-50.

McCarthy, J. E., & Perreault, N. D. (1990). *Basic marketing.* Boston: Irwin.

Michaels, C. (1992). Carondelet St. Mary's nursing enterprise. *Nursing Clinics of North America, 27,* 77-86.

Reddy, A. C., & Campbell, D. P. (1993 Winter). Positioning hospitals: a model for regional hospitals. *Journal of Health Care Marketing,* 40-44.

Appendix 22-A   Marketing Plan Worksheet

I. Mission Statement: _____

_____

_____

II. Market Audit
A. Target Markets
   1. _____ (Male/Female)

   2. _____ (Age)

   3. _____ (Socioeconomic Status)

   4. _____ (Education Level)
B. Community: (Immediate zip coded service area) *Obtainable by Dunn & Bradstreet
   1. Demographics
      a. _____
         (Immediate Service Area)

      b. _____
         (Secondary Service Area)

      c. _____

      d. _____
   2. Geographics: (Accessibility, i.e., transportation, roadways)
      a. _____

      b. _____

      c. _____
   3. Target Audience: (Aggregates, i.e., Senior Citizens, Smokers)
      a. _____

      b. _____

      c. _____

   4. Community Resources (Voluntary Services, i.e., American Cancer Society, American Heart Association)
      a. _____

      b. _____

      c. _____
   5. Professional Groups and Organizations (MD, RN, Women Bankers, Chamber of Commerce)
                    Internal
      a. _____

      b. _____

      c. _____

                    External
      a. _____
      b. _____
      c. _____
   6. Community Clubs and Organizations: (Better Breathers, AA)
      a. _____
      b. _____
      c. _____
C. Physicians Targeted
   1. _____
   2. _____
   3. _____
D. Business & Industry
   1. _____
   2. _____
   3. _____
   4. _____
E. Trends
   1. _____
   2. _____
   3. _____
F. Competition
   1. _____
   2. _____
   3. _____
   4. _____

III. Internal Analysis
A. Strengths
   1. _____
   2. _____
   3. _____
   4. _____
   5. _____
B. Weaknesses
   1. _____
   2. _____
   3. _____
   4. _____

C. Opportunities

1. _____

2. _____

3. _____

4. _____

D. Threats

1. _____

2. _____

3. _____

4. _____

IV. Develop the Plan

A. Product

1. _____

2. _____

3. _____

B. Promotion

1. _____

2. _____

3. _____

C. Placing

1. _____

2. _____

3. _____

D. Pricing

1. _____

2. _____

3. _____

4. _____

V. Resource Needs

A. Space (What kind and for what?)

1. _____

2. _____

B. Equipment (What kind and how expensive?)

1. _____

2. _____

C. Education

1. _____

2. _____

VI. Service Goals (Projected dates)

A. _____

B. _____

C. _____

VII. Service Outcomes (Admission, Revenue, Success Rates)

A. _____

B. _____

C. _____

Chapter 23

Implementing Nurse Case Management in a Rural Community Hospital

Sharon Jehle, MSN, RNC
Gail Terry, BSN, RNC
Margaret Murphy, PhD, RN

OVERVIEW

Nurses in a rural health-care system help the nurse case management model evolve from implementation through evaluation.

Having identified the need for a clearly defined client (patient) care delivery system, this rural referral center implemented the first case management model in Wisconsin. Case management offered an organized, common sense approach to deliver efficient, coordinated, quality client care while promoting professional development and satisfaction. The evolution of this nursing care model from implementation through evaluation was a long and complex process. Today, as the hospital network reorganizes to meet the future needs of its clients and community, plans are being made for the development of an even more responsive model of nurse case management.

Holy Family Memorial Medical Center, located on Wisconsin's east shore, is a rural referral center with an average daily census of 100 inpatients. This hospital employs over 800 people, 360 of whom are acute care nursing personnel. Its nursing department was the first in the state to select and implement a differentiated nurse case management model.

Typical of many hospital nursing departments in the late 1980s, Holy Family Memorial lacked a clearly defined client care delivery system. Although clients expressed a high level of satisfaction with the excellent care they received, the care responsibilities of nurses were often fragmented. Moreover, there was a lack of

congruence between basic nursing education and job expectations.

The RNs, the majority of whom are diploma or associate degree nurses, were prepared to use the nursing process. This meant nurses that were educated to be accountable and responsible for the well-being of a defined client group by using nursing diagnosis, outcomes, and a plan of care, including the evaluation of this plan from admission to discharge. This process, however, was not operationalized in the clinical practice setting. Rarely did RNs assume accountability or responsibility for total nursing care for a specific client.

Some of the reasons that the nursing process was not operationalized in the clinical practice setting included:

- Limited knowledge about the application of process in practice;
- Lack of role models; and
- Lack of opportunity to practice the use of nursing process in a task-oriented environment.

As a result, RNs poorly differentiated their role from other ancillary care providers and routinely performed non-nursing tasks such as client transport and supply pickup. Physicians were viewed by nurses as the primary coordinator of services with the nurse responsible for implementing a prescribed course of action. Because of this perception, true collaboration between the RN and physician was virtually nonexistent.

One additional area of concern facing the nursing department was the national nursing shortage. Although the turnover rate at Holy Family Memorial was only 5%, the vacancy rate remained constant at 11%. The nursing department leadership could ill afford to continuously orient RNs at an estimated cost of $2,500 per nurse. It has been shown that increased staff turnover and vacancy rates can be reduced if nurses are allowed to practice in a professional system (Edwards, 1988). Implementing a professional practice model, therefore, became a high priority.

For these reasons, the nursing department embarked on a path to identify a nursing care delivery system and assure that nursing turnover and vacancy rates would remain low. The strategic goal of the nursing department was to find a system that would:

- Establish a work environment that promoted staff involvement;
- Make nurses accountable and responsible (provide them with authority for their own practice);
- Improve the mechanism for documentation of nursing process;
- Promote maximal utilization of all nursing staff;
- Reduce vacancy and turnover rates (enhance recruitment efforts); and
- Promote cost-effective care by minimizing fragmentation and maximizing coordination of services.

RATIONALE FOR NURSE CASE MANAGEMENT

When selecting a delivery system, the vice-president of nursing made a decision to adopt the differentiated nurse case management model described by Dr. Peggy Primm (1987). He believed that this case management model had a strong nursing focus and that when implemented could achieve the nursing department goals. Furthermore, he decided that demonstration units would not be used. Rather, all nursing units including surgical, medical, oncology, obstetrics, pedi-

atrics, rehabilitation, critical care, emergency department, and home health care would participate fully in this project. This decision was made based on the belief that all nurses could benefit by education and the fact that it was less expensive to introduce the system to all units at once.

Differentiated nurse case management is based on a philosophy that focuses on the restructuring of roles and functions of nurses according to educational preparation and competence (McClure, 1991). The concept of differentiated nursing practice was developed in response to a need for common expectations of practice outcomes for future nursing education programs. The 1982-86 W.K. Kellogg-funded, Midwest Alliance in Nursing-sponsored project "Defining and Differentiating ADN and BSN Competencies" resulted in a nationally accepted model for differentiated nursing practice and education (Primm, 1987).

Dr. Primm, project director for Midwest Alliance in Nursing and progenitor of Differentiated Nursing Case Management model, incorporated a philosophy of differentiation of levels of practice that was based on complexity of decision making. Job descriptions for the nurse case manager and nurse case associate reflected the competencies of future graduates, baccalaureate degree, and associate degree graduates, respectively, and provided a mechanism for all currently practicing staff nurses to participate during the transition process.

IMPLEMENTATION OF NURSE CASE MANAGEMENT

The implementation phase, which lasted almost two years, involved a number of preparatory interventions including:

- Completing a Nurse Satisfaction Questionnaire by nursing staff;
- Establishing a steering committee and communication network;
- Introducing and completing factoring tool by all RNs;
- Providing education for nursing staff; and
- Conducting implementation data collection including chart audits.

Nurse Satisfaction

A new approach to the way nursing is practiced can alter the perception of satisfaction among the nursing staff (Slavitt, et al., 1978). Before implementation of the case management system, it was decided to measure the degree of nurse satisfaction. Each nurse was asked to complete a Nurse Satisfaction Questionnaire developed by Etta S. McCulloch (Ward, 1978). The specific purpose of the questionnaire was to measure the degree of satisfaction with various aspects of work adjustment to the hospital setting. Nurses answered the 120-item questionnaire by scoring on a 5-point Likert scale in which responses ranged from *not satisfied* to *extremely satisfied*. Factor variables that were measured were categorized as follows:

- Working conditions
- Professional consideration
- Professional preparation
- Compensation
- Emotional climate
- Supervision
- Social significance

Data were obtained the first year and the year after implementation of case management. Overall nursing staff satisfaction increased in the year after implementation, particularly in the areas of compensation, social significance, and professional consideration. From the results, the authors concluded that the case management implementation phase had a positive effect on the nurses' perception of job satisfaction.

Communication Strategies

The authors strongly believe, from a management orientation, that all successful implementation projects benefit from open discussion and a common vision shared by all persons involved. A complex communication network, therefore, involving all nurses at Holy Family Memorial Medical Center was established. This network included a steering committee, unit-based committees, and a staff network tree. In this system, all nurses received information and shared their thoughts about how to resolve issues.

An organization-wide steering committee, consisting of a unit nurse director, a staff nurse from each nursing unit, the vice-president of nursing, and a nurse educator-project coordinator met regularly. This committee was the driving force for implementation of case management and the center for discussion of issues, formation of policy, and communication of decisions including:

- Work schedule for case managers (float, low census, shift trading, and so forth)
- Clinical ladder appraisal system
- Job expectations for newly hired RNs
- Client transfers to other units

The unit-based case management committee consisting of unit members of the steering committee and staff from each shift met to identify and resolve issues specific to that unit with regard to case management implementation. Additionally, members on this unit-based committee were responsible for communicating information to other unit nurses who were assigned to them.

Through implementation of this communication network, nurse directors and staff nurses had input into decision making. As a result, all aspects of each issue were considered and the proposals generated were more readily accepted by the nursing staff, although implementation occurred slowly. Additionally, it was hoped that the ability to influence the environment and resources for practice would be a satisfier for nurses in our organization as it had been in others (Hinshaw et al., 1987).

To facilitate inter- and intradiscipline communication, an assignment board was hung in each nurse station. This board provided the key information to all caregivers, including the room number, client initials, case manager, caregiver, and physician's name "at a glance."

Factoring

Every RN was required to complete a "Job Description Factoring Tool" designed by Dr. Primm. The purpose of the tool was to assist the RN in selecting the case management job description (case manager or case associate) in which they would experience the most success. The factoring tool consisted of 50 practice characteristic statements, including 10 statements considered to be critical behaviors required of a case manager. The nurse indicated whether each statement was reflective of the nurse's current practice. Educational preparation was not a consideration of the factoring. With the nurse director, the RN agreed upon the job description (case manager, case associate) in which the nurse would practice for a three-month trial. If a nurse director decided the RN was a good candidate for the case manager role but lacked some necessary skill or experience, then the nurse director and the RN met to establish goals and learning activities with target dates to meet the job requirement.

Education

After each nurse had completed the factoring process and knew which job description role they would practice in for three months, the nurse was sheduled to attend a role-specific educational offering. The nursing department staffing mix ratio was 75% RNs to 25% LPNs. To achieve the department goal of maximal utilization of all nursing staff, attendance at educational sessions about nurse case management was required.

All nursing staff had initial inservice education sessions with Dr. Primm. RNs and LPNs were given case manager, case associate, and LPN job descriptions that detailed future role expectations. RNs received additional inservice education about the concepts related to applied nursing diagnosis. The cost of the educational offerings during this implementation phase was tracked. A total of 2,500 hours of education was provided for 230 nursing personnel.

Policy Development

The steering committee set policies addressing issues common to all nursing units. The first policy statement included the following key components:

- Within 24 hours of admission, every client (patient) will have a case manager with the exception of targeted populations and clients hospitalized less than 24 hours.
- The case manager is responsible for planning nursing care from admission to post discharge with client, family, and physician.
- RNs (whether case manager or case associate) provide direct care or delegate client care to other assistive personnel; LPNs deliver client care delegated by an RN.
- RNs and LPNs work together to facilitate health promotion and continuity of care.

The steering committee also established a set of charting expectations. This proved to be difficult to implement because documentation forms were different throughout the agency. After trying a number of proposals, the steering committee decided that key information had to be easily retrievable although the forms varied. Minimal information expectations included:

- Care plan with two- or three-part nursing diagnosis;
- Measurable, time-specific mutually set goals initialed by the nurse and the client and family;
- Time-specific, concise nursing interventions;
- Documentation indicating that all nursing orders were addressed;
- Daily case manager summary of client progress toward goal achievement; and
- Case manager discharge summary on day of or before client discharge.

The importance of established agreed-upon policy statements cannot be overemphasized. These policy statements, although seemingly concrete and simple, were accepted only after many hours of discussion.

Data Collection

Once factoring was completed and nurses were educationally prepared and working in their respective roles, data collection tools were introduced. The purposes of the tools were to:

- Reacquaint nursing staff with role expectations of case manager, case associate, and LPN positions;
- Provide opportunity for self-assessment;
- Identify staffing patterns;
- Identify staff development needs; and
- Collect data for research.

Case managers, case associates, and LPNs were asked to complete a self-assessment data collection tool for each shift over a six-week period. By scoring "yes" or "no" to questions asked regarding their completion of daily routine expectations, subsequent evaluations could focus on specific areas of concern.

The nurse directors of the involved units completed weekly summaries of information including total client census, number of case managed clients, and percentage of clients who were case managed. The standard, as set by the steering committee, was that all clients be case managed except those clients with less than a 24-hour length of stay.

Chart audits of case managed clients were regularly completed by the nurse educators. The audit criteria paralleled the newly specified documentation expectations and included such items as:

- Completed assessment using Gordon's functional health patterns;
- Two- or three-part nursing diagnosis;
- Time-specific, measurable mutual goals;
- Time-specific nursing orders;
- Case manager goal summary, including client and family progress toward goal achievement; and
- Documentation of all nursing orders by using focus charting format.

Results of chart audits provided meaningful feedback to case managers and nurse directors, thus demonstrating that documentation expectations were not always met. As a result of these findings, one-on-one feedback and education were provided to nursing staff.

EVOLUTION OF PROFESSIONAL PRACTICE
Shared Governance

As the nursing department continued to grow professionally, staff nurses expressed a desire to have more control over their practice. *Shared governance* has been identified in the literature as *a professional model that provides staff nurses with an organized and systematic way of governing themselves in activities that apply to nursing practice* (Allen et al., 1988). It acknowledges professionalism by allowing professional nurses to use their unique body of knowledge in making decisions regarding nursing practice and delivery within their practice environment.

After extensive investigation of various shared governance systems, the nursing department chose to implement a model consisting of a nursing cabinet, five staff councils (standards, practice, peer relations, quality assurance, and research), and one management council. Each nursing unit was represented on each of the six councils. As part of the reorganization process the agency steering committee for case management was dissolved and nurse case management, with all the issues and concerns surrounding it, became the responsibility of the practice council.

Merger

Three years after the implementation of case management, Holy Family Memorial Medical Center merged with an 87-bed community hospital. This merger raised issues and concerns about meeting the needs of nurses in the now "blended" nursing departments.

A nursing merger committee consisting of management and staff nurses from both facilities met to develop and implement plans to blend the best from both nursing departments including the nurse case management model used only at Holy Family Memorial Medical Center.

Thus, as part of their orientation, the nurses from the merged organization were introduced to the concepts of case management. Eight months later, RNs who were interested in functioning in the case manager role attended a formal education session. These sessions, conducted by nurse educators, contained the same content as programs originally presented at startup.

This merger and the attending issues related to blending nursing staffs with very different care delivery models brought all aspects of our current case management model into the forefront. With the spotlight pointed at nursing care systems, new questions were raised about the model and its efficiency.

EVALUATION OF NURSE CASE MANAGEMENT
Initial Evaluation

There were a number of advantages evident in the first two years after implementation of nurse case management. The reported advantages consistent with the goals of the nursing department included:

- Case managers had responsibility for client outcomes;
- Maximum utilization of all staff was achieved;
- Physicians expressed satisfaction to nursing vice-president;
- Care planning improved;
- Discharge planning improved;
- Communication network was established; and
- Nursing department moved toward shared governance model.

These early successes were shared with the nursing staff by means of letters to the units, articles in the nursing newsletter, and feedback within the communication network. Staff involvement was actively sought when outside agencies requested information about our case management model. The authors believed that the case managers and case associates themselves needed to articulate these advantages to others and thereby assume responsibility for the continuation of these advantages. Identified obstacles were viewed as opportunities to strengthen the case management

delivery system. Given the time and resources available, the authors chose to address the following:

- Lack of written standards
- Delegation issues related to the LPN
- Staff resistance to change

During the implementation phase, staff reported and chart audits verified that nurses were writing many of the same interventions for each nursing diagnosis, thereby increasing the time spent on charting. To decrease this unnecessary duplication, nurses on each unit developed written *minimum standards of care* based on commonly used nursing diagnoses. Thereafter, care plan interventions included the prewritten minimum standards of care and only those interventions individualized for a specific client were handwritten. Thus, the charting time and the amount of documentation were decreased and standardization of routine interventions was achieved.

A second issue related to LPN assignments was brought to light with the implementation of nurse case management. For many years, LPNs were assigned to provide direct care for clients with an RN caring for the clients as needed. In the new model, rather than receiving their own client assignment, LPNs were assigned to an RN who delegated certain aspects of care to the LPN. Although this change was subtle, the new emphasis was placed on active delegation rather than the LPN seeking the RN as needed. To prepare both the RNs and LPNs, workshops were planned and presented by the nurse educators. The workshops not only provided an educational offering to clarify roles for staff, but they also enhanced the open communication between RNs and LPNs on a sensitive issue.

The third obstacle addressed was the issue of staff resistance to change. This obstacle was closely tied to the need for nurses to work together as a team and to resolve conflicts in a constructive manner. To prepare the nurse directors to address this issue better, educational sessions were provided by an outside consultant who was an expert in teambuilding and conflict resolution. With the backdrop of the change process, nurse directors were guided through active participation exercises. Subsequent sessions on teambuilding and conflict resolution were conducted for nursing staff by trained facilitators together with nurse directors on their respective units. Immediate feedback from the participants by means of evaluation verified the recommitment to teamwork and a better working understanding of change process and conflict-resolution strategies.

Subsequent Evaluation

Change is a complex process that is best evaluated over time. Five years after the implementation of nurse case management, there was general agreement that this delivery system achieved a number of desired outcomes impacting the nursing department and ultimately care to clients. These desired outcomes included:

- Case managers had responsibility for client outcomes;
- All nursing staff was used to provide direct client care;
- All clients had a computerized care plan that was evaluated based on goal achievement;
- Nursing department minimum standards of care were developed;
- Critical pathways were developed;
- Turnover rate decreased from 5% to 4%, whereas vacancy rate decreased from 11% to 6%; and
- A shared governance model was implemented that promoted staff nurse involvement in clinical decision making.

These achievements were highly valued in light of the fact that the nursing department changed from a top-down decision-making system to one that promoted and shared ownership for decision making with the clinical nursing staff.

Improvements that were needed in this case management model were:

- Cost-effective means to minimize fragmentation of client care and maximize coordination of services; and
- Improved mechanism for documentation of the nursing process.

As a result of this evaluation, strengthening the case management process of delivering client care was identified as an important nursing department strategic goal. To accomplish this undertaking, a committee consisting of nurse directors, staff nurses from the Shared Governance Practice Council, and a representative from the utilization management department met on a regular basis. The goals of the committee were identified at this initial meeting and included the following:

- Strengthen the case manager's role
- Develop common outcome criteria
- Investigate charting tools and paper flow
- Strengthen the interdisciplinary team approach
- Incorporate and strengthen the critical pathways
- Develop a reporting system for variances
- Provide education regarding measuring of outcomes, cost containment, and quality
- Explore differential compensation for case managers

REDEFINITION OF THE NURSE CASE MANAGEMENT MODEL
Assessment of the Existing Case Management Model

The case management committee, which met over an eight-month period, spent much of the time assessing the existing model and planning for interventions to improve it. The committee identified that the case managers were unable to provide continuity of case-managed clients. It was learned that policies and procedures governing shift work did not take into consideration continuity in client care. For instance, all nursing staff were required to rotate unpaid days off (low census days) and to float to other units if client census warranted it. No consideration was given for the case manager's caseload or client requirements. In addition, some units found the lack of case manager continuity occurred more frequently because of scheduling patterns than as a result of the low census or float policies. Nurse directors, therefore, developed work schedules that allowed for consistency in scheduling.

To assess refinements needed to improve the success of the case management process further, the committee sought input from the case managers and case associates themselves. Two focus groups, one group consisting of case managers from each nursing unit and a second focus group of case associates from each unit, met independently of each other with a facilitator. Questions were sent out before the meeting so the case managers and case associates could get feedback from the other staff on their units. The questions included:

- What are problems for case management on your unit?
- What keeps case managers from being effective?
- What do you value in your present case management system?
- What makes case management work on your unit?
- What would be one or two suggestions to help case management function better on your unit?

The feedback received included observations of lack of continuity of care, inconsistency in meeting the expectations of the case manager role across units, and the excess amount of paperwork required. Nursing staff expressed mixed feelings about the nursing roles. The case managers expressed satisfaction and a feeling of autonomy and ownership over their practice along with collaboration with other health-care providers but felt they had a greater workload overall than did case associates. The case associates, conversely, reported feeling less valued yet doing the same work as the case manager.

The committee also networked with representatives from Sioux Valley Hospital, Sioux Falls, South Dakota, to discuss their case management model. New questions were raised concerning the role expectations of case managers and case associates and whether the standard that all clients need to be case managed was appropriate.

During this assessment phase, this cross-functional committee gained valuable insight into the reasons why the case management model was not achieving all the nursing department goals. It also was instrumental in implementing the strategies needed to refine the existing model to achieve the desired goals.

Development of the Action Plan

During the planning phase of the process of redefining the case management model, a common definition of case management was agreed upon: *Nursing was responsible for the management and coordination of all the client's (patient's) care from admission through discharge.* The case manager and case associate roles were redefined, and job descriptions were developed integrating some of the criteria from Sioux Valley. The case manager job description (Box 23-1) included responsibility to:

- Provide direct client care
- Identify and initiate appropriate referrals
- Initiate and complete discharge plan
- Collaborate with the physician
- Ensure that the critical pathway is followed or variances documented
- Involve the family in decision making
- Assess psychosocial needs
- Assess, initiate, and complete client teaching
- Individualize the client's plan of care, goals, and interventions
- Manage resource allocation
- Arrange scheduling and client assignments so the client would receive the fewest caregivers possible during the stay

The role description for the case associate was also revised by using some of the criteria from Sioux

---

BOX 23-1
CASE MANAGER JOB DESCRIPTION

Job Summary

Responsible and accountable for coordinating the care of patients (clients) (meeting case management criteria) across a continuum of care; ensuring and facilitating the achievement of quality, clinical and cost outcomes; negotiating, procuring and coordinating services and resources needed by the client and family.

Position Requirements

Education: Graduate accredited school of nursing. BSN preferred. Current license for State of Wisconsin.

Experience: 2-3 years minimum in area practicing.

Other: Excellent communication and organizational skills.
Must work minimum of 64 hours per pay period.

Responsibilities

In addition to staff RN responsibilities:

1. Utilizing the nursing process to facilitate the delivery of holistic care:
   a. Coordinates and/or provides direct/indirect care for the client meeting case management criteria.
   b. Analyzes and integrates complex data to develop specific nursing diagnosis and individualized interventions.
   c. Involves client and family in identifying their needs and expectations to develop mutual and realistic goals.
   d. Revises and adjusts on a daily basis the plan of care to fit the needs of the individual client based on continuing assessment of client's condition.

   e. Assumes responsibility and accountability for the care plan effectiveness and client outcomes.
   f. Initiates and follows through with early/appropriate discharge planning in collaboration with the health-care team.
2. Using interactive communication skills:
   a. Facilitates communication links among the different disciplines involved in the treatment plan.
   b. Collaborates on a daily basis with MD(s) regarding the client's progress and changing needs.
   c. Negotiates care provided with members of the health-care team, client and family to ensure timely and cost effective client outcomes.
3. Acknowledging the financial component of health care and practicing in a fiscally responsible manner:
   a. Coordinates and facilitates efficient use of resources.
   b. Identifies and/or controls variances in the client's condition to control costs.
   c. Controls duplication and fragmentation of care by assuring consistency, continuity, and coordination of care.
   d. Works closely with ancillary and support services to control and prevent inappropriate hospital stays.
   e. Maintains cost-effective care by monitoring proper utilization of interventions, supplies, and equipment.
   f. Utilizes knowledge related to DRGs and reimbursement procedures in developing plan of care.

Valley (Box 23-2). This role included responsibility to:

- Follow through with the teaching plan
- Follow through with the discharge plan
- Provide care for the same clients consistently
- Follow through with the nursing plan of care
- Evaluate client responses to nursing interventions
- Communicate pertinent goal-directed information to the case manager
- Provide direct client care for the shift worked

The committee recognized that the first step in moving toward strengthening the case management system was to develop a written action plan to include identified responsible parties for each step and target dates for implementation and completion. The plan included these actions:

- Redefining which client populations needed to be case managed;
- Determining the number of case managers needed for each unit;
- Developing job descriptions for the new case manager role and the new case associate role; and

- Developing new policies to address the issues of scheduling, client assignments, low census, and floating to other units.

To determine whether all clients or only specific client populations needed to be case managed, a survey tool was developed in checklist format (Box 23-3). During a one-month period of time, all clients admitted to each unit were assessed to determine their need for a case manager. It was learned that only a percentage of clients needed the expertise of a case manager, whereas other clients could be effectively cared for by a case associate. The percentages of clients eligible for case management ranged from 100% of the clients on the rehabilitation unit, to 60% of the clients on the medical units, 40% on the surgical unit, 20% on the orthopedic unit, and 10% on the pediatric unit. Nurses on all units currently use a survey tool (see Box 23-3) to determine the need for case manager involvement.

Based on the survey results, the medical, surgical, and oncology units determined a need for four case managers, whereas the orthopedic, pediatric, obstetric, rehabilitation, and mental health units found two case man-

BOX 23-2
CASE ASSOCIATE JOB DESCRIPTION

Job Summary

Responsible and accountable for direct nursing care for assigned patients (clients). The nurse functions within environments where the policies, procedures, standards and pathways for provision of health care are established. Client caseload reflects continuity of care.

Position Requirements

Education: Graduate accredited school of nursing.
            Current license for the State of Wisconsin.
Experience: No previous experience necessary.

Responsibilities:

In addition to staff RN responsibilities:
1. Utilizing the nursing process in managing and providing direct care:
   a. Completes assessment to identify nursing care needs.
   b. Organizes and analyzes data to select pertinent standard care plans with individualization as indicated.
   c. Establishes with the client short-term goals consistent with the overall plan of care.
   d. Implements an individualized plan of care using established standard care plan, policies, procedures, and critical pathways.
   e. Evaluates client responses and modifies nursing interventions as necessary to meet client needs.

   f. Initiates a discharge plan at time of initial assessment and evaluates progression during work period.
   g. Prioritizes the delivery of direct nursing care (using time and resources effectively and efficiently).
2. Using interactive communication skills:
   a. Establishes short-term goals with client, based on needs and expectations of client.
   b. Networks with health team members, to include MDs, by communicating pertinent data based on nursing diagnosis and critical pathways to provide continuity of care.
3. Ensures continuity by providing nursing care to same clients based on client needs.
4. If a client's condition changes and needs to be case managed, notifies case manager of need to pick up.

The case associate caring for case-managed clients during the case manager's off shifts or days off:
1. Provides direct nursing care according to the established plan of care.
2. Implements and evaluates responses to the established plan of care, documenting any variances.
3. Communicates pertinent goal-direct information to the case manager.
4. Notifies case manager of significant changes in the client that require immediate changes in plan of care.

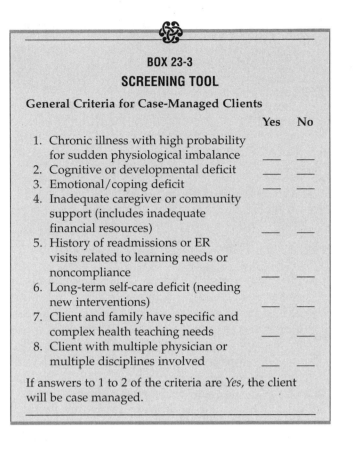

BOX 23-3

SCREENING TOOL

General Criteria for Case-Managed Clients

	Yes	No
1. Chronic illness with high probability for sudden physiological imbalance	___	___
2. Cognitive or developmental deficit	___	___
3. Emotional/coping deficit	___	___
4. Inadequate caregiver or community support (includes inadequate financial resources)	___	___
5. History of readmissions or ER visits related to learning needs or noncompliance	___	___
6. Long-term self-care deficit (needing new interventions)	___	___
7. Client and family have specific and complex health teaching needs	___	___
8. Client with multiple physician or multiple disciplines involved	___	___

If answers to 1 to 2 of the criteria are *Yes*, the client will be case managed.

agers to be sufficient for their case management-eligible client census. An average caseload for a case manager providing direct care was established at three clients. Additional cases would be carried by a case manager if a case associate or licensed practical nurse were providing the direct care and the case manager assumed responsibility for managing and coordinating care. During times of peak client census or vacations, the case manager might be required to carry a maximal caseload of five clients with a case associate or a licensed practical nurse providing the direct care.

Policy guidelines for case manager position eligibility required that the nurse:

- Work a minimum of 64 hours per pay period;
- Work shift hours that best accommodate making contacts with clients, families, physicians, and other health team members;
- Exhibit skills needed as case manager, such as communication skills and critical thinking skills;
- Be scheduled for consecutive days to allow for continuity;
- Transfer the caseload if off more than two days; and
- Is exempt from float or low census policies unless the caseload was low.

Implementation of the Action Plan

When the nursing department originally established case management as its delivery system, the selection process for filling the case manager positions included the desire of the RN to be a case manager and the completion of a factoring tool. The revised selection process for the position of nurse case manager included these tasks:

- Post the case manager position according to hospital policy;
- Complete an application and return it to the human resource department;
- Interview with the nurse director of the unit (for future applicants, case managers would be involved in the interview process);
- Check for satisfactory previous job performance; and
- Sign an agreement stating a commitment to carry out the job expectations.

When a large-scale change process is introduced, it is imperative that top management support is visible. For that reason, the vice-president of nursing held meetings for staff nurses to explain not only the roles of the new case manager and case associate but also the rationale for changing the roles. He specifically emphasized the shift in the philosophy holding that all clients needed to be case managed to one holding that only certain high-risk and complex clients needed to be case managed.

The proposed changes in the case management model were met with mixed feelings. Nurses who had been case managers and were now ineligible because of the number of hours they preferred to work felt devalued. A number of individual discussions were held in an attempt to explain further the difference between managing a client's care and being a case manager as well as to emphasize that all clients deserved and would receive excellent nursing care no matter how predictable or complex their situations. Emphasis was placed on the belief that the client's needs should receive first priority and the staff's needs a close second, but second.

Educational sessions were planned that would enable all case managers to learn the additional skills needed for the new role of case manager. Eleven months after the case management committee met to evaluate case management, the education sessions began for case managers.

The introductory session, Segment I, was an eight-hour inservice with case managers divided into three groups. The topics addressed included (Cohen & Cesta, 1993):

A. Concepts of case management
  1. Delivery systems and other health-care trends
  2. Client care delivery systems
  3. Components of case management
    a. Client identification
    b. Individual assessment and diagnosis

c. Planning and resource identification

d. Linking clients to needed services

e. Service implementation and coordination

f. Monitoring service delivery

g. Advocacy

h. Evaluation

4. Definitions of case management

B. Role of the case manager in relation to other members of the health-care team

1. Professional image

2. Case manager job description

3. Case manager criteria

4. Accountability versus responsibility

5. Collaborative relationships

C. Documentation of the plan of care in the case managed client

1. Care plans

2. Critical pathways

3. Standards of care

D. Discharge planning process

1. Assessment and planning

2. Referrals

E. Costs and reimbursement

1. Diagnosis related groups (DRGs) and length of stay (LOS)

2. Payment sources

3. Assertive utilization management

The formal presentation of the educational material was followed with a time for a practical application of this information by using a case study method.

The next education sessions were scheduled as one four-hour session held every three weeks. The objective of Segment II was to improve the use of communication techniques for the case managers. This session addressed how to use negotiation skills, conflicting management skills, and problem solving skills effectively to achieve improved client outcomes (quality, costs, and satisfaction). In Segment III, the case managers reviewed the process and principles of adult learning. This segment used techniques for adult teaching and learning that could be applied to client education to achieve desired client education outcomes.

Two educational sessions were planned especially for case associates because they care for those clients who are not case managed, that is, 60% to 70% of the hospital's client population. In the first session, emphasis was placed on issues surrounding health-care costs and reimbursement, inluding the length of stay for the top DRGs at our hospital compared with the national averages and the actual costs versus the reimbursement received by Holy Family Memorial Medical Center. As a result of this presentation, the case associates were better able to understand the importance of their role in caring for the noncomplex client population.

A second educational session for case associates reinforced the need for effective communication strategies such as assertive communication, negotiation, delegation, and planned confrontation. These techniques were then used by the case associates to become more effective in communicating with clients, physicians, ancillary services, and other health-care providers.

Revision of the Redefined Case Management Model

To evaluate the success of our redefined model of case management, data were collected and assessed in four areas:

- Effective assessment and documentation of client needs
- Early and complete discharge planning
- Effective communication with other members of the health-care team
- Case manager and case associate satisfaction with their new roles

Chart audits were conducted to evaluate the assessment and documentation of client needs and the completeness of discharge planning. The results of the audits identified some continuing deficiencies in these areas. Feedback from the case managers indicated that the required documentation was time consuming, redundant, and did not reflect the discharge planning process. The existing documentation system did not meet the needs of the redefined case management model.

Based on the analysis of the problem, a decision was made to develop a documentation format that would be less time consuming and easier to document the needed information. Various charting formats were evaluated, and it was decided to develop a charting by exception format to include specific areas for documentation of discharge needs and learning needs. Moreover, additional clinical pathways were developed with a multidisciplinary approach and included specific discharge planning and client outcome criteria.

To improve the communication between the case managers and discharge planners, a committee consisting of case managers, discharge planners, and staff from utilization management and social services met to improve the discharge planning process. The purpose of the committee was to define more clearly the obstacles to effective discharge planning and identify ways to improve the overall discharge planning process and meet the needs of the clients better. It further provided both groups with the opportunity to discuss openly and resolve issues that continued to surface.

The committee began its work by flowcharting the discharge process. Through this process, both groups were better able to understand the complexity involved in discharge planning and the importance of each person's role in the process. As a result of this committee's work, client discharge needs are identified and communicated in a more timely manner. An improved documentation process within the computer system allowed for follow-through of the discharge plan. Daily staffing conferences on clients provided an opportunity for all members of the health-care team to have input into the plan of care and discharge plan while the case manager retained the coordination role.

CONCLUSION

The preceding description of the development, implementation, and evaluation of a nurse case management model in a rural community hospital details the evolutionary process and the impact of the process on organizational infrastructure. The reader who is considering such an undertaking needs to realize that a number of key characteristics positively influenced the trajectory of this evolution. Of primary importance to this project was the active participation of a vice-president of nursing who believed in the importance of the nurses' role. Through his vision and leadership, a nursing department culture evolved that promoted empowerment of the staff nurse in organizational and clinical decision making.

Another key characteristic to the success of this project was the value placed on education. The nursing department at Holy Family Memorial not only values the importance of learning but has dedicated resources necessary to support this value. The services of a nurse consultant were used to initiate this project beginning with staff education. Through educational sessions, nurses were exposed to new ideas that expanded their knowledge base and helped them to begin to view their practice differently. Ongoing educational support was provided by a strong, capable education department staff with hours devoted to this project. Additionally, as part of its benefit package, the medical center offered tuition reimbursement for nurses pursuing advanced degrees. Since beginning this project, the percentage of baccalaureate-prepared nurses has gone from 15% of the nursing staff in 1988 to 27% currently.

Simultaneous institution of a *shared governance model* helped to formalize the role of staff nurse involvement in organizational decision making. In this model, decision making is deliberate and is based on data collected. Through participation in shared governance, all staff nurses are invited to share their knowledge, ideas, and clinical expertise to assist the nursing department and ultimately the medical center to achieve its goals.

One last key characteristic that influenced the direction of this project was the value placed on risk taking. When this process began, there were few institutions implementing nurse case management. Consequently, little concrete data were available in the nursing literature. It was the nursing department culture that valued "cutting edge" thinking that encouraged risk-taking behaviors to begin exploring and integrating this model. Through creative problem solving and persistence, the *nurse case management model* has evolved at Holy Family Memorial Medical Center.

Throughout the evolution of case management, the authors learned that change is a complex process and that plans for the next step of the process evolve over time as a new model is developed. The authors are confident that the nursing staff will continue to work in partnership with management to develop creative solutions that will ultimately lead to achieving optimal client outcomes, financial integrity, and staff satisfaction.

REFERENCES

Allen, D., Calkin, J., & Petersar, M. (1988). Making shared governance work: a conceptual model. *Journal of Nursing Administration, 18* (1), 37-43.

Cohen, E. L., & Cesta, T. G. (1993). *Nursing case management: from concept to evaluation.* St Louis, MO: Mosby.

Edwards, D. (1988). Interviewing staff autonomy: a key to nurse retention. *Journal of Pediatric Nursing, 3* (4), 265-8.

Hinshaw, A., Smeltzer, C. H., & Atwood, J. R. (1987). Innovative retention strategies for nursing staff. *Journal of Nursing Administration, 17* (6), 8-16.

McClure, M. L. (1991). Introduction. In *Differentiating nursing practice into the twenty-first century.* Kansas City, MO: American Academy of Nursing.

Primm, P. L. (1987). Differentiated practice for ADN and BSN prepared nurses. *Journal of Professional Nursing,* July/August, 218-225.

Slavitt, D. B., Stamps, P. L., Piedmont, E. B., & Haase, A. M. (1978). Nurses' satisfaction with their work situation. *Nursing Research, 21* (2), 114-120.

Ward, M. J., & Lindeman, C. A. (1978). *Instruments for measuring nursing practice and other health care variables.* Washington (vol. 1&2) Washington, DC: U. S. Department of Health, Education and Welfare Publication (HRA), 8-54.

Chapter 24

Differentiated Practice within and beyond the Hospital Walls

S. Jo Gibson, MS, RN, CCM

OVERVIEW

Differentiated nursing practice establishes a system of nurse case management that fosters interdependence, trust, and collegiality.

Clients range all along the health-care spectrum. In this era when acute care episodes continue to shorten and care transcends the hospital lines, the greatest challenge of case management programs will be to work effectively throughout these same ranges.

This chapter describes case management through a differentiated practice model that links the inpatient stay with other settings along the health-care continuum. The model promotes a seamless, integrated transition for clients that ensures continuity of care once the client returns to the community and when rehospitalized. Development of collegial relationships and collaboration with the appropriate members of the interdisciplinary as well as interagency team are paramount.

WHY COLLABORATE?

The beauty of case management is the diversity in which it can be applied in various settings and customized to meet the unique needs of individualized institutions (Cohen & Cesta, 1993). To its detriment, case managers are starting to collide as the race is on to determine who reigns as the primary case manager. Various disciplines (physicians, nurses, social workers, therapists, pastoral counselors, dentists, funeral directors) in a variety of settings (hospitals, home care, clinics, insurance companies, nursing homes, and local, state, and national government) are using case management terminology and integrating their version of the case manager role into practice. The professional turf guarding and inconsistent implementation strategies based on disciplinary differences are creating segregated, ineffec-

tive models (Sowell & Meadows, 1994). Integrated, multisite approaches to case management are critical.

Opposite this perplexing, disjointed health-care system are the consumers whose lives have no lines or dichotomies. Clients range all along the health-care spectrum. Health-care system networks and alliances, which operate from a managed care-competition perspective, are promoting a seamless, unified integration of services. The concept implies that continuity will occur without a break even though the location of environment changes for the clients. These integrated systems of health-care delivery cannot, however, operate in a vacuum. As Ruffolo and Nichols (1994) point out, the most difficult task for the case manager may indeed be to get the system to look at the clients as people. Nurses have traditionally focused on the whole person and on the ill—not the illness. The reality of having a nurse case manager to coordinate services for complex clients nears the horizon and will bring numerous benefits.

THE ART OF COLLABORATION

Webster defines *collaboration* as *the act of working jointly with others especially in an intellectual endeavor.* The nursing literature described by Nugent (1992), explains that collaborative practice is "not dictatorial, but includes a cooperative venture between the health care consumer and the members of the health care team" (pp. 107-108).

The underlying philosophy of collaboration is best represented in a metaphor about the emergency landing of *United Airlines* Flight 232 on July 19, 1989. The flight crew radioed down to the nearest control tower but were told that the mechanical problem was not listed in the emergency instruction manual. Without the luxury of emergency guidelines to direct the complicated landing, the captain promptly pulled together the resources that were available at 30,000 feet. This team included the first officer, flight engineer, and a passenger who happened to be a pilot. The captain calmly instructed the flight attendants to prepare the passengers for an emergency landing. Together, the flight crew determined the best course for the crippled DC-10 and made a creative landing in a Midwestern cornfield, thus saving 178 lives. They did it *collaboratively.*

Similarly, case management requires a collaborative team effort. Various disciplines are, however, scrambling to claim ownership over case management (Williams, 1992). If the primary goal of case management is to provide high-quality, cost-efficient care over the continuum, then the primary challenge is to get the interdisciplinary team and systems to work together.

The old system of leadership through hierarchy, control, and dependence will need to be replaced with a new, integrated system where a shared vision, joint decision making, and individual autonomy are recognized through guiding principles and common goals (Koerner, 1992; Wheatley, 1992). Translated into case management terminology, this new heterarchial model places the nurse case manager in the pivotal role of unifying the interdisciplinary group. The role of case manager is to coordinate the appropriate resources, thus bringing the diverse talents and contributions of others to the table. Empowerment is recognized: members of the team are awarded a speaking voice and develop a vested interest in becoming part of the process. Teamwork requires that members value contradiction and honesty. It is no longer enough that the team collaborates—it must be done collegially.

CASE MANAGEMENT THROUGH DIFFERENTIATED NURSING PRACTICE

Sioux Valley Hospital has utilized differentiated practice as the client care delivery model for more than seven years (Koerner & Karpiuk, 1994). The roles of associate, primary, and advanced practice nurse provide the clinical foundation for the model. Nurses choose their role based on competency, skill, desire, and education.

Associate Nurse Role

Associate nurses are responsible for shift-to-shift client care during an episode of illness. Integrated Clinical Pathways (ICP) are utilized as tools to guide and manage client care and expedite the intershift report. Accountability is based on a vertical focus of client care activities within the shift of care.

Primary Nurse Role

Primary nurses are responsible for coordinating client care from admission to discharge during an episode of illness. Clients are screened and assigned a primary nurse if they are integrated clinical pathway (ICP) outliers or if they have complex discharge planning, educational, or psychosocial needs. A major focus for primary nurses is the coordination of resources and discharge planning to facilitate quality outcomes for the client and an appropriate length of stay. Primary nurses are geographically based with accountability based on a horizontal focus for the entire hospital stay.

Advanced Practice Nurse Role

Advanced practice nurses, including clinical nurse specialists (CNSs) and nurse practitioners (NPs), are responsible for continuum care that extends beyond geographic boundaries and encompasses all health-care settings. The master's-prepared CNS case manages chronically ill clients whose high resource utilization and readmission patterns create financial risk for the hospital (Gibson, et al., 1994). The CNS also fulfills the traditional role components of expert clinician, consultant, educator, researcher, and change agent. Most recently, the advanced practice nurse has dual preparation in the CNS and NP roles. The focus is acute care case management by subspecialty in which the CNS and NP are responsible for a population of clients, such as cardiovascular surgery clients (Vaska, 1993), and are accountable for managing the entire spectrum of care into all health settings for acute and chronic clients. The preeminent focus is to empower clients to adjust their lifestyle to chronic illness, to maximize their self-care capabilities, or to prepare them for a peaceful death with dignity.

Figure 24-1 depicts the model of case management through differentiated nursing practice at Sioux Valley Hospital. Boundaries are obscure, but overlapping is

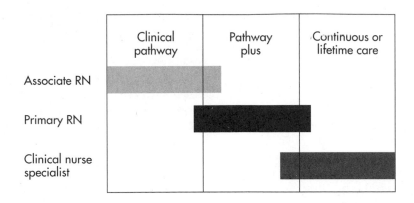

	Clinical pathway	Pathway plus	Continuous or lifetime care
Associate RN			
Primary RN			
Clinical nurse specialist			

FIG. 24-1   Case management through differentiated nursing practice (Adapted from Koerner, et al.: Differentiated practice: the evolution of a professional practice model for nursing service. In Flarey, D. (Ed.): *Redesigning nursing care delivery: transforming our future,* 1994, Philadelphia: JB Lippincott Co.)

necessary to avoid fragmentation and to address each client's health-care needs. In association with the philosophy of *shared governance,* the differentiated practice model at Sioux Valley Hospital facilitates mutual valuing, respect, and an enhanced understanding of these complementary roles. A milieu of interdependence, trust, and collegiality has been fostered as nurses freely consult one another. Blue et al. (1994) makes a distinction about the evolution of differentiated nursing practice at Sioux Valley Hospital:

> *No longer is the nursing practice looking at vertical and horizontal patterns of consultation, but rather at a transformation into a complex matrix of intradisciplinary and interdisciplinary collaboration as practice partners. This is a transformation by design (p. 210).*

Differentiated practice has elevated nursing from a supportive to a collaborative level with other disciplines. The only prerequisite was to start from "within" the distinguished profession of nursing.

CLINICAL PATHWAYS: AN ACUTE EPISODE TOOL

Clinical pathways are being widely used as tools to map client care through acute episodes of illness. These tools guide the identification of client outcomes, time frames, and necessary resources by case type (Lyon, 1993). Numerous beneficial outcomes have been identified, including reduction in length of stay and charges, improved quality of care indicators, and unchanged complication and recidivism rates.

Definition

The development on integrated clinical pathways began in January 1992 at Sioux Valley Hospital. An *integrated clinical pathway* (ICP) is defined as *a map or outline of care*

on a timeline that is specific to a medical diagnosis, surgical procedure, or presenting sign(s) or symptom(s). Pathways are physician- or physician-group–specific to reflect personal practice patterns. An interdisciplinary approach is used and resources are coordinated to achieve a cost-efficient and timely discharge with expected client outcomes. Various timelines have been used including:

1. *Day-by-day* for routine and predictable cases such as surgical and less complex medical diagnoses. Figure 24-2 reflects the clinical pathway for diabetes and insulin management for adults.
2. *Steps or stages* for complex medical diagnoses such as the premature neonate (stage by diagnosis and gestational age) and for stages of labor and care in vaginal deliveries (six-hour blocks post delivery).
3. *Presenting signs or symptoms* for emergency room clients (such as chest pain) and clients admitted without a definitive diagnosis (such as severe pain or febrile neutropenia in the oncology client).
4. *Across settings* for expanding the episode of illness beyond hospitalization to include the physician's office at preadmission, and home health or long-term care post discharge.

Process

The planning process for ICPs began with the establishment of a nursing task force with two representatives from each unit: one associate and one primary nurse. Others who served as consultants to the task force included clinical nurse specialists, a nursing administrator, a unit director, a staff educator, a quality review manager, a nurse researcher, a computer expert, and a clinic nurse. The goals for developing and implementing pathways at Sioux Valley Hospital were fourfold: (1) to promote interdisciplinary collaboration, (2) to streamline the documentation system, (3) to enhance client and

INTEGRATED CLINICAL PATHWAY

DIABETES AND INSULIN MANAGEMENT FOR ADULTS
Physician Group:
Attending MD:
DRG: 294
Primary RN: _____
Date Reviewed by MD/RN/Patient: _____
Advance Directive: Yes _____ No _____
Code Status: _____

MEDICAL HISTORY			
Admit Date	ICU Date	Transfer Date	Allergies:

Present problem: _____

Past history: _____

Surgical & special procedures: _____

Physician Consults:

Date	Physician	Reason	First visit	Signed off

Phone Numbers:
Name _____
Relationship _____
Home _____
Work _____
Name _____
Relationship _____
Home _____
Work _____

DISCHARGE PLANNING

Discharge Destination	Initiated D/C Plan Date/Initial	D/C Outcome Date/Initial	Community Services	Initiated D/C Plan Date/Initial	D/C Outcome Date/Initial	Transportation	Initiated D/C Plan Date/Initial	D/C Outcome Date/Initial
Home alone/family	/	/	Dept. social services	/	/	Family	/	/
Home w/	/	/	Senior companion	/	/	Wheelchair service	/	/
Home w/home health ____	/	/	Homemaker	/	/	Paratransit	/	/
Home w/public health nurse __	/	/	Respite care	/	/	Ambulance	/	/
Nursing home, skilled ____	/	/	Meals on wheels	/	/	Indian health services	/	/
Nursing home, intermediate__	/	/	Lifeline	/	/	State penitentiary	/	/
Nursing home,			HEARTH	/	/	Other _____	/	/
assisted living	/	/	Hospice	/	/			
Rehab _____	/	/	Wellness center ____	/	/	Equipment	Date/Initial	Date/Initial
Swing bed: _____	/	/	Cardiac rehab ____	/	/	Home oxygen	/	/
VA hospital	/	/	Vascular rehab ____	/	/	Home IV therapy ____	/	/
Hospice cottage	/	/	Support group ____			Assistive devices ____	/	/
State penitentiary	/	/						
Hotel _____	/	/	Other _____	/	/	Other: _____	/	/
Other_____	/	/						

Initials/Signature: _____ / _____ _____ / _____ _____ / _____
_____ / _____ _____ / _____ _____ / _____

OFF PATHWAY   ☐ YES   **If pathway discontinued, chart summation note as to reason why discontinued.**
DATE _____ / _____ / _____   01/95 CHART FORM   © 1992 Sioux Valley Hospital, Sioux Falls, South Dakota. All Rights Reserved.

FIG. 24-2   Integrated clinical pathway: diabetes and insulin management for adults (From Sioux Valley Hospital, Sioux Falls, South Dakota)

DAY/DATE	Day Admit Date _____	Day 1 Date _____
CONSULTS	Contact diabetes educator (pager 1359) Dietician	
LABS X-RAY OTHER	Daily FBS, 11, 4, 10 (one touch) CBC, UA, lytes	Daily FBS, 11, 4, 10 (one touch) Can use patient's meter if readings are within 20% of labs x 3
TREATMENTS/ PULMONARY	Order glucose meter	
MEDICATIONS/ IVs	Insulin	Insulin
NUTRITION	_____ cal ADA	_____ cal ADA
ACTIVITY/PT SAFETY	Up ad lib	Up ad lib
DISCHARGE PLANNING	Complete assessment tool Initiate data base	Review data base Discuss home arrangements
NURSING DX/ INTERDISCIPLINARY FOCUS	Knowledge Anxiety Potential hypoglycemia Hyperglycemia Fluid volume	Knowledge Anxiety Potential hypoglycemia Hyperglycemia Fluid volume: resolve

KEY NURSING
ACTIVITIES/
TEACHING
	Record B.S. on diabetes flow sheet
	VS routine, I & O, Wt
	Assess LOC and S&S hypo/hyper q 4 hrs
	Push fluids
	    Education emphasis
	    1. Provide diabetes folder/film list ___
	    2. B & S hypoglycemia/hyperglycemia ___
	
	KEY
	A = Pt/family verbalize understanding
	B = Pt/family need reinforcement
	C = Pt/family not available
		VS routine, I & O
		Assess LOC and S & S hypo/hyper q 4 hrs
		Push fluids
		Record BS on flow sheet
		Attends DB classes/watches films
		    Education emphasis
		    1. Blood glucose meter ___
		    2. Hypoglycemia ___
		    3. What is diabetes ___
		    4. Nutrition ___
		    5. Reinforce education ___
		
		KEY
		A = Pt/family verbalize understanding
		B = Pt/family need reinforcement
		C = Pt/family not available

KEY PATIENT
OUTCOMES
	1. Verbalizes S & S of hypoglycemia
	2. Begin looking at diabetes folder
	3. Assessment within normal limits (WNL) for patient
		1. Demonstrates *One Touch* meter
		2. Verbalizes basic understanding of diabetes,
		    hypoglycemia and nutrition
		3. Assessment WNL for patient; no s/s of
		    hypo/hyperglycemia

SHIFT RN SIGNATURE	D. N.	D. N.
INITIALS/ SIGNATURE	_____/_____ _____/_____	_____/_____ _____/_____

FIG. 24-2   *Continued*

Day 2 Date _____	Day 3 Date _____	Day 4 Date _____
		DISHCARGE
Daily FBS, 11, 4, 10 (one touch) Can use patient's meter if readings are within 20% of labs x 3	Daily FBS, 11, 4, 10 (one touch) Can use patient's meter if readings are within 20% of labs x 3	Daily FBS, 11, 4, 10 (one touch) Can use patient's meter if readings are within 20% of labs x 3
Insulin	Insulin	Insulin
_____ cal ADA	_____ cal ADA	_____ cal ADA
Up ad lib	Up ad lib	Up ad lib
Review plans, revise as needed	Review plans, revise as needed Confirm home arrangements	Finalize discharge plans
Knowledge Anxiety Potential hypoglycemia Hyperglycemia: resolve	Knowledge Potential hypoglycemia Anxiety	Knowledge: resolve Potential hypoglycemia: resolve Anxiety: resolve
VS routine, I & O Assess LOC and S & S hypo/hyper q 4 hrs Push fluids Record BS on flow sheet Attends DB classes/watches films Pt administers own pm insulin Education emphasis 1. Insulin/medication ___ 2. Nutrition ___ 3. Exercise ___ 4. Emotions ___ 5. Reinforce education ___ KEY A = Pt/family verbalize understanding B = Pt/family need reinforcement C = Pt/family not available	Pt administers own insulin VS routine, I & O Assess LOC and S & S hypo/hyper q 4 hrs Push fluids Record BS on flow sheet Attends DB classes/watches films Education 1. Sick day/ketoacidosis ___ 2. Diabetes complications ___ 3. Home management, community resources and accessing care ___ 4. Reinforce education ___ KEY A = Pt/family verbalize understanding B = Pt/family need reinforcement C = Pt/family not available	Pt administers own insulin Reinforce education Finalize discharge teaching and provide written instructions Education 1. Community resources and accessing care ___ 2. Home management ___ KEY A = Pt/family verbalize understanding B = Pt/family need reinforcement C = Pt/family not available
1. Demonstrates & administers insulin 2. Verbalizes understanding of diet 3. Verbalizes understanding of effect of exercise 4. Demonstrates glucose meter 5. Verbalizes feelings regarding diabetes 6. Assessment WNL for patient, no s/s of hypo/hyperglycemia	1. Demonstrates & administers insulin 2. Discuss sick day management/ ketoacidosis 3. Verbalizes measures to prevent complications 4. Verbalizes home management of diet, exercise, insulin, and B9M and hygiene 5. Demonstrates glucose meter 6. Assessment WNL for patient, no s/s of hypo/hyperglycemia	1. Demonstrates & administers insulin 2. Verbalizes understanding of discharge instructions 3. Demonstrates glucose meter 4. Assessment WNL for patient, no s/s of hypo/hyperglycemia
D. N.	D. N.	D. N.
_____/_____ _____/_____	_____/_____ _____/_____	_____/_____ _____/_____

Special Orders

KEY 1. Initialed in red = ordered 2. Black line = not ordered 3. Circled in black = exception	_____ _____ _____ _____ _____ _____	_____ _____ _____ _____ _____ _____	_____ _____ _____ _____ _____ _____

FIG. 24-2   *Continued*

family involvement in care, and (4) to reduce length of stay and charges without jeopardizing quality of care.

Interdisciplinary Collaboration

Interdisciplinary involvement in the development of pathways is essential for successful implementation. Diverse talents and abilities are recognized through interdisciplinary interaction. These diverse abilities need to be complementary for the pathway to provide a unified comprehensive approach to client care (Nugent, 1992).

Integrated clinical pathways are jointly developed by nurses, physicians, and all disciplines who interface with the selected client population to outline the interventions and expected outcomes. Nurses, by virtue of their constant presence with clients in all settings, are pivotal in the development and implementation of pathways. Primary nurses, in collaboration with associate nurses and clinical nurse specialists, draft the pathway to reflect the medical and nursing aspects of care. The primary nurse then coordinates an interdisciplinary team meeting to review and modify the drafted pathway before implementation. The final pathway reflects a comprehensive plan of care with each discipline's contributions in achieving expected client outcomes. Once implemented, pathways require constant surveillance by primary nurses. Appropriate revisions are made as patterns evolve (American Health Consultants, 1993).

Active physician participation is salient in the development of these written guidelines. Starting with progressive, influential physicians who efficiently manage client care proved to be a successful strategy at Sioux Valley Hospital. Also, clinical nurses who have established credibility and professional relationships with physicians made the initial contact. Favorable responses resulted by having expert primary nurses and CNSs meet with the physicians rather than department directors or unfamiliar staff (Gibson & Thomas, 1994). At Sioux Valley Hospital, pathways are developed specific to physician or physician groups to reflect personal practice patterns and avoid the accusation of "recipe" medicine.

Streamlined Documentation

A burdensome maze of paperwork is not uncommon in hospitals but can be streamlined through the use of pathways. A prerequisite is that the pathways be established as part of the permanent record so integration can occur. A comprehensive review of the documentation system, preferably by all disciplines, is necessary to determine where duplication and nonessential charting forms exist and what can be eliminated or meshed.

Integrated clinical pathways are designed as the comprehensive plan of care which incorporates the medical, nursing, and other disciplines treatment interventions. Specifically, nursing diagnoses, interventions, and expected client outcomes are listed to reflect the standard of care for the specific diagnosis. A separate nursing care plan is, therefore, eliminated. Only identified client needs that are not already listed on the pathway are required to tailor and individualize care. The client-specific nursing diagnosis, interventions, and expected client outcome are written by the primary or associate nurse directly on the pathway to address the specialized need.

Assessment by exception flow sheets and focus charting have been adopted and have significantly reduced the documentation time for associate nurses. Focus notes are only written if the client is unable to achieve an expected outcome on the pathway. Significant events such as substantial changes in assessment are also recorded as focus notes. The primary nurse writes an initial focus note reflecting the discharge plan and provides a periodic update of the client's progress.

Various forms have been eliminated by integrating information onto the pathway or assessment flow sheet. These forms include the Kardex, nursing discharge summary, client education forms, skin assessment, and fall risk assessment flow sheets.

An acuity rating system has also been integrated with pathways. The total acuity points accrued for each day of the pathway have been trended and staged into categories. Clients whose courses are following the pathway as outlined are now easily assigned an automatic acuity rating by the associate nurse, thus eliminating the time-consuming steps of the traditional computerized methodology. This concept can be readily applied to routine, predictable populations such as obstetrical deliveries and uncomplicated surgical or medical cases.

Other members of the interdisciplinary team document significant interventions and outcomes directly on the pathway. The importance of communicating valuable information to the team that is readily retrievable was identified through a "shared interventions" concept. Incentive spirometry is one such example of an intervention in which both respiratory therapy and nursing are responsible. Respiratory therapy may complete the initial teaching and establish important baseline parameters for incentive spirometry which need to be communicated for nursing to follow through. Similarly, nursing may identify client-specific strategies that optimize spirometry performance that need to be communicated back to respiratory therapy, such as pain medication 30 minutes before treatments, or splinting techniques.

Client and Family Involvement

Active participation of the client and family in the plan of care is readily achieved by using the pathway and individualizing identified needs. The primary nurse reviews the pathway initially and on a daily basis so clients and families understand the expectations. Pathways provide the mental preparation necessary for clients to achieve a timely discharge and recovery. To avoid the medical jargon and acronyms that can be confusing, primary nurses and clinical nurse specialists have developed client versions of pathways in lay terminology. Orthopedic, surgical, and obstetrical client pathways are currently in place (Refer to Table 24-1 for an orthopedic client pathway).

Clinical and Fiscal Outcomes

Integrated clinical pathways clearly define the expectations by all members of the interdisciplinary team so quality of care can be enhanced. These valuable orientation tools outline the plan of care to augment continuity of intershift care as well as across unit boundaries. The pathway is used for communication during the primary-to-primary and associate-to-associate nurse report as the client enters a new unit.

Satisfaction has improved for clients who now understand the course of care and expectations based on the pathway. Physicians find favor with pathways by having clients cared for according to their practice preferences. Nurse satisfaction has increased through decreased charting time and comfort in having pathway guidelines when caring for unfamiliar client populations.

Documentation has become more reflective of the client's progress in terms of expected outcomes. With the pathway as the central focus, documentation is now viewed as a means to communicate with other team members and not merely separate plans and charting for each discipline. With the pathway as the focal point for communication, the team has become the focal point for care delivery. An interdisciplinary approach enhances communication and avoids fragmentation and duplication of services.

Fiscal awareness by the interdisciplinary team has dramatically improved. Lengths of stay and charges have decreased overall without an increase in complication, recidivism, morbidity, or mortality rates. Data have been compared for pathway and nonpathway clients of the same diagnosis related group (DRG) over the first 24 months since implementation. As a result of managing 6,265 clients by pathway for 140 physicians, a total of 1,275 hospital days and $4.4 million have been saved (Gibson & Thomas, 1994).

Accountability

It is important to remember that the pathway is only an organizational tool consisting of words on paper. The challenge of proposing and developing pathways is minimal compared with the challenge of making them work successfully. Professional accountability is significant in making the pathway a functional, working document, that is, one from which all team members can benefit.

The underlying philosophy of pathways in relation to accountability can be represented in a metaphor about a musical score. Beethoven's classic *Fifth Symphony* can be beautifully performed to please the listener. The score, however, is only musical notes on a piece of paper. The challenge of the conductor is to choose the musical score and to persuade the orchestra to believe in and value the content. The challenge of the orchestra is to fill in the outline and be in tune with the goals of the other instruments. The conductor coordinates communication so the orchestra can work in harmony for the optimal outcome—a resounding performance.

Similarly, the primary nurse is the conductor who coordinates communication and convinces the physicians and other disciplines to see the value in the pathway. The other disciplines, like the individual orchestra members, are not told how to perform but are encouraged to complete the outline so that it is complementary and in harmony with the goals of the other team members and most importantly, the client. Although each discipline is independent in its clinical decision making, it is interdependent with other elements within the organization (Etheredge, 1989). Each discipline must define and defend what they do and value the contributions of each team member.

The most rewarding benefit of pathways is the clinical sophistication that is packaged and brought to the bedside without the expert team members having to be physically present at all times. Pathways steer the team to focus on one mutual purpose for its being—the client. Professional accountability has improved with the client as the central focus. All members of the team unite as partners to meet the needs of the client—another resounding performance.

Expanding Pathways Beyond Hospitalization

Although inpatient services are dwindling to only a small segment of care, the emerging community-based continuum is rapidly expanding. It is becoming vain to focus on the short portion of care that occurs in the tertiary setting. The many benefits recognized by using pathways in the hospital need to expand to encompass the entire episode of illness. Physician clinics, home care, transitional and subacute care, nursing homes, and other community support services must be included to ensure success.

Short-stay mastectomy pathway. Sioux Valley Hospital is currently piloting a short-stay option for mastectomy clients. The pathway begins in the physician's office, continues in the hospital with surgery and a 24-hour stay, and is completed with two home visits provided by a surgical primary nurse (Gibson, Thomas, & Burnette, 1994).

TABLE 24-1   Total hip replacement (your pathway to recovery)

Thank you for selecting Midwest Orthopedic Center and Sioux Valley Hospital as your choice for health care. You have a very important job . . . recovering from total hip surgery. Within 6 days after surgery, you will be discharged from the hospital. The following pathway (or plan) describes the day-by-day expectations. Your discharge goals will be independent transfers and walking with a walker. Please bring a pair of walking shoes, comfortable fitting clothes, and a walker if you have one.

If you feel you will be unable to go home at this time by yourself, please discuss the following options with your family, physician, and nurses.

Option 1: Home with Family Members

Arrangements for a visiting nurse, homemaker services, or Meals-on-Wheels can be made by your nurse to assist you and/or your family.

Option 2: Sioux Valley Hospital Rehabilitation Unit

This is a unit where you will receive extensive therapy to become more independent. You could be transferred to this unit on the 4th day after surgery.

Option 3: Temporary Placement

Arrangements can be made for you to go to a small hospital or a nursing home until you are independent enough to go to your own home.

DAY/DATE	DAY OF SURGERY	DAY 1	DAY 2
Activity *Goal:* To progress to walking with walker or crutches	▪ Bed rest Harris (traction that holds your surgical leg in proper position)	▪ Up in chair twice a day ▪ Harris when in bed	▪ Up in chair 2-3 times a day ▪ Discontinue Harris. Hassock placed between legs while in bed. (Blue rectangular pillow) ▪ Physical therapy by tilt table (cart that allows you to stand up and walk)
Pain control *Goal:* To be able to tolerate activity or therapy with pain pills	▪ PCA pump or IM medications ▪ Tell nurses about your pain	▪ PCA pump or IM medications ▪ Tell nurses about your pain	▪ Discontinue PCA pump/IM medications ▪ Switch to pain pills ▪ Take every 3-4 hours as needed ▪ Ask for pain pills 1/2 hour before therapy and at bed time.
Elimination *Goal:* To progress to independent bowel and bladder functions	▪ Bed pan or urinal ▪ Catheter for urine if needed	▪ Bed pan or urinal ▪ Catheter for urine if needed	▪ Bed pan or urinal ▪ Remove catheter
Breathing *Goal:* To keep lungs clear	▪ Cough and deep breathe every hour while awake ▪ To use Volurex (a breathing device) 10 times every hour while awake	▪ Cough and deep breathe every hour while awake ▪ To use Volurex (a breathing device) 10 times every hour while awake	▪ Cough and deep breathe every hour while awake ▪ To use Volurex (a breathing device) 10 times every hour while awake
Eating (diet) *Goal:* To progress to previous diet	▪ Clear liquid diet	▪ Full liquid diet	▪ Advance as tolerated ▪ Drink fluids
Bathing/Dressing *Goal:* To progress to independent bathing and dressing with O.T. equipment	▪ Self bath	▪ Towel bath in bed	▪ Assist with bathing while in a chair
TED hose *Goal:* To apply independently with O.T. equipment	▪ Off 1 hour	▪ Off 1 hour twice a day	▪ Off 1 hour twice a day

From Sioux Valley Hospital, Sioux Falls, South Dakota.

DAY 3	DAY 4	DAY 5	DAY 6	NOTES
■ Up in chair ■ Physical therapy twice daily ■ Walk to bathroom and hall with walker or crutches	■ Up in chair for meals ■ Physical therapy twice daily ■ Walk to bathroom in halls 2-3 times a day with walker or crutches	■ Up in chair for meals ■ Physical therapy twice daily ■ Walk to bathroom in halls 2-3 times a day with walker or crutches	■ Up in chair for meals ■ Physical therapy twice daily ■ Walk to bathroom and in hallway 3 times daily	
■ Pain pills ■ Take every 3-4 hours as needed ■ Ask for pain pills 1/2 hour before therapy and at bed time	■ Pain pills ■ Ask for pain pills 1/2 hour before therapy and at bed time	■ Pain pills ■ Ask for pain pills 1/2 hour before therapy and at bed time	■ Able to maintain pain control and tolerate activity	
■ Walk to bathroom with assistance of walker	■ Walk to bathroom with assistance of walker	■ Walk to bathroom with assistance of walker or crutches	■ Walk independently to bathroom with assistance of walker or crutches	
■ Cough and deep breathe every hour while awake ■ To use Volurex (a breathing device) 10 times every hour while awake	■ Cough and deep breathe every hour while awake ■ To use Volurex (a breathing device) 10 times every hour while awake			
■ Soft diet ■ Drink fluids	■ Regular diet ■ Drink fluids	■ Regular diet ■ Drink fluids	■ Regular diet ■ Drink fluids	
■ Assist with bathing while in a chair	■ Self-assisted bath while in a chair ■ Occupational therapy for dressing	■ Self-assisted bath	■ Self-assisted bath	
■ Off 1 hour twice a day	■ Assist with TED hose application and removal with O.T. equipment ■ Off 1 hour twice a day	■ Assist with TED hose as needed ■ Off 1 hour twice a day	■ Application and removal of TED hose independently	

Before the pilot, the usual length of stay for mastectomy clients was three days. The surgeons quickly pointed out that eliminating the last two days of hospitalization and providing the postsurgery care in the client's home would constitute acute care and require the expertise of an acute care nurse, not a generalist home care nurse. Surgeons were adamant that the "expert" primary nurse be the one to provide the two follow-up visits.

The primary nurses were cross-trained for these speciality home care visits and worked cooperatively with the home health agency. A home pathway was developed to include measurable outcomes and the last two days of the integrated clinical pathway were recreated to reflect the two home visits (Figure 24-3). After the second visit, the primary nurse makes appropriate referrals (such as home care, CNS case management, and support group involvement) for progress to continue. A client version of the pathway in lay terminology accompanies the hospital pathway used by the interdisciplinary team and the home care pathway used by the primary nurse.

Outcomes. Continuity of care is enhanced by having the primary nurse coordinate care from preadmission through hospitalization and into the home. Client responses have been favorable with a shorter period of time spent in the hospital and follow-up in the privacy and comfort of home.

An unexpected finding was that a significant number of clients who chose the short-stay option did not require follow-up home visits. These clients were knowledgeable and had supportive caregivers at home who were willing to assist with care that the client could not complete because of limited mobility of the affected arm. Another unexpected finding was that a few clients, with limited income and no insurance, elected to have same-day surgery. The follow-up home visits by the primary nurse have been crucial in these isolated instances (see Case Study).

The estimated savings when comparing charges of a three-day stay versus the short-stay option, including home visits and supplies, is $1,500 per case. The estimated savings when comparing charges of a three-day stay and same-day surgery, including home visits and supplies, is $4,500 per case. These nontraditional methods are valuable for hospitals that are under capitation and looking for economical approaches to care.

Future Pathway Challenges

It is anticipated that a successful pilot with the mastectomy population will lead to expansion of pathway completion in the home with other client populations and other primary nurses. Obstetrical primary nurses at Sioux Valley Hospital are currently providing expertise in the terbutaline therapy management for high-risk obstetrical clients to prevent preterm labor. Primary nurses at Sioux Valley Hospital, and nurses in general, are being called upon to be flexible and competent in adapting to the anticipated massive shift to outpatient and community practice. If physicians know that highly specialized nurses are cross-trained and available, they will be more likely to discharge clients earlier or order the technical necessities and home nursing care instead of an admission.

Education and cross-training of the primary nurses will be required. Problems surrounding staffing and coverage of clients during the primary nurse's absence caused by home visits will need to be addressed. Rural clients living at extended distances from the hospital will need to be evaluated to determine the costs and benefits of traveling to provide home care. Limits and alternate care methods will need to be established. Telemedicine, rural outreach, and strategically positioning community health nurses into identified geographic rural areas are potential options.

Pathways need to be expanded into nursing homes and swing beds for subacute and skilled needs of short duration. Sioux Valley Hospital is currently collaborating with an area nursing home to provide a continuation of the pathway for orthopedic clients. It is anticipated that these pathways will be developed according to the client's functional abilities and expectations rather than by diagnosis and that primary nurses or CNSs will provide follow-up in the nursing home.

The home care pathway as a methodology to plan care and monitor outcomes needs to be explored. The potential that home pathways could streamline the complex Medicare documentation requirements could be revolutionary. Primary and home care nurses are working collaboratively to evaluate the feasibility of an integrated documentation system.

Automation of pathways will become critical for efficiency purposes and tracking variances. Development of a functional, efficient manual system is a prerequisite. Information systems within the hospital as well as into clinics and other agencies will need to be developed and linked so clinical and fiscal information is readily available.

CASE MANAGEMENT ON A CONTINUUM FOR HIGH-RISK CLIENTS

A small percentage of clients are being identified as having support and coordination of care needs beyond the acute episode of illness. Unlike episode-based care that has a finite beginning and end, case management on a continuum is less definitive and predictable. Similarly, the strategies and design used to manage these two groups need to be different.

DAY/DATE	VISIT 1 Date _____	VISIT 2 Date _____
CONSULTS	Oncology nurse beeper #1022 Office nurse	VNA/Home health nurse

TREATMENTS/
PULMONARY
	Change incision dressing 4 x 4 daily
	JP site care using H$_2$O$_2$ Q-tip apply 4 x 4 dressing
	  (betadine for specific MD)
		Change incision dressing 4 x 4 daily
		JP site care using H$_2$O$_2$ Q-tip apply 4 x 4 dressing
		  (betadine for specific MD)

MEDICATIONS/ IVs	Review home medications Complete schedule of medication as necessary	PO pain medications
NUTRITION	Regular as at home	Regular as at home

ACTIVITY/PT
SAFETY
	Up ad lib
	Instruct on no stretching, straining or lifting
	Sponge bath - reinforce reason for no tub/shower
	  while JP in
		Up ad lib
		Reinforce activity teaching
		Sponge bath - reinforce reason for no tub/shower
		  while JP in

NURSING DX/ INTERDISCIPLINARY FOCUS	Comfort Knowledge Coping Tissue perfusion	Comfort - resolve Knowledge - resolve/refer Coping - resolve/refer Tissue perfusion - resolve

EDUCATION
CLASSES
	DISCUSSION
	
	Describe surg. proc ____ Perm breast prosthesis ____
	SVH instruct sheet ____ Lymphedema ____
	Pre-op teach ____ Infection ____
	Appearance ____ Home: Diet ____
	Function (child bearing) ____ Activity ____
	Sexuality ____ Self care ____
	Cancer ____ Milk JP ____
	Avoid injury arm/hand ____ When to call Dr ____
	Avoid restrictive clothing ____
	When to do exercise ____
	Monthly SBE ____
	
	KEY
	A = Pt/family verbalize understanding/
	  no review
	B = Pt/family need reinforcement
	__ = Pt/family not ready/available
	
	VIDEO
	POST MASTECTOMY
	CARE & RECOVERY,
	keep video overnight
	as pt desires
		DISCUSSION
		
		Describe surg. proc ____ Avoid restrictive clothing ____
		SVH instruct sheet ____ When to do exercises ____
		Pre-op teach ____ Monthly SBE ____
		Appearance ____ Perm breast prosthesis ____
		Function (child bearing) ____ Lymphedema ____
		Sexuality ____ Infection ____
		Cancer ____ Home: Diet ____
		Avoid injury arm/hand ____ Activity ____
		    Self care ____
		    Milk JP ____
		    When to call Dr ____
		
		KEY
		A = Pt/family verbalize understanding/
		  no review
		B = Pt/family need reinforcement
		__ = Pt/family not ready/available

KEY INTERVENTIONS	1. VS X 1 (BP, P, R, Temp) Call abnormal to office 2. Multisystem assess x 1 3. Assess incision & drains 4. Milk drain tubing daily with dressing change 5. Monitor pain control IV/ po meds 6. Teach pt care of drain and incision 7. Obtain node pathology report from office & review w/patient	1. VS (BP, P, R, Temp) Call abnormal to office 2. Multisystem assess x 1 3. Assess incision & drains 4. Milk JP tubing daily with dressing change 5. Monitor pain control IV/po meds 6. Review care of incision & drain w/pt 7. Review node report w/pt 8. Assist pt in making follow up appt as necessary

KEY PATIENT
OUTCOMES
	1. VS stable
	2. Assessment WNL for pt
	3. Incision well approximated w/o s/s infection,
	  drains patient to suction as ordered
	4. Drains functioning properly, drains patient
	  w/o s/s infection
	5. Pain controlled w/ po med
	6. Verbalizes understanding incision care, JP site
	  care emptying of JP drain, milking of tubing
	7. Verbalizes understanding of node report &
	  follow up if node report positive
	8. Tolerates diet w/o n/v
	9. Activity tolerated w/o complications
	10. Working toward outcomes
		1. VS stable
		2. Assessment WNL for pt
		3. Incision well approximated w/o s/s infection,
		  drains patient to suction as ordered
		4. Drains functioning properly, drains patient
		  w/o s/s infection
		5. Pain controlled w/ po med
		6. Verbalizes understanding incision care, JP site
		  care emptying of JP drain, milking of tubing
		7. Verbalizes understanding of node report &
		  follow up if node report positive
		8. Appointments made
		9. Toleratess diet w/o n/v
		10. Activity tolerated w/o complications
		11. Outcomes met

SHIFT RN SIGNATURE	D. N.	D. N.
INITIALS/ SIGNATURE	_____/_____ _____/_____	_____/_____ _____/_____

FIG. 24-3   Integrated clinical pathway: mastectomy home ICP (From Sioux Valley Hospital, Sioux Falls, South Dakota)

INTEGRATED CLINICAL PATHWAY

MASTECTOMY HOME ICP
Name: _____
Primary RN: _____
Advance Directive: Yes _____ No _____
Date Initial Visit: _____

Assess and observe each visit:
1. Complete assessment including: VS, multisystem physical assessment, incision drain:
2. Teach wound/drain care as Dr. orders:
3. Assess pain control with po medications:
4. Assess emotional status:

Standard of care:
1. Comfort:
2. Knowledge:
3. Coping:
4. Tissue perfusion:

Patient outcomes:
1. Pain controlled with po pain medications:
2. Patient's physical assessment and VS are normal for post op mastectomy surgery:
3. Pt/significant other will demonstrate understanding of disease process, self-care management and treatment plan:
4. Tissue perfusion will be maintained:

Recommended frequency—2 visits total:
It is anticipated that some patients may stabilize and learn more quickly with all outcomes met by the end of 2 visits some patients, however, will require additional visits to be furnished by the Visiting Nurses Association or the home health nurses, as the patient chooses. The number of these visits will be determined by the contracted agency as the patient outcomes are met. These visits will be used to assess, evaluate and complete, the education not yet accomplished.

Initials/Signature: _____   _____ /_____   _____ /_____
_____ /_____   _____ /_____   _____ /_____

OFF PATHWAY   ☐ YES
DATE _____ /_____ /_____   01/95 CHART FORM   © 1992 Sioux Valley Hospital, Sioux Falls, South Dakota. All Rights Reserved.

FIG. 24-3   *Continued*

Why Advanced Practice Nurses?

Case management on a continuum requires flexibility and mobility in terms of time and geography to coordinate and negotiate services efficiently. Success also requires collaboration with multiple agencies and disciplines with which the case manager is not immediately connected. Effective communication between all members of the team is critical and hinges upon who assumes the pivotal role of case manager.

Because nurses take a holistic approach and are involved in all aspects of the client's care, nurses are logical choices and function well as case managers (Cohen & Cesta, 1993). What academic preparation and credentials are necessary is the present debate.

The American Nurses Association (ANA, 1988) states that the minimal education for a case manager is a baccalaureate degree. Given the extensive knowledge and skills required, however, the ANA acknowledges that baccalaureate education may not be adequate. Ethridge and Lamb (1989) found that nurses prepared at less than the BSN level "were unable to predict and document measurable outcomes within the time frame necessary for reimbursement" (p. 32).

CASE STUDY

Mastectomy: Expanding Pathways into Home

Lynn Thomas, RNC, Primary Nurse
Surgical Unit
Sioux Valley Hospital

Ms. G. is a 53-year-old white female diagnosed with breast cancer by mammogram. She underwent a right modified radical mastectomy as a same-day surgery patient.

Ms. G.'s support system is limited. She has been divorced for five years and has five grown children. Contact with her children is minimal. She has been in abusive relationships in the past. She has few friends, and social contacts include a weekly visit with one of her children and occasional business contacts; she has withdrawn from church. After elimination of her job last year, her finances are limited. She is now self-employed as a seamstress in her own home working "18-hour days." She does not have insurance and therefore is personally responsible for all medical bills.

Ms. G. was introduced to the home mastectomy program concept in the physician's office. Preoperative teaching including the discharge plan was completed by the office nurse and the surgical primary nurse. On the day of surgery, the primary nurse met with Mrs. G. to arrange a time for the first home visit, provide home instructions, and a contact person (the charge nurse of the surgical unit) to call the first night at home if needed.

Once the preoperative visit was made, a referral was made to social services who assisted the client with finances and emotional support. Social services also assessed whether a home visit by a social worker was necessary.

Postoperatively, the primary nurse made two home visits. The first visit was the first day after surgery and focused on client education, including pain control, diet management, and emotional support. The surgeon was called for the node report in the primary nurse's presence. Ms. G. and the primary nurse rejoiced as they learned together that the report was negative and would not require referrals to the oncology physician and staff. The dressings were changed and the client was instructed on incision and drain cares. A mastectomy videotape was left overnight for the client to view so the primary nurse could reinforce education on the second home visit. The amount of time spent at the first visit equaled two hours.

The second visit on the second day after surgery was to reinforce previous teaching, provide incision and drain cares, continue with emotional support, and answer additional questions. The primary nurse then evaluated the outcomes listed on the pathway, available support services, whether further visits were needed by a home health care nurse, and whether other community support services were necessary. The amount of time spent on the second visit was one hour.

The care of Ms. G. by the primary nurse was completed with a follow-up phone call made 48 hours after the second visit. The major concern for Ms. G. at this time was financially based. The primary nurse referred her mammogram bill to "Friends Against Breast Cancer" for payment and a referral was made to the American Cancer Society for assistance with breast prosthesis when fitting was available. The primary nurse referred Ms. G. to Sioux Valley Hospital's Breast Health Institute who contacted her by phone to discuss available support groups including the "ABC Program."

Ms. G. has made an expeditious recovery. She and the surgeon verbalized not only satisfaction with the home experience option but recommend it to other clients.

Cronin and Maklebust (1989) report that BSNs expressed frustration and felt ill prepared to case manage effectively because they "lacked confidence in their ability to collaborate and delegate" (p. 38). The findings were based on a differentiated practice pilot project sponsored by the Midwest Alliance in Nursing (MAIN) in which associate degree nurses functioned as case associates and baccalaureate nurses functioned as case managers. The qualities and characteristics that nurses with advanced educational degrees bring to the role of case manager include the ability to:

1. Assess and evaluate complex clinical situations
2. Practice autonomously
3. Critically think and problem solve
4. Function from an interdisciplinary, organizational perspective
5. Effectively communicate and work with groups
6. View and negotiate complex systems (Herbage Busch, 1993; Pappenhausen, 1990; Sporacino, 1991)

These skills need to occur within as well as beyond the comfort of the case manager's own staff and institutional walls.

Case management literature cites several programs that use CNS case managers (Cronin & Maklebust, 1989; Gaedeke Norris, 1991; Holdren Mann, et al., 1993; Nugent, 1992). Building on Sioux Valley Hospital's model, the CNS role was selected to develop case management on a continuum and to expand differentiated practice at the advanced clinical practice level.

Definition

Case management on a continuum at Sioux Valley Hospital involves coordination of the entire spectrum of client's care, unlimited by setting or time span. The CNS collaborates with multiple health-care providers across service settings to access and coordinate care in a timely, efficient, and economical manner.

Process

Case management on a continuum at Sioux Valley Hospital is designed to address the needs of select clients who have continuous and comprehensive health-care needs beyond the acute episode of illness. The program began in 1992 as a demonstration project with time allocated to formalize the structure and process.

Collaboration. Early in the developmental stages, it became evident that dialogue and networking needed to occur within the institution as well as into the community. A hospital-wide case management task force, led by the vice-president of patient services at Sioux Valley Hospital, was organized to address the need for a seamless, integrated system across all health-care settings (Koerner, et al., 1994). Having nurse executive support is critical to empower case managers among other administrative professionals. Nurse executives' active involvement and promotion of the profession prevents other professionals from dictating nursing practice that ultimately reduces nursing autonomy (Gaedeke Norris & Hill, 1991) and coordinated client care. The task force established steering committees to address three areas: acute care, outpatient and community, and prevention and health maintenance. Representatives from home care, wellness center, social work, pharmacy, ambulatory care, therapy and rehabilitation, senior administration, primary nursing, and the clinical nurse specialist group made up the steering committees. Consultants to the steering committees included the department directors for finance, reimbursement, information systems, quality resource management, medical records, and marketing. Physicians were consulted for practice issues specific to client populations.

Having the appropriate disciplines and departments involved from the beginning intercepted potential obstacles and calmed turf issue debates. Because no professional can successfully work in isolation, all departments and disciplines were recognized for their distinct and valuable contributions that would make case management a success. The design team recognized that a full and accurate portrayal of the clinical and financial picture was possible with all resources actively involved.

Objectives. The major objective for case management on a continuum was to promote coordinated, integrated care and diminish fragmentation and replication of services. Projected outcomes included:

1. High quality care
2. Appropriate use of health-care dollars
3. Decreased length of stay
4. Decreased readmission rates
5. Decreased acuity upon readmission
6. Appropriate use of resources
7. Enhanced interdisciplinary and interagency collaboration
8. Client and family, physician, and nurse satisfaction

The CNS case manager focuses on health restoration, maintenance, and prevention, and educates the client to make informed choices. As advocate, the CNS emphasizes the importance of empowering clients to maximize self-care capabilities or to achieve a peaceful death with dignity (Gibson, et al., 1994).

Client selection. In the beginning, the CNSs worked closely with medical records and data processing to generate lists of potential candidates for case management. Specifically, persons with frequent inpatient admissions of three or more in one year were screened. Consideration was also given to persons who had frequent emergency department visits. More specific criteria developed and used by the CNS included:

- Chronic illness or catastrophic event (e.g., high-risk pregnancy);
- Frequent inpatient admissions or emergency visits;
- Fixed financial resources (e.g., Medicaid, Medicare, self-pay);
- Absent or inadequate caregiver support;
- Cognitive or developmental deficit; and
- Decreased coping capacity or emotional support.

The CNSs used these criteria for all clients across the life span but soon recognized that a majority of clients could potentially meet the selection criteria. Presently, each CNS case manager works closely with the primary and associate nurses, physicians, social workers, and other appropriate team members to redefine the selection criteria for targeted populations. Referrals have become more appropriate and timely.

The CNS selects clients on an individualized basis within the specialty practice. In the beginning, the CNS group was selective in case managing clients within a 60 mile radius. Sioux Valley Hospital, however, frequently absorbs clients from rural communities of up to 250 miles. The case study depicts how rural clients can efficiently benefit from CNS case management.

CNS case manager role. The operationalization of case management exists within the context of the nursing process. The CNS assesses, plans, implements, and evaluates each client's care through the continuum.

The CNS begin with completing a baseline assessment by using advanced physical assessment skills. The CNS also possesses advanced expertise in assessing the human response to illness, functional abilities,

CASE STUDY

Premature Neonate: Transitioning from Acute Care to Rural Home

Sharon Martin, RN, MS, NNP
Neonatal/Pediatric CNS Case Manager
Sioux Valley Hospital

Annie is a two-year-old Caucasian female who was born at 29 weeks gestation with severe intrauterine growth retardation and weighing 550 grams. She spent the first six months of her life in the intensive care and extended care nurseries. She had multiple problems associated with prematurity, with the primary problem of severe bronchopulmonary dysplasia. Because of her lung disease, Annie was oxygen dependent and required frequent nebulizations and medications. She also had feeding problems, developmental delays, recurrent upper respiratory infections with otitis media, and failure to thrive. Annie also had rickets as a result of complications from prematurity.

Annie's parents are married and live in a rural area 250 miles away from the tertiary hospital and follow-up clinics. They both have college educations and are employed in health-care fields. Annie's parents are intelligent, nurturing and supportive, and have a reliable supportive family and community.

At four months of age, the Intensive Care Nursery (ICN) primary nurse and primary nurse practitioner referred Annie to CNS case management because of her high risk for readmissions and complications. The CNS case manager collaborated with the ICN primary nursing team, social worker, attending neonatologist, hometown family pediatrician, home health agency, DME provider, hometown school district, insurance case manager, state Medicaid/SSI office, and family to develop a comprehensive discharge plan for Annie based on King's Theory of Goal Attainment with mutual goal setting.

Annie was discharged at six months of age with the appropriate sources and services in place including home oxygen, apnea monitor, nebulizer treatments, and medications. The CNS case manager and the family developed a plan to keep close communication by telephone, phone voice mail, or pager. When the CNS case manager was on vacation, coverage was provided by an ICN CNS case manager familiar with Annie. The family has kept in close contact with the CNS case manager when questions or concerns arise about Annie's care. Also fielded were concerns the parents had about their daughter which required the CNS to consult with pediatric subspecialty physicians including a pediatric pulmonologist, endocrinologist, and gastroenterologist.

Because of the many expenses accrued for Annie's care, the parents were not able to make their student loan payments, and their private insurance had to be supplemented by Medicaid SSI. The CNS case manager contacted the student loan officer requesting the loans be placed on hold without accumulation of interest until the parents were more financially stable. The loan payments are now on temporary hold. The CNS case manager also arranged travel reimbursement through the Department of Social Services whenever the parents were required to make the 250-mile (one way) trip for Annie's follow-up clinic appointments or rehospitalizations. With these financial stressors alleviated, the parents were able to focus their energy on Annie's needs.

Annie frequently required steroids during her recurring episodes of upper respiratory infections and ultimately developed reactive airway disease. She continued to have many respiratory setbacks and required six rehospitalizations during her first year after discharge from her initial hospitalization. During one of those hospitalizations, Annie had a feeding gastrostomy placed due to failure to thrive secondary to her chronic lung disease and subsequent oral aversion. The parents were taught G-tube feedings with the use of a Kangaroo pump.

Although Annie finally had established weight gain, she continued to have significant reactive airway disease. Because this occurred at home and subsided during hospitalization, a thorough evaluation suggested sensitivities to her home environment. The CNS case manager collaborated with Annie's hometown pediatrician and the pediatric pulmonologist. Children's Miracle Network was contacted to provide financial assistance for thorough cleaning of the home, including purchasing an air cleaner, to eliminate the allergens in Annie's environment.

Annie has had a total of seven readmissions to date. Through the CNS collaborating with the entire health-care team, Annie has been rehospitalized not only less frequently, but more importantly, less acutely ill. This is evidenced by her readmissions to general pediatrics rather than ICU. Also important is that her length of stay averaged two weeks per admission for the first four hospitalizations and now averages less than one week per admission.

An important factor for Annie was referral to the local school district for coordination of developmental therapies including speech therapy to correct her oral aversion. The CNS case manager communicates on a regular basis with the interagency coordinator for early childhood education regarding Annie's progress. Shared education between the health care and educational system fosters early intervention and the desirable outcome for Annie eventually to be mainstreamed into the public school system. The CNS case manager also works closely with the DME and home health agency and has successfully educated the parents to wean from home health services gradually.

The CNS case manager provides support from an educational, advocacy, financial, and spiritual dimension. The parents have been successfully empowered to assume the role of case manager in the form of parenting.

developmental stage, family dynamics, community resources, and financial resources. The CNS either performs reassessments directly or coordinates a system to monitor relevant and critical assessment data efficiently. For example, the cardiology CNS at Sioux Valley Hospital established a program for home dobutamine infusions and developed a standardized assessment tool to assure documentation of significant data by primary and associate nurses. This was essential not only for communication within nursing but also provided longitudinal data for the physician and staff. The CNS provided this along with a weekly summary report to the cardiologist.

Individualized planning occurs as the CNS analyzes all assessment data and collaborates with the client and family, physician, primary nurse, and other client specific team members. Individualized, realistic, and measurable outcomes are established and prioritized through mutual goal setting with the client and family.

Implementation of the plan involves procurement, delivery, and coordination of services. The CNS allocates and arranges human and material resources outlined to achieve the identified client outcomes. To illustrate, transfer of a ventilator-dependent client to a subacute nursing home bed required that the pulmonary CNS at Sioux Valley Hospital not only procure a ventilator and other necessary supplies but also educate the nursing home staff on how to care for a client with these high technological needs.

Monitoring and evaluation of the client's progress in relation to established outcomes are an ongoing process for the CNS case manager. The CNS collaborates with the client and family, physician, primary nurse, and other team members to evaluate goal progression or achievement and whether modifications need to be made within the plan. The CNS also monitors the care to assure quality and evaluates the cost effectiveness of the care. As a researcher and consultant, the CNS is instrumental in identifying cost-effective strategies (Gaedeke Norris & Hill, 1991). For example, the nutrition support and metabolic CNS at Sioux Valley Hospital was consulted by a rural affiliate hospital to facilitate alternate methods of care for a client with complex feeding needs (Case Study).

The CNS case manager functions in the traditional roles of expert clinician, educator, consultant, and researcher. Added dimensions of communication liaison, managerial role, and change agent have also been identified.

Implementation. CNS case management began in early 1993 with a demonstration project. Because positive clinical and fiscal outcomes were recognized within six months of the demonstration project, the program has continued to evolve.

A database was developed and is generated for all case management clients to track information on selected demographics, admission patterns, charges and reimbursement, CNS hours of service, and referral sources. A documentation system was created for recording progress notes, including the plan of care. Activities of daily living (ADL), instrumental activities of daily living (IADL), and caregiver strain scores were completed when appropriate.

The medical records department keys the CNS case manager's social security number into the client's abstract file. Data processing then generates a daily report to alert each CNS of any admission activities of the case managed clients including inpatient, emergency, and outpatient services.

Role clarification for the CNS, primary nurse, home health nurse, and social worker were priority areas to be addressed. The CNS group networked and dialogued with these and others in the hospital and community. Role modeling and actual client experiences proved to clarify the CNS case manager role and to define supportive and complementary roles of others.

Satisfaction surveys and interview questions were implemented after CNS case management was well established. The data from these surveys and interviews were used to evaluate perceptions of care from clients, family, physician, staff, and CNS perspectives.

Outcomes of Case Management on a Continuum

A descriptive analysis of data was completed for all clients who underwent case management for six months. A six-month time frame was identified as the mean time for active case management activities. The majority of clients either achieved desired outcomes and were placed on inactive status after six months or expired within six months.

A total of 43 clients met at least two of the selection criteria. Eight of these expired before the six-month time frame and were, therefore, excluded from analysis. The remaining 35 clients were included in the data.

The mean age was 44 years (range 8 months to 82 years; the median age was 41 years). Greater than half of the clients were female (60%). Equal percentages of clients were married or single (44%), 11% were widowed, and 3% were divorced. The majority of clients were white (94%), which is reflective of the community demographics. Only a small percentage of clients represented minority groups (6% Native American).

Medicare was the primary insurer for the majority of clients (40%), followed by Medicaid (31%), and private insurance (29%). None of the clients was a self-payor.

Case management referrals came from a variety of sources. Primary nurses referred the majority of

CASE STUDY

By Referral: Collaboration with a Rural Facility

Carol McGinnis, MS, RN, CNSN
Metabolic/Nutrition CNS Case Manager
Sioux Valley Hospital

The Center for Case Management received a referral from an affiliate rural hospital regarding a 58-year-old female Medicaid patient. She reports multiple episodes of illness over much of her life requiring intermittent hospitalizations. She was recently diagnosed with celiac sprue, a malabsorption disease, and reports numerous food intolerances, which have been present as long as she can remember. Because of the numerous reported food intolerances and exhibited symptoms of malnutrition, parenteral nutrition was initiated several months before the CNS consult. The client, who was also a nontraditional college student, began to receive her parenteral nutrition on an outpatient basis. She attended class during the day and received intravenous nutrition while she slept at the hospital every night. This was necessary because the state Medicaid system only reimbursed for this very expensive nutrition if it was delivered in the hospital setting. This made home therapy prohibitive for this client.

The major concern the staff in the rural institution had was dealing the "manipulative" and occasionally inappropriate behavior this client exhibited. The client was believed to be totally dependent on the parenteral nutrition. Because reimbursement for this costly therapy in the home was impossible, a prolonged inpatient stay with daily passes was anticipated. The physical and emotional concerns of the client were taxing the entire staff. They began to question their ability to help in this complex situation. To complicate matters, the client identified the staff as her sole support system.

The CNS case manager with nutritional and metabolic specialization was consulted. She visited with the physician, dietitian, social worker, and the nursing staff at the rural facility 60 miles away. The visit with the staff exceeded five hours as they ventilated extreme frustration in dealing with this client's "manipulative" behavior. A visit with the client also revealed a very distraught person. Her frustrations with food intolerances had not been validated, and she verbalized feelings of isolation from an early age. She spent much of her time dwelling on her illness at the expense of wellness-focused behavior.

The CNS case manager consulted with physician subspecialists, a clinical pharmacist, the nutrition support dietitian, as well as other CNS case managers at Sioux Valley Hospital. Formal recommendations to the client and hospital staff included suggestions to maximize the nutritional benefit of the current solutions and minimize the related physical finding, such as elevated liver function tests. After establishing gut function, the CNS suggested means to reintroduce specific foods gradually and taper parenteral nutrition. Psychological intervention was encouraged, and a counseling student was found with whom the client agreed to work. The CNS suggested that the counselor network with the staff to focus on wellness aspects and positive client reinforcement.

With continued CNS follow-up by telephone, the client was able to wean from parenteral nutrition and return home. Although she tried more foods than she would have ever consented to previously, the physical discomforts associated with celiac sprue, including severe diarrhea, persisted and gradually worsened. The CNS recommended trial of an elemental nutritional product, which the client chose to drink throughout the day. The patient felt stronger, gained weight on the 2,000 to 2,400 calories of the enteral form of nutrition, and no longer experienced the physical discomforts from other oral nutrition. The enteral product is quite expensive for the client who has a very limited income and resources. With the encouragement of the CNS, the client worked with the product company to provide the oral nutrition at a discount rate. For promotional purposes, the client currently receives free enteral nutrition from the product company. Reimbursement from second-party payors is being sought at this time by the CNS.

A tremendous cost savings can be realized by these interventions, in addition to the benefits for the client who is able to function in her own home with oral intake. An estimated cost for continued parenteral therapy as it was before CNS intervention was conservatively $331,000 per year, shared by Medicaid and the hospital. Costs of current nutritional therapy are currently free secondary to two generous medical nutritional companies. The estimated cost for the enteral product is $10,700 annually. The CNS is working with the reimbursement specialist and the state Medicaid system to cover the enteral product and also to consider parenteral therapy in the home should this client ever require it in the future as well as for other clients. This is significantly less than the costs of malnutrition, repeat hospitalizations, and the previous parenteral therapy as an inpatient.

Interactions between the CNS, clients, and rural hospital staff now transpire through a newly implemented telecommunications network between the rural hospital and the large urban hospital. The rural hospital has asked the CNS and the Sioux Valley Hospital Center for Case Management for guidance in implementing case management at their institution. This, as well as inservices in related areas, has been provided to the rural hospital by the telecommunications network as a result of this case management experience. It is anticipated that the CNS case managers in the tertiary hospital will continue to provide consultation and assist with complex clients in rural areas.

clients (60%), followed by CNS case manager and data processing finds (23%), others including affiliate rural hospital staff, childbirth educator, and pulmonary rehabilitation (11%), and physicians (6%).

An attempt was made to establish a control group to serve as a matched sample for comparison purposes with the case managed group. This proved to be unfeasible because of differing comorbidities and individual client variables. Case managed clients were, therefore, used as their own control. Preintervention data for six months before CNS case management were compared with six months of postintervention data.

Dramatic results were achieved. The CNS case managed clients demonstrated a 27% decrease in hospital admissions (Figure 24-4), a 66% decrease in inpatient days and mean length of stay (Figures 24-5 and 24-6), and a 79% decrease in charges (at the time of the study a cost accounting system was unavailable). Reimbursement remained essentially the same, which is representative of the Medicare and Medicaid payment systems for the majority of clients (Figure 24-7). The costs for the CNS case managers were cal-

culated to include the time spent in direct or indirect contact with clients, consultation with physicians and other team members, documentation, and travel. The overall financial impact was a difference of $552,666—a 79% decrease in loss over six months for 35 clients (Table 24-2).

The CNS spent an average of 2.0 hours per client per month on individual case management activities. This is somewhat lower than other models and is attributed to the sophisticated differentiated practice model at Sioux Valley Hospital. Having a plan in place at all times and having the CNS work closely with the primary nurse upon readmission facilitates a timely discharge. Home health is also fully developed to allow the CNS to manage care efficiently via telephone, thus decreasing direct client contact and travel time. These two components have built a solid foundation with the CNS spending the majority of time coordinating, brokering, monitoring, and advocating on behalf of the client rather than providing the direct skilled care. In many instances, the traditional hands-on care is delegated and reserved for the expert acute

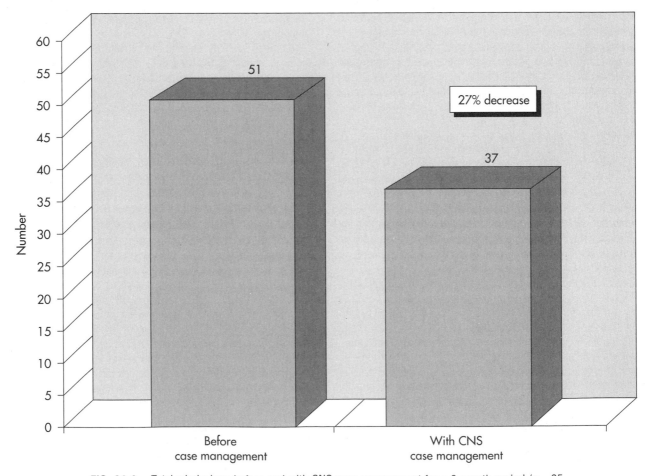

FIG. 24-4   Total admissions before and with CNS case management for a 6-month period (n = 35 patients)

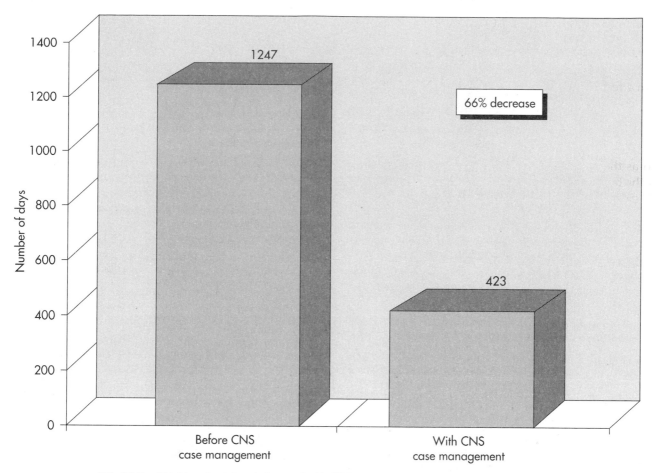

FIG. 24-5   Total inpatient days before and with CNS case management for a 6-month period (n = 35 patients)

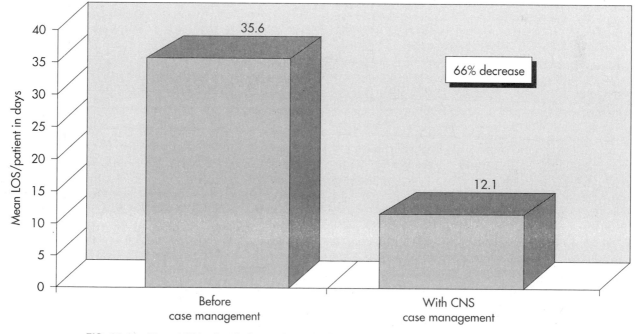

FIG. 24-6   Mean LOS/patient before and with CNS case management for a 6-month period (n = 35 patients)

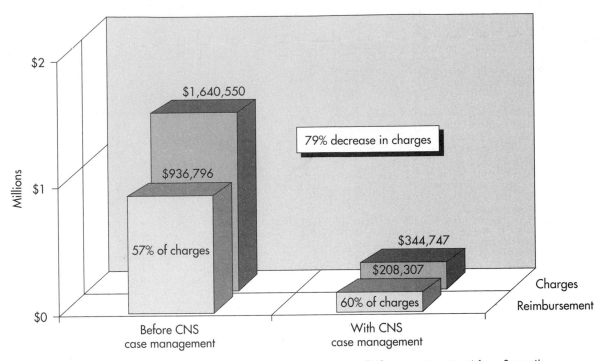

FIG. 24-7   Total charges and reimbursement before and with CNS case management for a 6-month period (n = 35 patients)

TABLE 24-2   CNS Case management financial outcomes—6-month study period (n = 35 patients)

	Before CNS case management	With CNS case management	Total variance (%)
Total charges	$1,640,550	$344,747	79%
Total reimbursement	936,796	208,307	78%
% of charges reimbursed	57%	60%	3%
Total CNS hours	0	418.5	
Mean CNS hrs/pt/mo.	0	2.0	
Total CNS cost	0	14,648	
Mean CNS cost/pt	0	419	
Financial impact	−703,754	−151,088	79%

care nurses, home care nurses, and other less expensive ancillary staff. Efficient and economical management of care results with a decrease in fragmentation and replication of services.

The use of critical care days was also calculated and significantly decreased with CNS case management. The critical care units included the adult, coronary, pediatric, and neonatal units. Before case management, 10 of the 35 clients used a total of 257 critical care days. With CNS case management, 3 of the 35 clients used a total of 10 critical care days. The resulting 96% decrease in critical care days reflects the primary goal of prompt and early identification of the causative factors contributing to exacerbation.

Teaching clients their unique triggers and warning signs facilitated early intervention to bypass unnecessary admissions or a timely hospitalization at a lower acuity. By avoiding costly critical care stays, the DRG dollars were not immediately consumed and a greater percentage of reimbursement was achieved.

Perceptions and Satisfaction

A sampling of clients and family members was interviewed by a member of the CNS group practice who was not the case manager for the clients. Common themes for which the clients and families expressed satisfaction with the CNS case manager included:

1. Having the same nurse who knows the unique situation for the client and family;
2. Comfort, independence, and knowing limitations in caring for self or loved one;
3. Being informed and knowledgeable about the disease process, progression, and options for care; and
4. Comfort with contacting and confiding in the CNS at any time.

Physicians were asked to complete a questionnaire which yielded a 25% response rate. These physicians expressed their gratitude for having the CNS coordinate and facilitate the client's care. Having the work speak for itself through direct, positive case-management experiences has resulted in favorable physician comments. Physicians have recognized time efficiency with fewer inappropriate and nonmedical phone calls, especially at night, from anxious clients and family members for which the CNS is prepared to facilitate. Routine and more frequent telephone contacts have been initiated by either the CNS or client and family during the day to anticipate needs, answer questions, and bypass preventable crisis situations. For terminally ill clients, quality-of-life discussions, including code status, living wills, durable power of attorney, and advance directives, are encouraged by the CNS during stable, nonemergent times. The client and family then discuss this with the physician and a final decision is frequently made before a crisis event.

Nurses, social workers, pharmacists, dietitians, and other members of the team stated that communication improved, and the CNS case manager promoted an interdependent and collaborative practice. Primary nurses, specifically, stated the support of having follow-up provided for labile, high-risk clients was comforting. Having the CNS provide feedback on the client's progress in relation to the discharge plan was also rewarding for the primary nurses.

The CNS case managers unanimously highlighted the autonomy in actualizing practice the way that nurses have been taught and yearned for since the profession's inception. The CNS case managers also appreciated the opportunity to participate actively in clients' lives and to develop professional relationships more fully on a continuum. Having clients exposed to nurses in this model, as opposed to traditional nursing, may heighten public awareness of the unique contributions nurses bring to health care beyond traditional hospital nursing.

The CNSs at Sioux Valley Hospital have diverse specialties ranging from the premature neonatology to geriatrics. Having the CNSs work closely on this project resulted in a formalized group practice. Case management provided the common thread for bonding the group and creating a united front. Building on the existent *shared governance model* at Sioux Valley Hospital, the CNS group practice now operationalizes the work through four councils. Advisors to the group include a nursing administrator, the director of home health and hospice, and the vice-president of patient services. The CNS group also routinely meets with nurse managers, nurse administrators, educators, and other advanced practice nurses to discuss corporate issues.

CONCLUSION

Future work with case management includes research with a focus on outcomes, continuous quality improvement, and the differentiated practice model. Consumer involvement and marketing the role of nurse case manager to the public is critical. As aggressive political action plan needs to be instituted to assure proper legislative and regulatory support for advanced practice nurses within the state (Koerner, et al., 1994). Fee structures can then be established. Nursing needs to become actively involved with hospitals and business contracts to ensure that the nurse case management component is an integral part of the managed care negotiation process.

Active involvement of consumers and decentralization of nursing at a community level is urgent. This includes the infusion of nurses at work sites, churches, schools, retirement communities, homes, and other residences.

Focusing on prevention and wellness and having a greater number of advanced practice nurses in the primary care role are essential for a viable future. Establishing advanced practice nursing centers and wellness clinics, which emphasize the importance of empowering clients to maximize their potential for well-being, will appropriately place nursing in a prevention and teaching capacity (Koepsell, et al., 1994).

Finally, automation within institutions and into physician's offices and other connected agencies will be essential. With all appropriate information systems connected, clinical and fiscal reports will easily be compiled and accessible. Development and linkage of a computerized universal database for case management will strengthen outcome data.

Whatever the future holds, it will require collegial collaboration. Differentiated nursing practice is actualizing this by advocating how roles can complement one another and enhance client outcomes. Case management is a contact sport that requires active participation by each member of the interdisciplinary team, including the client. Then, and only then, can we stand back in awe at what we have created.

ssociation. (1988). *Nursing case management.* American Nurses Association.

.. Consultants. (1993). As case management ...ves, pathways may need revision. *Hospital Case Management, 1* (5), 88, 93.

Blue, R. J., Bunkers, L. B., McGinnis, C., McMahon, L. J., & Newstrom, P. (1994). Consultation. In J. G. Koerner, & K. L. Karpiuk (Eds.). *Implementing differentiated nursing practice: transformation by design.* Gaithersburg, MD: Aspen Publishers, Inc.

Cohen, E. L., & Cesta, T. G., (1993). *Nursing case management: from concept to evaluation.* St Louis, Mosby.

Cronin, C. J., & Maklebust, J. (1989). Case-managed care: capitalizing on the CNS. *Nursing Management, 20* (3), 38-47.

Etheredge, M. L. S. (1989). *Collaborative care: nursing case management* (pp. 63-64). New England Medical Center Hospitals: American Hospital Publishing, Inc.

Ethridge, P., & Lamb, G. (1989). Professional nursing case management improves quality, access, and costs. *Nursing Management, 20* (3), 30-35.

Gaedeke Norris, M. K., & Hill, C. (1991). The clinical nurse specialist: developing the case manager role. *Dimensions of Critical Care Nursing, 10* (6), 346-353.

Gibson, S. J., Martin, S. M., Johnson, M. B., Blue, R., & Miller, D. S. (1994). CNS-directed case management: cost and quality in harmony. *Journal of Nursing Administration, 24* (3), 45-51.

Gibson, S. J., & Thomas, L. (1994). Hospital saves $4.4 million with critical paths over two years. *Hospital Case Management, 2* (11), 188-192.

Gibson, S. J., Thomas, L., & Burnette, J. (1994). Atypical pathway sends mastectomy clients home early. *Hospital Case Management, 2* (7), 117-120.

Herbage Busch, A. M. (1993). Is the CNS as house staff an option? *Clinical Nurse Specialist, 7* (6), 287.

Holdren Mann, A., Hazel, C., Geer, C., Meaker Hurley, C., & Podrapovic, T. (1993). Development of an orthopaedic case manager role. *Orthopaedic Nursing, 12* (4), 23-27, 62.

Koepsell, P. A., Jensen, R., Reisdorfer, J. T., Slack, C., Young, S., Weber, A., Fjerstad, T., Gibson, S. J., & Paulson, N. J. (1994). Continuity. In J. G. Koerner, & K. L. Karpiuk (Eds.). *Implementing differentiated nursing practice: transformation by design* (pp. 167-168). Gaithersburg, MD: Aspen Publishers, Inc.

Koerner, J. (1992). Differentiated practice: the evolution of professional nursing. *Journal of Professional Nursing, 8* (6), 335-341.

Koerner, J., Bunkers, L., Gibson, S. J., Jones, R., Nelson, B., & Santema, K. (1994). Differentiated practice: the evolution of a professional practice model for nursing service. In D. Flarey (Ed.). *Redesigning nursing care delivery: transforming our future.* Philadelphia: J. B. Lippincott Co.

Koerner, J. G., & Karpiuk, K. L. (1994). *Implementing differentiated nursing practice: transformation by design.* Gaithersburg, MD: Aspen Publishers, Inc.

Lyon, J. C. (1993). Models of nursing care delivery and case management: Clarification of terms. *Nursing Economics, 11* (3), 163-169.

Nugent, K. E. (1992). The clinical nurse specialist as case manager is a collaborative practice model: bridging the gap between quality and cost of care. *Clinical Nurse Specialist, 6* (2), 106-111.

Pappenhausen, J. L. (1990). Case management: a model for advanced practice? *Clinical Nurse Specialist, 4* (4), 169-170.

Ruffolo, M. C., & Nichols, N. (1994). Satisfaction and role performance of case managers in the mental health system. *Journal of Case Management, 3* (1), 36-42.

Sowell, R. L., & Meadows, T. M. (1994). An integrated case management model: developing standards, evaluation, and outcome criteria. *Nursing Administration Quarterly, 18* (2), 53-64.

Spoaracino, P. S. A. (1991). The CNS-case manager relationship. *Clinical Nurse Specialist, 5* (4), 180-181.

Vaska, P. L. (1993). The clinical nurse specialist in cardiovascular surgery: a new twist. *AACN Clinical Issues, 4* (4), 637-644.

Wheatley, M. J. (1992). *Leadership and the New Science.* San Francisco: Berritt-Koehler Publishing Company.

Williams, R. (1992). Nurse case management: working with the community. *Nursing Management, 23* (12), 33-34.

Chapter 25

The Influence of Reimbursement on Nurse Case Management Practice: Carondelet's Experience

Phyllis Ethridge, MSN, RN, CNAA, FAAN
Suzanne Johnson

OVERVIEW

Nurses expand and improve the delivery of health-care services to people as reimbursement methods and policies change.

At Carondelet Health Care, services have been reimbursed in many ways, from fee-for-service under contract to discounted fee-for-service and capitation. Each type of reimbursement has influenced both the referrals to our practice and our practice itself. Moreover, the sharing of risk and fiscal incentives between nurse case management and Carondelet as well as between Carondelet and payors is also an influence. A sample contract for formalizing a relationship between nurse case management services and the payor concludes the chapter.

Professional nurse case management at Carondelet Health Care Corporation of Southern Arizona will soon celebrate a decade of services to the community. Originally, the case management program was established because nurses and physicians were frustrated at the decrease in length of stay that occurred after the Medicare diagnosis related groups (DRG) payments were implemented. Clients were being sent home at higher acuity levels. This was especially a concern when the client was frail, elderly, and chronically ill. For Medicare clients who had been referred to home care, Rusch et al. (1985) evaluated the education received in the hospital. Eighty-five percent of the clients could not remember what they had been taught, even though the education was well documented in the client's record.

Although the clients and families remembered the nurses giving them certain instructions, it was determined that the hospital was not the best environment for learning because of the anxiety associated with being a client. Without the self-management education, hospital readmission rates began to increase. One solution to improve the quality and cost of care was professional nurse case management offered along the continuum of care.

CASE MANAGEMENT AS CRISIS INTERVENTION—REVENUE PROTECTION

In the late 1980s, the finance departments within hospitals became more sophisticated, looking primarily at inpatient volume. Individuals' hospital stays were classified by DRG as a profit or loss. Product line management committees were formed to identify opportunities for improvement. Hospital executives sought ways to change their DRG mix to survive in the future. The chronically ill, frail elderly were determined to be the highest risk and the greatest loss to the hospital's bottom line. These clients had the longest length of stay in hospitals. Critical pathways became the popular managed care process to gain efficiencies within the hospital walls.

Utilization review departments began to flourish. Nurses were asked to review the records of all Medicare beneficiaries who were hospitalized and make sure each individual met the specific criteria published by the Health Care Financing Administration (HCFA). If clients did not meet a specific criteria for hospitalization, they were either discharged or asked to assume monetary liability for further hospital services. Home care visits increased; however, many of the chronically ill older adults did not meet the established criteria to acquire assistance. HCFA began to penalize hospitals for clients readmitted with the same diagnosis within a given period of time. Many clients, nurses, families, and physicians began to complain that some individuals were being sent home before being capable of coping with recovery.

During the first few years, the clients referred to professional nurse case management were seen as noncompliant, forgetful, anxious, living alone or with an overburdened caregiver, or known to the staff on a first-name basis because of their many admissions to a specific unit. Although numerous physical, psychosocial, and environmental issues were identified by the case managers caring for these clients, there were several common examples. Clients trying to live solely on social security could not always afford to refill their medications in a timely manner and were therefore labeled noncompliant. Others would run out of food the last week of the month and be readmitted for malnutrition or dehydration. Some clients would be fearful of dying at home alone, become anxious, and call 911. If they were chronically ill and frail, they usually could get admitted to the hospital and, if not, at least get an emergency department visit. Nurse case managers were challenged to minimize these psychosocial and environmental issues and to provide ongoing education and support through regular monitoring of clients and referral to community services.

At this time, professional nurse case managers were not reimbursed for their services by payors. Nevertheless, hospitals could improve their profits or decrease their losses from Medicare if clients were not readmitted within a 14-day cycle for the same diagnosis. On the case management learning curve, this period is often referred to as crisis management.

After three years of professional nurse case management along the continuum, Carondelet nurses began to see a decrease in length of stay as well as fewer readmissions and hospitalizations. The meaning? Professional nurse case management was impacting the length of stay by earlier access to care. Clients who were experiencing an exacerbation of chronic illness were quickly assessed and, if necessary, referred to a physician's office, emergency room, or admitted to the hospital at a low severity of illness. Therefore, either a hospitalization was avoided or clients were admitted earlier in their illness, thus bypassing critical care and being able to leave the hospital sooner and stronger.

THE FIRST CASE MANAGEMENT CONTRACT—DISCOUNTED FEE FOR SERVICE

In 1988, the first professional nurse case management contract was negotiated with an Arizona Health Care Cost Containment System (AHCCCS) provider, which is Arizona's Medicaid managed care plan. The contract based reimbursement on a discounted fee-for-service requiring authorization for case management visits. Fee-for-service is the lowest risk contract for a provider, and a discounted fee-for-service is considered a second step toward midlevel risk for services. Under this contract, the professional nurse case manager agreed to summarize the first ten cases in writing for quality and cost effective review by the payor. This client population under contract was younger than Medicare beneficiaries, but extremely complex. The payor authorized nurse case management for clients who already were costing the plan large amounts of money or had the potential for costly complications. All teenage pregnant women who were determined to be high-risk because of drug use, alcohol use, or a secondary chronic illness were referred to a case manager specializing in maternal and child health. Other types of individuals referred were homeless clients who had major illnesses and terminally ill young clients whose parents may or may not have been working. In one instance, the client was on Medicare disability and was the sole supporter of the household; therefore, all heroic measures were continued regardless of this client's wishes.

With professional nurse case management the savings to the plan were tremendous; however, any low-cost service that might have assisted families and clients toward a healthy lifestyle was usually never authorized, for example, bereavement, assisted living, day care, and heating or cooling for the home. The professional nurse case managers, although concerned and limited in the number of visits allowed, did acknowledge the differences in their practice due to the shift from crisis management to more planned intervention.

NURSING HMO—CAPITATION

In July, 1989, a senior-care health maintenance organization (HMO) began services in Tucson. Many of the Medicare beneficiaries being case managed became interested in enrolling because of the financial savings. Medications were $5.00 a prescription for a 30-day supply. Physician office visits were $10.00 per visit. No supplemental insurance was necessary and the annual $500.00 self-pay deductible did not exist. Entering into a contract with this senior HMO, Carondelet Hospital Administration negotiated global per-diem reimbursement for all inpatient services and discounted fee-for-service for outpatient services. Global per diem is a flat reimbursement for hospital services, per day, no matter what the nature of the services. Hence, the hospital would be reimbursed $750.00 per day for a client having open heart surgery or a client admitted for back pain. This contract type has a moderate amount of risk, higher or lower depending upon the hospital case mix and encourages administrators to decrease the cost of inpatient care in order to meet guaranteed volume. Today, per-diem contracts are no longer negotiated globally but according to such specific services as critical care or obstetrics. Per-diem reimbursement encourages providers to admit clients to the hospital and keep them longer. Further, it does not encourage the use of community services. Under per-diem reimbursement, fewer clients were referred to professional nurse case management, and the nursing division was eager to evaluate their entire community nursing network of services. It seemed, therefore, appropriate to accept a home-care capitated contract of $2.20 per senior enrollee per month with the Medical HMO. Capitation allowed nursing to render services in the community according to client need. No authorization from the payor was necessary. Capitated contracts place the provider at the highest risk, shifting emphasis from illness to health monitoring and disease prevention. In June 1990, the community contract was finalized, and the first nursing HMO was established.

Capitation enabled nurse case managers (NCMs) to match client need with community nursing resources. With this flexibility, they had the opportunity to improve practice in two major ways. One way was moving nursing assessment beyond client need identification to pattern recognition. Margaret Newman, PhD, RN, a visiting nursing theorist, helped the NCMs to discern patterns of health and illness and to build meaningful connections between discrete needs. This, in turn, led to a second improvement in practice intervention. NCMs began working with clients to identify patterns that exacerbate illness. One specific intervention was hospice care. Without time for these services, caregivers could only fall back on the hospital for respite, an often-seen pattern of response to the caregiving burden. Under the capitated contract, respite-services became essential for quality, cost-effective care.

The nursing capitated contract supported a health focus and continuity of care which simplified the relationship between Carondelet's community nursing services and the medical HMO. It also, however, created a different incentive for the hospital and nursing. The hospital was still on a per-diem contract, and the nursing HMO was capitated. Hospital administration was reimbursed when a person was hospitalized. With a predetermined amount of money per month, the nursing HMO had an incentive to avoid or minimize hospital use to demonstrate effective services. Nevertheless, the values, mission, and philosophy of the hospital and nursing HMO were identical. After 17 months of the HMO, the hospital administration negotiated a capitated risk contract for inpatient, outpatient and community services, with an emphasis on caring for clients in the community.

After functioning as a nursing HMO for one year, 700 clients had received services within their home. Approximately 2,500 were being cared for in the community nursing centers. The average number of enrollees in the senior plan was 15,000. The admissions to hospitals per 1,000 enrollees was 1,311. This was approximately 200 less than expected and 500 less than national Medicare figures. The professional NCMs were accountable to assess all senior plan admissions to the hospital, determine necessary nursing services before discharge, monitor all community services being rendered, and continue to care for the client in the community if necessary.

Further in-depth evaluation indicated high client satisfaction, increased symptom management, and increased ability of clients to be case managed toward self-care responsibility. From a cost-effectiveness standpoint, findings indicated fewer readmissions to the hospital and fewer emergency room visits when clients were enrolled in the nursing HMO.

This first capitated system risk contract excluded home health. The medical HMO provider started its own home-care program. This impaired the flow of communication among services. The referrals to case management started to decline, especially if the HMO enrollee was eligible for home care. The senior HMO seemed interested in making a profit from their home-care program, as opposed to providing support and recognizing patterns that may exacerbate an individual's chronic illness and avoid or minimize a possible hospitalization. There was a definite conflict in philosophy. The progress made toward a seamless community delivery system halted. Admissions to the hospital began to increase. In fact, during the 1994 fiscal year, a 17% increase was noted.

Carondelet hospital administration was also successful in negotiating a second captitated senior HMO contract for both inpatient and outpatient services and community services. This contract included home health but on a discounted fee-for-service basis. This method of reimbursement guarantees an increase in volume, which allows the fixed cost to be spread over more business, therefore decreasing the cost of care for all clients. Usually, a 10% to 15% discount from charges or a cost-plus-10% contract is negotiated. With this reimbursement, each client receiving services had their care authorized by the HMO. In essence, the hospital does not have the control of home care services, once again disrupting the seamlessness of community services. Other community services not included in the capitated payment were durable medical equipment, respiratory therapy, and IV home infusion services.

Professional NCMs are the client advocates for needed services. If the payor does not think that the equipment or service is required, the case manager must file a justification or assist the client through the grievance process. Often the client is readmitted to the hospital because services were delayed or equipment was determined to be an unnecessary cost by the payor. Hospitals negotiating capitated contracts should insist upon the inclusion of all services along the continuum to control costs and prevent unnecessary hospital admissions.

COMMUNITY NURSING ORGANIZATION—RISK-ADJUSTED CAPITATED DEMONSTRATION PROJECT

The Community Nursing Organization demonstration project, or CNO, is a program for Medicare clients which expands services within the community. Using much of the data and information from the Nursing HMO, Carondelet applied to the Health Care Financing Administration for the moneys allocated for the CNO by legislation passed in 1986. Carondelet was one of four sites selected.

Within the CNO, emphasis is placed on health promotion and disease prevention. Each individual enrolled in the program is assigned a nurse partner. For people at high risk for managing their health concerns, this partner is a professional NCM. Enrollees can be monitored by nurse partners in nursing centers, ambulatory care settings, or in other community environments depending upon the acuity of the individ-

ual. Reimbursement is allocated on a capitated payment according to age, sex, assessment of activities of daily living (ADL) limitations, and previous use of home care services. This type of payment promotes creativity and allows flexibility in caring for enrollees along a continuum within nursing and with the other disciplines that provide outpatient therapies.

Challenges and opportunities exist for keeping individuals healthy and assisting caregivers to help clients toward self-care responsibilities, while maintaining their own health. Although this project is in its infancy, professional NCMs who are participating are excited about the impact this program has had on expanding their practice.

CONCLUSION

As health-care executives plan to survive in a future managed care environment, capitated risk contract for services are inevitable. Advanced-practice nurse case managers will have numerous opportunities to assist individuals along a continuum of care. They will be pivotal in all areas of a seamless integrated delivery system. Identifying needs in community services that will improve quality and reduce the cost of care, defining those services, and negotiating methods of reimbursement will be a challenge for all group practices. Communications between provider and payors is essential for efficient services, which are enhanced when the risks and incentives are shared.

REFERENCES

Rusch, et al. (1985). Unpublished evaluation of retention of client education from hospital to home.

SELECTED READINGS

Health Services Advisory Group, Interqual, I.S.D. (1994). Criteria (revised).
Ethridge, P. (1991). A nursing HMO: Carondelet St. Mary's experience. *Nursing Management, 22,* 22-27.
Community Nursing Contract with Senior HMO.
Newman, M., Lamb, G. S., & Michaels, C. (1991). Nurse case management: the coming together of theory and practice. *Nursing & Health Care, 12,* 404-408.
Burns, L. R., Lamb, G. S., & Wholey D. (Submitted for publication). *Impact of integrated community nursing services on hospital utilization and cost in a Medicare risk plan.*
Carondelet Readmission Rates '91 through '94 of Original Senior HMO contract, to be published.
Papenhausen, J. (1995). *The effects of nursing case management intervention on perceived severity of illness, enabling skill, self-help, and life quality in chronically ill older adults.* Dissertation Abstracts International, Ann Arbor, Mich.: University Micro Films International.

Sample Contract
Proposal

to

*_____

from

Carondelet Community Health Services

INTRODUCTION

Carondelet Health Care Corporation of Arizona is submitting this proposal for consideration. Carondelet proposes to provide community health services to the *_____ Health Plan enrollees in *_____ counties:

1. Home Health Care
2. Home IV Therapy
3. Nurse Case Management for chronically ill or complicated clients
4. Step-down (SNF) services
5. High-risk maternal-child case management
6. Home immunizations for children 0-5 years of age
7. Selective behavioral health outpatient interventions periodic case management and counseling services
8. Respite care for caregivers at home
9. Diabetic community education and outreach
10. DME/RT services
11. Hospice services

In addition, neighborhood-based community health centers are available. Proposed costs are listed in Appendix.

BACKGROUND

Carondelet Community Health Services, a division of Carondelet Health Care Corporation of Arizona, has provided health care for the people of Tucson and southeastern Arizona for over a century. Under the continued sponsorship and support of the Sisters of St. Joseph's of Carondelet, Carondelet has maintained a strong commitment to its communities and has expanded its services to respond to changes in the health-care delivery system. Carondelet hospitals provide a full spectrum of health services, which are integrated into a system of care that spans the health-care continuum. Services include acute care inpatient services, extended care and long-term care services, home care services, hospice services, ambulatory care services, and nurse-managed neighborhood health centers. Professional nurse case managers coordinate care of clients who are physiologically imbalanced, are emotionally challenged, have caregivers with a knowledge deficit, only qualify for home health for a short period of time, but need private services, homemaker and/or respite services and choose to stay in their own homes, or consistently utilize the emergency room or the hospital for immediate health-care needs. The Carondelet Philosophy is to treat the whole person—body, mind, spirit— and to that end, Carondelet integrates behavioral wellness and treatment at every point of contact promoting self-care and empowerment. Carondelet is committed to health promotion services and the prevention of illness, utilizing all resources to promote optimal health of the family within the community setting, while decreasing costs of expensive acute care.

PROPOSED PROGRAMS

A. Home Health Care

Carondelet Home Health Services has been in operation since 1983. There has been a two-fold increase between 1989 and 1994 in number of home health units provided by Carondelet Home Health Services from just under 12,000 to over 35,000 visits. The fiscal health of Carondelet Home Health Services is a reflection of the increase in its gross margin from $100,000 in FY 1989 to over $1,100,000 in FY 1994. Carondelet Home Health Services has had experience in providing all or selected home health services in Pima, Santa Cruz and southeastern Pinal counties, as follows:

1. *Fee-for-service* for SEAGO for provision of Home Health R.N., Home Health Aide and Housekeeping services on a per-unit (60 minutes) basis to the residents of Santa Cruz County, Arizona.
2. *Fee-for-service* between 1989 and present for the Arizona Long-Term Care Services (ALTCS) Home and Community-based Programs Division, providing RN home visits and home health visits.
3. *Fee-for-service* for Mercy Care, an AHCCCS provider for home health services in Pima and Santa Cruz counties of Arizona.
4. *Capitated* arrangements for Family Health Plan (FHP) between June 1990 and July 1991 to provide home health services, nurse case management, infusion care, and respite services to enrollees in FHP's Medicare Risk Plan.
5. *Fee-for-service* for Intergroup Commercial and Senior Plan for the past three years for Home Health Services in Pima and Santa Cruz Counties.
6. Selective Adult Med/Surg complicated cases for Pima Health AHCCCS Plan.
7. Eastern Pinal County: Case management and three Promatores who are health-care Hispanic residents who visit the ill and refer or provide necessary services to local residents and Diabetic education and counseling. We are currently renovating a building in Mammoth to provide primary care services, as well as all home health DME/RT and IV Therapy care, besides current services.

B. Home IV Therapy

Carondelet Home IV Therapy Program has been in existence for two years. Our primary goal as a service-intensive health-care company is to deliver superior quality, therapeutic services and products to nonhospitalized clients requiring sophisticated infusion and related therapies under the supervision of a physician.

C. Case Management of Chronically Ill or Complicated Clients

Carondelet hospitals have provided Nurse Case Management to at-risk and high-risk elderly, pregnant women, and neonates since 1985. In 1990, Multiple Sclerosis clients were case managed through a contract with the Multiple Sclerosis Society. Nurse Case Managers work across service settings to assist clients to manage their health concerns and access services in a timely and effective way. Carondelet's Nurse Case Management Program has received extensive national attention. Carondelet has had experience providing nurse case management:

1. As part of a three-year Flinn Foundation funded *demonstration* project for improving coordination and access to health services for frail elderly.
2. Under a *fee-for-service* arrangement with Mercy Care Plan of AHCCCS to provide Nurse Case Management to high-risk AHCCCS member, particularly high-risk elderly and high-risk pregnant women and neonates.
3. Under *capitation* with two Medicare risk plans for seniors to provide home health services, Nurse Case Management and respite services to enrollees in FHP's and Intergroup's Medicare Risk Plan. Nurse Case Managers design a service plan that best matches individual needs for recovery from acute illness or adapting to unstable chronic diseases.
4. Under *fee-for-service* to Pima AHCCCS Health Plan for high-risk maternal and child clients for the past three years.
5. Most recently, Carondelet was chosen as a demonstration site by HCFA to manage the community services for Medicare enrollees.

A nurse case manager:
- Assesses client's needs holistically;
- Assesses client's health, safety and functional status, including need for preventive services;
- Identifies goals collaboratively with the client and family;
- Designs a plan of care collaboratively with the client, which may include needs for self-care, education, monitoring, community services and additional resources;
- Arrange for provision of services, equipment identified in the plan;
- Follows up to assure that services have been initiated;
- Reassesses client at regular intervals to identify changes in needs, health and functional status and if nurse case management coordination should be continued;
- Refers to appropriate community resources;
- Acts as advocate for the client, encouraging self-responsibility, self-care, and appropriate utilization of the health-care system, avoiding fragmentation of services; and
- Coordinates with primary care physicians as indicated.

Outcomes of goals will be regularly evaluated and documented and integrated across the continuum of care—hospital and community. Achievement of needs satisfaction will determine the completion of the service plan. Any difficulties reoccurring for the client will be evaluated and assistance provided toward resolution.

Stabilized clients may be referred to Carondelet's community health centers, which are neighborhood based, if there is a continued need for monitoring, health maintenance, health promotion, and screening. Nurse case management services would be reinstituted if clients' needs dictate.

Multiple quality and cost outcomes have been evaluated. All research and publications are attached or available upon request.

D. Step-down Skilled Nursing Facility (SNF) Services

Carondelet Holy Family in Tucson and Holy Cross SNF in Santa Cruz are extensions of the Carondelet Health Care system's continuum of care—offering a broad spectrum of skilled and rehabilitative services. Holy Family was built in 1987 as an alternative health-care facility, serving people from all faiths and from all walks of life. Holy Cross SNF has been in existence for many years and is the only facility available in Santa Cruz County.

Both facilities are licensed by the Arizona Department of Health Services and are currently rated as *substantially exceeding* licensure standards. They are also Medicare-certified facilities, meeting strict OBRA guidelines and standards for quality of care.

1. *Services:* Both facilities offer services that range from convalescence following hospitalization to permanent long-term care needs.

Nursing service provides care to residents requiring various fluctuating levels of care:
   a. *Intermediate* care (moderately independent, self-feeder, continent) to
   b. *Skilled* (more staff dependency, needing assistance with mobility, feeding, transfers, episodes of incontinency), or
   c. *SNF/Sub-acute* (total dependency on staff to meet all needs). Experienced nursing staff also provides care to those in need of IV therapy, trach care, colostomy/ileostomy care, central lines and hyperalimentation and compassionate care to HIV and MRSA clients.

   Carondelet SNF facilities provide on-site physical therapy programs to improve functional skills, strength, range of motion, balance, and gait. Occupational therapists, as well as Speech therapists, complete the rehabilitation team. Therapy is offered twice daily, six days a week in our modern, well-equipped therapy department. The gently but firm and consistent guidance of the therapists motivates the client to greater degrees of independence and freedom, which improves and enhances self-esteem and confidence.

Other support services are also provided by Carondelet staff: social services, dietary, activities, chaplain services, housekeeping. All act in concert to provide a therapeutic environment with essential social, physical, psychological and spiritual components in an atmosphere which emphasizes the dignity and worth of each individual.

  2. *Fees:* Carondelet SNF facilities are interested in contracting with you on a fee-for-service basis. All pharmaceuticals for *_____ clients shall be provided for by a *_____ contract vendor who shall bill *_____ directly. Under these terms, Carondelet SNF facilities would be willing to discount our services to this group of clients. Carondelet proposes a 10% discount off of all gross charges.

E. Selective Maternal/Child Health and Prenatal Case Management
Carondelet's Nurse Case Management program has been providing Maternal/Child Health management, including prenatal case management, for the past 4½ years. Contracts have included the AHCCCS Mercy Care Plan and Pima Health Plan. Each assessment and recommendations are shared with the health plan.

  1. *High-risk criteria for obstetric clients* have included: teenage pregnancy, pregnant clients over 40 years of age, chemical addiction of drugs or alcohol, chronic illness (especially diabetes, asthma, renal problems), developmentally disabled, seizure disorder, preterm labor, pregnancy-induced hypertension, homeless, multiple fetuses, depression, and psychotic mental illness.

  2. *High-risk criteria for pediatric clients* have included preterm less than 37 weeks or in hospital over five days, small for gestational ages, congenital anomalies, hypoglycemia, chronic illness, juvenile diabetes, asthma, failure to thrive, high environmental risk factors, addicted clients, violence in home, overcrowding, homelessness, and addiction.

  3. *Neighborhood wellness centers:* Carondelet proposes that, in addition to home visits with a 1:1 relationship, prenatal group educational classes (6-10 clients) be provided in high-risk neighborhoods. Teenage counseling could also take place.

F. Home Immunization for Children 0-5 Years of Age
Immunization could be given in two settings with communication by letter or by phone to the primary care physician for documentation:

  1. At home for one or more children within a family where family tends not to participate in community programs.

  2. At a neighborhood wellness center where space is borrowed, such as a church. Cost is decreased for this method.

G. Selective Behavioral Health Outpatient Intervention and Periodic Case Management
Carondelet Behavioral Health reflects the philosophy that brief behaviorally specific treatment interventions are the most advantageous approach to behavioral health needs of a vast majority of the populations. Brief courses of treatment allow for skill development on the part of the client, while avoiding unnecessary dependency on others or institutions. Empowerment of the individuals to solve their current issues, while developing the sense of competency to solve future challenges, is the hallmark of this approach. To that end, Carondelet possesses a continuum of care with behaviorally specific time-limited approaches that allow for the least restrictive level of care to be applied at the appropriate time. These include:

  1. *Acute Inpatient Psychiatric Stabilization:* Time limited brief hospitalization, oriented toward emergency stabilization and reentry into this community. Carondelet has expertise in converting AHCCCS clients to ACCM-eligible clients.

2. *Detoxification (Inpatient):* Detoxification for complex medically unstable issues of addiction that require medically monitored detoxification protocols.

3. *Partial Hospital:* Time limited partial hospitalization structured program designed to increase skill acquisition to prevent rehospitalization and develop self-reliance skills and resiliency.

4. *Evening Outpatient Chemical Dependency Group:* Design includes weekly modules for skill acquisition, rehearsal of new behaviors and relapse prevention, all provided in weekly capsules.

5. *CHOICES Group:* Design includes weekly modules to provide increased skills for situational depression, victimization, and codependency symptoms.

6. *OPTIONS (Individual Outpatient):* Brief strategic therapeutic model oriented toward one to six sessions, provided in an individual or family modality.

7. *Case Management:* Case management of at-risk behavioral health clients oriented toward the most cost-efficient outcome-oriented results.

H. Respite Care

Respite care is provided for the caregiver by a home health aid through Home Health. Services are available by the hour and provided in blocks of four hours, once or twice a week to allow caregivers necessary time to socialize to continue on-going caregiving responsibilities 24 hours a day. (If this is not offered, the client is usually admitted to the hospital to accomplish respite for caregivers.)

I. Diabetes Care

The Diabetes Care Centers located at Carondelet St. Mary's Hospital and at Carondelet St. Joseph's Hospital are the sole providers of quality diabetes education as recognized by the American Diabetes Association. Additional services are available through our Diabetes Care Center in Nogales, Arizona through Carondelet Holy Cross Hospital's Home Health Department. These unique programs meet the prescribed national standards and are staffed by Certified Diabetes Educators. It is a model program patterned after the successful multidisciplinary teams in the recent Diabetes Control and Complications Trial.

J. DME/RT Services

In the interest of expanding the services along the Carondelet continuum of care, Carondelet opened its full-service DME/RT division in 1994. Offering a broad base of quality product and service combinations to home clients is Carondelet's primary strength. Maintaining a high level of clinical support to clients with the greatest need is the single most important objective of Carondelet's clinical management team. A dedicated full-time staff helps maximize the client's home experience. Carondelet has committed over $1,500,000 to facilities and home medical equipment to meet the needs of its clients at home.

K. Hospice

Carondelet Hospice Services is designed to provide specialized care for terminally ill clients and to support their families and caregivers. Although the focus of the hospice concept is home care, designated units and specially trained staff at Carondelet St. Joseph's Hospital, Carondelet St. Mary's Hospital, and Carondelet Holy Cross Hospital in Nogales provide short-term inpatient care for symptom control and respite care.

QUALITY ASSURANCE

Carondelet Health Care Corporation has an active Quality Improvement (QI) program to enable it to systematically monitor and evaluate the quality and appropriateness of health services to its customers, to solve identified problems and to pursue opportunities to improve services. Each of the service components has its own QI plan. Currently, each of the Carondelet programs follows the JCAHO guidelines for quality improvement. In current programs, structure, process and outcomes of care delivery are monitored and evaluated.

FISCAL NEGOTIATIONS FOR EACH SERVICE

All services have been individually costed out for the purpose of accepting a capitated payment. Fiscal agreement will be on an individual basis. The following pages depict a proposed fee schedule for each service.

Proposed Fee Schedule Unless Capitated

HOME HEALTH CARE

Registered Nurse, per visit	$55.00
Physical Therapist, per visit	65.00
Occupational Therapist, per visit	65.00
Speech Therapist, per visit	65.00
Home Health Aide, per visit	30.00
Social Work (MSW), per visit	75.00

HOME IV THERAPY (PER DIEM)*

TPN 1 liter	$135.00
2 liter	165.00
3 liter	195.00

ENTERAL NUTRITION

Category #1 Basic milk & soy based	25.00
Category #2 Specialized high nitrogen	45.00
Category #3 Hydrolized protein amino acid	55.00
Antibiotic Therapy	
AWP of Medication plus	60.00
Pain Management	
AWP of Medication plus	60.00
Chemotherapy	
AWP of Medication plus	60.00
Hydration	
AWP of Medication plus	40.00
Central line catheter care	20.00
Aerosolized Pentamidine	195.00

*The above per-diem rates include the following:

—All administration and ancillary supplies necessary to administer therapy
—Delivery
—Nursing assessment and coordination, client training, initial home visit and set-up
—Ongoing 24-hour per day clinical pharmacy and IV nursing services availability
—One follow-up nursing visit per week, as needed.

CASE MANAGEMENT OF CHRONICALLY ILL OR COMPLICATED CLIENTS

Initial Visit	$70.00
Return Visits	55.00

STEP-DOWN (SNF) SERVICES   90% OF GROSS CHARGES

Selective Prenatal Case Management	
Initial Visit	$70.00

Return Visits	55.00
Neighborhood Wellness Center Group Education (10 hours)	60.00

HOME IMMUNIZATIONS FOR CHILDREN 0-5 YEARS

Per Visit	$55.00
Neighborhood Wellness Center/per staff member, per hour or $5.00 for each child's immunization	50.00
Selective Behavioral Health Outpatient Intervention and Periodic Case Management	
Acute Inpatient/day	$450.00
Detox (chemical dependency)/day	450.00
Partial Hospital with 10 clients/group, per day, 4-5 hours	80.00
Evening Outpatient Chemical Dependency with six clients/ group, 3 hours × 4 days (flexible) – per day	50.00
CHOICES with 4 clients/group, 3 hours × 4 days – per day	50.00
Case Management	
Office setting/phone	25.00
Initial Home visit	70.00
Follow-up home Visits	55.00

DIABETES CARE

Basic Diabetes Self Management Skill	$74.00
Diabetes Consultation	85.00
Diabetes Exercise Rehab	78.00
Diabetes Exercise Therapy	130.00
Diabetes Therapy Program	420.00
Fingerstick Blood Glucose	19.10
Gestational Diabetes Therapy	387.00
Glucose Meter Rental	55.00
Glycated Hemoglobin	30.00

DURABLE MEDICAL EQUIPMENT/RESPIRATORY THERAPY

Rentals:	*Per Month*
Hospital bed, manual w/rails & mattress	$50.00
Hospital bed, semi-electric w/rails & mattress	75.00
Overbed table (included with bed rental)	N/C
Continuous Positive Airway Pressure	75.00
Pressure pad, alternating w/pump	20.00
Oxygen, "E" system	10.00
IPPB, AP-5	50.00
Oximeter, Nonin 8500M	50.00
Nebulizer w/compressor	25.00
Trapeze	20.00
Oxygen, concentrator	150.00
Oxygen, liquid system	75.00
Suction pump, home model, portable	30.00
Tens, four lead	25.00
Tens, two lead	25.00
Client lift	25.00
Wheelchair, standard, DDA, DFR	25.00
Wheelchair, standard, DDA ELR	25.00
Wheelchair, fully reclining, DDA, DFR	40.00
Wheelchair, heavy duty, DDA, DFR, 20" wide	40.00

Wheelchair, hemi, DDA, DFR	35.00
Wheelchair, ltwt, DDA, DFR	35.00
All other rentals	40% off list

Sales:

Liquid oxygen (per pound)	$.90
"E" cylinder refill	8.00
Nebulizer, w/compressor	90.00
Maintenance fee (per hour)	35.00
All other sales	20% off list

Hospice Services	*Per Day*
Routine Home Care	$88.00
Continuous Home Care	25.00
Respite Care	92.00
General Inpatient	394.00

Chapter 26

Discovering and Achieving Client Outcomes

Judith Lynne Papenhausen, PhD, RN

OVERVIEW

A nurse researcher concludes that establishing partnerships is the nurse case manager intervention associated most closely with improved client outcomes.

Recent cost-containment trends in health-care delivery include increasingly restrictive private and federal reimbursement policies, restraints on institutional length of stay, and constrictions of the range of reimbursement for health-care services, which have the potential to influence the quality of health-care delivery negatively. Additionally, the appraisal of health-care quality has become progressively driven by the use of evaluation criteria associated with specific client outcomes. These trends have forced effective health care to be balanced between the cost and quality of care outcomes. Although it is generally accepted that cost and quality interact, the identification of clear indicators of acceptable standards of where these outcomes emerge or intersect is in the process of discovery. This chapter examines the nature of nurse case management interventions and resulting client outcomes when nurse case managers practice via the Professional Nurse Case Manager (PNCM) model developed at the Carondelet Hospital and Health Center in Tucson, Arizona.

Cost-containment methods have altered the distribution of health care and have been shown to have a negative influence on persons who are least likely to be able to afford private payment (Pegels, 1988; Strumpf & Knibbe, 1990). Among those most impacted are persons in high-risk categories such as the chronically ill, whose labile health-care status requires frequent monitoring and periodic interventions and who may require multiple hospital admissions. These clients are often discharged from acute care facilities early in the recuperative and restorative phases of their illnesses. Increasingly, lower cost alternatives are being chosen, including early transfer to extended care facilities, or returning home with or without the support of informal caregivers, and home health care. Often these alternatives are used before the formulation of a comprehensive health-care plan, which includes the development of a support network of multidisciplinary health professionals and services to meet health-care needs (Hicks, Stallmeyer, & Coleman, 1992; Olivas, Del Togno-Armanasco, Erickson, & Harter, 1989a, 1989b; Zander, 1990a). This restrictive economic climate has fostered a redefinition of advanced nursing practice roles and the development of increasingly autonomous nursing practice strategies that are cost effective and guided by client outcomes. This situation has created an opportunity for the evolution of the role of the Nurse Case Manager (NCMr) and the development of Nurse Case Management (NCM) models to serve selected client populations (Bower, 1992; Ethridge & Lamb, 1989; Zander, 1988). The purpose of this chapter is to examine the nature of NCM interventions and the resultant client outcomes when NCMrs practice in the Professional Nurse Case Management (PNCM) model developed at Carondelet Hospital and Health Center in Tucson, Arizona.

CLIENT OUTCOMES AND THE DEVELOPMENT OF ROLE OF THE NURSE CASE MANAGER

Increasingly, professional nurses are performing the case manager role with selected client populations. Because of the diversity of their needs and the complexity of the existing health-care delivery system, chronically ill clients particularly require professional guidance in coordinating, executing, and evaluating their health-care plans. The effective management of chronic illness requires time-intensive coordination of multiple health-care professionals and services, operating under common outcome goals. The direction of these services is provided by a case manager who facilitates and evaluates the usage of the complex health-care system (ANA, 1988; Bower, 1992). The legitimacy of the role of the nurse case manager is strongly supported by the literature. Many authorities support the view that nurses are the logical candidates to become case managers for clients having acute and chronic physiological health problems. More than any other health-care agent, professional nurses have a generalist background with a broad knowledge of the physiological and psychological ramifications of specific health conditions. Through their practice, nurses gain experience in assessing, diagnosing, and treating client responses to disease and disability. Historically, their practice has also afforded them an opportunity to participate in the implementation and monitoring of medical protocols in acute care and community health settings (Bower, 1992; Ethridge & Lamb, 1989; Fralic, 1992; Zander, 1990a, 1990b). Case managers require knowledge and skill in three general areas:

- Clinical expertise relative to the client's health-care needs.
- An ability to determine client resources and to negotiate for health-care services.
- An ability to implement the steps in the process of case management.

Further, many authors agreed that nurse case managers should have advanced academic preparation and previous experience in clinical practice (Brockopp,

Porter, Kinnaird, & Silberman, 1992; Fralic, 1992; Hinton-Walker, 1993; Lynn-McHale, Fitzpatrick, & Shaffer, 1993; Petryshen & Petryshen, 1992; Rogers et al., 1991; Sherman & Johnson, 1994; Tahan, 1993, Trinidad, 1993).

THE PROFESSIONAL NURSE CASE MANAGEMENT (PNCM) MODEL

The PNCM model, which blends the elements of acute care and community models, has been the focus of several studies. This model allows for the continuity of a single nurse case manager who designs a multidisciplinary plan of care that is initiated during the client's hospitalization. The case manager follows the client into the home setting and continues to execute and monitor the plan of care (Bower, 1992; Ethridge, 1991; Ethridge & Lamb, 1989; Michaels, 1992; Rusch, 1986). The PNCM model at Carondelet Hospitals and Medical Centers was an outgrowth of a centralized home health-care service implemented in 1983.

Based on a pilot program to evaluate outcome benefits, the role of the professional nurse case manager and the PNCM model evolved over a five-year period (Box 26-1).

Qualifications and Education of the NCMrs Practicing the PNCM Model

At Carondelet St. Marys, all NCMrs complete a common NCMr educational program and internship, share common job descriptions and are exposed to the same case management philosophy and practices. In general, NCMrs must be graduates from accredited BSN programs and have had at least two years of professional nursing experience in an acute care or community setting. Newly hired NCMrs attend a mandatory inservice education program that consists of a clinical internship with a case manager preceptor and comprehensive review of the orientation manual. Each

---

BOX 26-1

SCOPE OF THE NURSE CASE MANAGER

- Assessing the client and family
- Establishing a nursing diagnosis
- Developing a plan for nursing care
- Delegating nursing care to associates
- Activating interventions
- Coordinating and collaborating with the interdisciplinary team
- Evaluating outcomes
  (Ethridge & Lamb, 1989)

new employee is teamed with an experienced case manager for a period of one to two months. In addition to the clinical internship with the NCMr, mandatory home visits are made with home health nurses, social workers, and hospice nurses. The clinical internship is terminated by mutual consent once role understanding and comfort has been achieved.

NCMr meetings are held regularly to exchange information concerning their practice, and daily communication is common among the members for the purpose of informal consultation and sharing of client information. Because NCM services are available 24 hours a day, a case manager is always on call. At Carondelet Hospitals and Health Care Centers, Tucson, Arizona, the NCM intervention practiced by the NCMrs is guided by the PNCM model. The NCMr "forms partnerships with the

people at high risk and moves across the spectrum of health care to assist them in learning to live with one or more chronic diseases" (Michaels, 1992, p. 79). The goal of the professional case manager is to identify high-risk clients, establish a therapeutic relationship, and to coordinate the entire spectrum of care across settings, for an extended period of time (Ethridge, 1991, Ethridge & Lamb, 1989).

Fiscal Outcomes of the PNCM Model

The fiscal advantages of the PNCM model, when used with elderly chronically ill clients, have been documented and are summarized in Table 26-1. Ethridge and Lamb (1989) compared cost data on length of stay (LOS) between total hip replacement clients who were and were not case managed and for recidivistic clients

TABLE 26-1   Fiscal outcomes of the professional nurse case management model

Description of study	Variables measured					
Ethridge & Lamb (1989) compared LOS of total hip replacement clients who received NCM services and those who did not.	**LOS** Without NCM — With NCM 10.2 — 8.1					
Ethridge & Lamb (1989) compared institutional averages on COPD clients in the year before NCM services with the year post-NCM services.	**LOS** Without NCM — With NCM 12.4 — 4.3		**COST LOSS VS GAIN/CASE** Without NCM — With NCM −$3,291 — +$1,553			
Ethridge (1991) compared variables 15,000 members of a senior managed care plan with national Medicare per 1000 member averages. Of the total members, 5% to 6% were receiving NCM services.	**NUMBER OF ADMISSIONS** Medicare — Senior Plan 319 — 242		**LOS** Medicare — Senior Plan 7.5 — 5.8			
Rogers, Riordan, & Swindle (1991) compared 38 chronically ill (*M* age = 75) on fiscal variables pre- and post-NCM services. Cost of NCM service was an average of $962 per client at a rate of $36.00/hour.	**ADMISSIONS** Pre-NCM — Post-NCM 2.2 — .79		**LOS** Pre-NCM — Post-NCM 10.7 — 5.3		**COST OF CARE** Pre-NCM — Post-NCM $261,638 — $6,885	
Weyant (1991) compared 130 chronically ill clients (*M* age = 75) on fiscal variables pre- and post-NCM services.	**ADMISSIONS** Pre-NCM — Post-NCM 3.05 — .88		**LOS** Pre-NCM — Post-NCM 9.2 — 6.3		**COST OF CARE** Pre-NCM — Post-NCM Per client $9,483 — $845 Overall cost $1,232,776 — $109,804	
Gibson et al. (1994) compared cost 6 months prior and 6 months during NCM services on 22 chronically ill subjects and the cost of NCM services was $9975 or an average of $453 per subject.	**ADMISSIONS** Pre-NCM — Post-NCM 41 — 22		**LOS** Pre-NCM — Post-NCM 36.1 — 9.4		**COST:REIMBURSEMENT RATIO** Pre-NCM $928,997/$467,795 Post-NCM $190,601/$133,936	

with Chronic Obstructive Pulmonary Disease (COPD). For case managed clients, the average LOS was lower than the average LOS for those clients who were not case managed. In addition, the COPD population, before NCM services represented a net loss to the medical center of $3,291 per case, (average $ per case less average reimbursement). After NCM services, the COPD population represented a net profit to the medical center of $1,552 per case. These investigators concluded that this financial impact was attributed to the ability of the nurse case managers to intervene earlier in an acute exacerbation of the respiratory illness.

Ethridge (1991) reported cost savings in a group of 15,000 healthy and medically disabled seniors who were enrolled in a per capita senior plan contract. The impact of nurse case-managed services, admission rates per 1,000 members, yearly hospital bed days, and length of stay data were compared against national Medicare averages. This comparison revealed that in all categories the total group of enrollees demonstrated improved fiscal outcomes, determined by decreased admission rates, yearly hospital bed days, and length of stay. Ethridge concluded that nursing case managed services were responsible for these results and stated "each patient day saved reflects a cost savings of approximately $900.00" (1991, p. 26).

Using the PNCM model in a midwestern medical center, other researchers found similar financial advantages (Rogers et al., 1991; Weyant, 1991). The first evaluation was based on data using 38 frail chronically ill Medicare clients with a history of frequent readmissions, extended lengths of stay, numerous complications, and multiple morbidities (Rogers et al., 1991). The second evaluation was based on data from an additional 92 subjects who participated in the program during 1990 (Weyant, 1991).

In the first study of 38 clients, the decrease in number of admissions and length of stay are depicted in Table 26-1. Cost of care savings are also noted.

Additional data were obtained from subjects who entered the NCM program in the year following the first study (Weyant, 1991). These data revealed that after NCM services, mean number of admissions per client and the average LOS were decreased by 71% and 31%, respectively. The total health-care cost in an equal period decreased by 91% (see Table 26-1). No measurement of quality outcomes were made in these studies, but Rogers et al. (1991) offered "the most efficient inpatient care and excellent discharge planning may be in place, but if there is no one to implement, assess, modify, and otherwise make the plan work, such high-risk patients return to the hospital over and over again" (1991, p. 31).

The PNCM model was also implemented in a northern, midwest state (Gibson et al., 1994). Twenty-two chronically ill subjects who were nurse case managed over a six-month period demonstrated reduced admissions and LOS when compared with a six-month period before NCM. As with other studies, the subjects demonstrated high rates of recidivism and represented a major source of financial loss to the hospital before NCM. The total health care was decreased by 86% during the NCM period which included the cost of the NCM services (Gibson, et al., 1994).

On the basis of these data, these investigators concluded that nurse case management has had a financial impact on the cost of hospitalization. This cost savings was achieved both at the end of the stay, by lowering the average LOS, and at the beginning of the stay, by earlier admission of clients at a lower acuity level (Ethridge & Lamb, 1989).

The fiscal advantages of the PNCM model have been supported in three separate geographic locations and in five comparisons of financial data. Clough and Thomas (1992) stated, "Why does our hospital pay these nurses for these services which presently are not reimbursable? Because it's cost effective. In a high Medicare/managed care environment the hospital realizes benefits through reduced admissions and lengths of stay" (p. 1). Many researchers have proposed that the fiscal outcomes are linked to quality of care outcomes which are embedded in nurse case management interventions (Ethridge, 1991; Ethridge & Lamb, 1989; Rogers et al., 1991). Michaels (1992) offered:

As nurses, we believe other outcomes are significant, nursing-related patient outcomes like self-care status, empowering and well-being. Conceptually, we have translated these outcomes into broader health care outcomes, using hospital discharges, bed days, and emergency department visits as a reflection of our work. In general, we assume that the more seniors accept responsibility for managing their health concerns, be it through their own effort or by accepting the help of others, the lower will be their severity of illness when hospital services are sought (p. 83).

The PNCM model has demonstrated impressive reductions in the cost of providing health care to chronically ill, elderly clients. Investigators suggested that the explanation for these cost benefits was embedded in the process and the resultant client care outcomes of the experience. Central to the process of the PNCM model is the formation of a therapeutic nurse client relationship from which mutually driven client outcomes emerge.

THE PNCM MODEL: BUILDING THE RELATIONSHIP

The PNCM model was developed based on a belief that if high-risk, chronically ill clients could be identified early during an acute hospitalization, the NCM could establish a continuous nurse-client-family therapeutic relationship and coordinate the entire spectrum of care in both settings for an extended and indefinite period of time. It was anticipated that both cost and quality outcomes such as reduced recidivism, more appropriate service utilization, improved chronic illness management, and increased client satisfaction would result. Perhaps the central difference that distinguishes the professional nurse case management approach from acute care models lies in the context of the professional relationship between the client and the NCM. Several authors (Mound et al., 1991; Rheaume et al., 1994; Sowell & Meadows, 1994; Wadas, 1993; Wagner & Menke, 1992) have commented on the nature and importance of the nurse-client relationship which develops when the NCM works closely with the client across the health-care continuum. An important aspect in assisting persons to meet their goals was the personal quality and continuity of the NCMr-client relationship (Gibson et al., 1994; Mound et al., 1991; Wagner & Menke, 1992) and the formation of a partnership based on trust (Sowell & Meadows, 1994). Wadas (1993) offered that through the PNCM, the nurse case manager "establishes goals with the patient and begins a long-term caring relationship" (p. 41). Rheaume et al. (1994) observed that "a special type of relationship must be established for nurses to become successful in healing and promoting their client's health" (p. 32).

Newman, Lamb, and Michaels (1991) explored the process and the nature of nurse case management interventions that are unique to the PNCM model. They characterized the philosophical and professional orientation of the NCMr, the dimensions of the professional relationship, and the relationship to hospital staff. The philosophic orientation was described as holistic, caring, and closely tied to "the spiritual dimension of person and the environment and all other aspects" (Newman et al., 1991, p. 405). The professional orientation was described as a nonhierarchical model of group practice, with each nurse case manager having a loosely designated area of individual expertise. Newman et al. (1991) noted that the title "case manager" was inconsistent with the subjects' philosophy. NCMrs did not attempt to control or manage the client's situation but rather worked to build self-reliance and facilitate informed choices. Because of the mutuality of the relationship, the NCMr has the obligation to discuss options and explore alternatives but must ultimately respect the client's choice. The focus of the NCMr was on the process of the nurse-client relationship, the length and intensity of which was governed by client need and readiness. Newman et al. (1991) offered, "The nurse-client relationship is rhythmic, and timing is important: when to connect and when to separate" and "freed from usual bureaucratic time constraints, the NCMr and the client can orchestrate their interactions to match optimal times for growth and change" (Newman et al., 1991, p. 406). Building the client-nurse relationship, therefore, is central to NCM services and the discovery and achievement of client outcomes.

Core Practice Components and Client Outcomes of Nurse Case Manager Interventions

Client outcomes resulting from NCMr interventions were examined from both a quantitative and qualitative perspective to determine if these interventions increase the self-care responses in elderly clients with chronic illness. The purpose of the study was to measure client outcomes before and after three months of NCMr intervention. The outcomes measured were clients' perceived severity of illness, general self-efficacy, life quality, and self-help abilities. In addition, the qualitative statements of clients were examined. Areas addressed concerned their perceptions of differences in self-care and illness management abilities they believed were the result of NCMr interventions.

The outcomes were defined as follows: (1) severity of illness was the client's perception of the level of severity of the chronic illness judged by the fluctuation or stability of the symptom pattern and the treatment effectiveness; (2) general self-efficacy was the client's perception of ability to adequately perform an activity and a belief that adequately performing the activity would produce a desired result; and (3) life quality was the clients' perception of satisfaction with overall life situation. Self-help abilities were defined as the client's perception of (1) physical disability judged by ability to perform basic activities of daily living (ADLs) such as grooming, dressing, bathing, and ambulation and instrumental activities of daily living (IADLs), such as shopping and household activities; (2) social satisfaction judged by level of participation and satisfaction in social activities with family and friends, and in hobbies and external social events. This also included a self-assessment of the degree to which the activities were satisfying; and (3) the ability to control and manage symptom distress which included a sense of mastery over the frequency of the symptoms and the degree to which the symptoms disrupted lives.

Characteristics of Client Population for the Study

A convenience sample of 76 nurse case managed chronically ill adults were identified for the study. These clients demonstrated most of the following high-risk selection criteria:

- Elderly, over 60 years of age
- Limited family support

- Chronically ill
- A high probability for physiological instability
- Qualified for home health care for a short period of time and chose to remain at home
- Consistently utilized the emergency room of the hospital for immediate health-care needs
- Voluntarily agreed to participate in the nurse case management program

The selected population were between the ages of 60 and 95 years and a median age of 78. The majority were female (59.2%), either married (40.8%) or widowed (40.8%) and lived alone (47.4%). Most were white or Caucasian (89.5%). Additional characteristics of the client selected group are found on Table 26-2.

In addition, a sample of 12 was selected from the main sample for an interview relative to their outcome experiences resulting from interaction with a NCMr. These subjects were interviewed within 90 to 105 days following initial intervention. Clients were selected to represent the widest variety of respondents with a variety of chronic illness diagnoses.

Intensity and Frequency of Nurse Case Manager Activities

Thirteen nurse case managers (NCMrs) provided NCM services for the 76 clients in this study. To describe the nature of NCM interventions, NCMrs were asked to complete a log of NCM activities (Figure 26-1) which included date, length of home visit including travel and documentation time, and estimated the percentage of time that was spent on the intervention categories of (a) assessment and monitoring, (b) teaching and informing, (c) supporting and sharing, (d) exploring alternatives and goal setting, and (e) direct service including treatments, medications, wound care, and other related tasks. Additionally, the NCMrs recorded the time and amount of activities related to monitoring progress, service coordination, and professional consultation, which included telephone conversations and additional meetings with clients, family, and other health-care professionals.

The average number of home visits and telephone contacts are found in Table 26-3 along with average time to complete each activity.

At the end of each home visit NCMrs recorded on the subject logs the estimated percentage of time which was spent on the specific intervention activities (Table 26-4). The greatest amount of time was spent on assessment/monitoring (29.71) followed by supporting/sharing (23.46).

It is interesting to note that the nature of the client-nurse relationship in acute care settings is more focused on curing rather than caring behaviors (Hinton-Walker, 1993; Wadas, 1993). Watson, Lower, Wells, Farrah, & Jarrell (1991) used observers to examine the type and time required to perform nursing functions in an acute care facility in the Midwest. The results revealed that out of each three-hour time period, staff nurses devoted 4.55 minutes to providing information and 3.84 minutes to providing psycho-emotional support to patients and families. By contrast the paramount purpose of the NCMr relationship is to provide emotional support and client education and is most probably the key difference in NCM's practice focus from that reported above in the acute care setting.

Collectively, acute care nurses studied by Watson et al. (1991) reported slightly less than 5% of each hour spent on emotional support and education, whereas NCMrs in this study devoted 51% of each hour of care to these interventions. These findings support the previous view held by Cohen and Cesta (1993) that the focus of the NCMr-client relationship is on self-care education, client advocacy, counseling, and emotional support, and is consistent with the themes in NCM generic goals that include education, support and enhancement of the client's self-care capability, quality of life, sense of autonomy, and self-determination (ANA, 1988; Bower, 1992). These data also support observations made by Newman et al. (1991) that a component of NCMr practice operationalizing the PNCM model was building self-reliance, discussing options, and facilitating informed choices. These findings are also consistent with those of Lamb and Stempel (1991, 1994) who identified interventions which were designed to promote the client's sense of self-worth and to provide emotional support in the working and changing phases of the NCMr/client process and with Lamb (1992) who found an increase in self-care skills and illness management and an increase in the sense of well-being in clients followed by NCMrs.

Results of the Quantitative Data

The MANOVA statistic was used to determine the differences in the collective subject scores on all depen-

TABLE 26-2   Client characteristics

% of Total selected population of 76	
Retired	69.7
Disabled	22.4
Provides own care (unassisted)	84.4
Illness diagnoses	
Acute coronary heart disease	14.5
Chronic coronary heart disease	31.7
Chronic obstructive pulmonary disease	21.1
Diabetes mellitus	9.2
Other	23.5

NURSE CASE MANAGER LOG OF HOME VISITS

Client _____ NCM _____ NCM# _____ Medical Record # _____

Date _____ Length of total visit _____ Treatment time _____ Documentation time Notes _____ Data entry _____ Other (specify) _____ _____	Nature of NCM interventions	% time
	Assessment and monitoring	
	Teaching or informing	
	Direct service facilities	
	Supporting and sharing	
	Exploring alternatives and goal setting	
	Other (specify) _____ _____ _____	

Date _____ Length of total visit _____ Treatment time _____ Documentation time Notes _____ Data entry _____ Other (specify) _____ _____	Nature of NCM interventions	% time
	Assessment and monitoring	
	Teaching or informing	
	Direct service facilities	
	Supporting and sharing	
	Exploring alternatives and goal setting	
	Other (specify) _____ _____ _____	

CONSULTATION/SERVICE ARRANGEMENT LOG

TELEPHONE CONSULTATIONS			CONSULTATION MEETINGS			OTHER ACTIVITIES		
Date	Person contacted	Time	Date	Person contacted	Time	Date	Person contacted	Time

FIG. 26-1   Sample logs of nurse case manager activities. (**A**) Nurse case manager log of home visits. (**B**) Consultation and service arrangement log.

dent variables before and after nurse case management intervention. The Wilk's Lambda multivariate test of significance indicated an overall significant difference. Paired two-tailed t-tests examined the variables separately (Table 26-5).

The results showed significant differences for decreased perceived severity of illness after NCM interventions. Significant differences were also seen in three of the four measurements of client's self-help abilities, namely, decreased perceptions of physical disability, decreased number of reported symptoms, and decreased perceived symptom distress. Significant differences were not found for the variables of perceived general self-efficacy, perceived quality of life, and perceived participation in socially satisfying activities.

TABLE 26-3 Average number and length of nursing case management home visits and telephone contacts self-reported by nurse case managers (N = 76)

Variable	n	Range
Average number of home visits*	7.84	2.67-15.36
Average number of telephone contacts**	4.17	1.67-7.40

Variable	M	Range
Average length of home visits in minutes*	53.93	31.88-83.63
Average length of telephone contacts in minutes**	7.49	3.00-11.20

*Data missing for one subject

**Data missing for two subjects

TABLE 26-4 Average percentage of time of home visits devoted to specific intervention activities self-reported by nurse case managers (N = 76)

Intervention activities*	%
Assessment or monitoring	29.71
Teaching or informing	16.52
Direct service	6.89
Supporting and sharing	23.46
Exploring alternatives and goal setting	11.12

*Data missing for one subject

Results of the Analysis of the Interview Data

The main purpose of collecting the interview data from the selected sample of 12 clients was to identify subjective client statements that were indicative of the six dependent outcomes of this study and to identify any new categories of outcomes resulting from NCM interventions that were not measured by the quantitative instruments. Three expert reviewers were given the transcribed interview data and used client phrases as the basic unit of analysis. For any phrase to be considered indicative of a dependent variable, reviewers had to reach an interrater agreement of 66.6% or higher. All reviewer judgments related to new outcomes were examined and collapsed into categories.

An analysis of the interview data revealed subjects' phrases indicating of all six of the study's outcome variables. Exemplars were identified for the three indicators of self-help, (i.e., decreased perception of physical disability, increased perception of social satisfac-

TABLE 26-5 Paired two-tailed t-tests of the dependent variables of severity of illness, general self-efficacy, quality of life, and the self-help measures of physical disability, social satisfaction, number of reported symptoms, and symptom distress (N = 71)

Variable	M Time 1	M Time 2	T	P
Severity of illness	287.85	229.75	3.87	0.000*
General self-efficacy	58.40	57.20	0.92	0.361
Quality of life	520.55	532.93	–0.70	0.484
Measures of self-help				
Physical disability	22.85	21.29	2.52	0.014*
Social satisfaction	14.04	13.62	1.28	0.204
Number of symptoms	4.92	40.4	5.49	0.000**
Symptom distress score	11.99	9.94	3.64	0.001**

*$p < 0.05$

**$p < 0.001$

tion, and symptom management), and for decreased severity of illness, increased general self-efficacy, and increased quality of life.

Exemplars of Clients' Statements Representative of Increased Self-Help Activities

There were client statements that represented all three indicators of increased self-help activities. The statements representing a perceived increased level of the ability to perform basic and instrumental activities of daily living such as grooming, dressing, bathing, ambulation, cooking, and performing household activities. Two clients described an increased ability to exercise by walking and an overall increased exercise tolerance. The statements indicating a perceived increase in socially satisfying activities were descriptive of interactions with family and friends, interactions with their NCMrs, and external social events. In the statements indicating perceived increased ability to control and manage symptom distress, clients conveyed a sense of mastery over the frequency of the symptoms and the degree to which symptoms disrupted their lives. Selected examples of these statements are presented in Boxes 26-2, 26-3, and 26-4.

Exemplars of Clients' Statements Representative of Increased Quality of Life, Increased General Self-Efficacy, and Decreased Severity of Illness

Exemplar statements indicating a perceived increase in quality of life included the clients' level of satisfac-

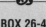

BOX 26-2

EXEMPLAR OF CLIENTS' STATEMENTS INDICATING PERCEIVED DECREASED PHYSICAL DISABILITY

"Well, [my NCMr] suggested that I walk. When I first started out I couldn't walk very far at all. You know, I was getting problems. So then [the NCMr] took me for a walk. [The NCMr] went along side me and we didn't go all the way around the park by any means. That started it, but then [the NCMr] wasn't here all the time to do it. So every night then I would go and I would try to go a little farther each night 'til I got that I could go around twice."

BOX 26-3

EXEMPLAR OF CLIENTS' STATEMENTS INDICATING INCREASED SOCIAL SATISFACTION

[Speaking about her NCMr and the benefits she gets from the visits] "Well, not only professional but socially. Cause I don't have a lot of company or a whole lot of friends. And [the NCMr] is such a friendly, as long as you're a professional person, [the NCMr] is such a friendly person, you can't help it. To enjoy [the NCMr]."

BOX 26-4

EXEMPLAR OF CLIENTS' STATEMENTS INDICATING INCREASED SYMPTOM MANAGEMENT ABILITY

[In reference to her perception of why her diabetic symptoms are more stable] "because I just, I'm just, I'm not hyper, I'm more settled. There for a while, until [my NCMr] started coming and getting me, more conscious of my blood sugar and my blood pressure. [The NCMr] brought out different subjects that made me realize I wasn't paying enough attention to my needs. And [the NCMr] would bring it out and try to tell me how to take care of myself and not let this bother me or if something health-wise bothered me, to try to get it out and work on it, you know, to see what I could do about it. But, I mean [the NCMr] brought out different things that made me realize that I wasn't doing that. I was just going through each day like a bull in a jewelry store. But [the NCMr] brought out different subjects that made me think."

tion with their present personal situations. Client statements indicating their perceived increased general self-efficacy including a perceived increased ability to adequately perform an activity and a belief that performing the activity would produce a desired result. Other exemplars included the clients' perceived decreased severity of illness including a perceived increased stability of the symptom patterns and treatment effectiveness. Selected examples of these client statements are presented in Boxes 26-5, 26-6, and 26-7.

Qualitative Exemplars of Additional Outcome Categories

The expert reviewers also identified clients' statements that represented six additional outcome categories of decreased hospital admissions, increased utilization of other health-care resources, increased monitoring of health status, increased understanding of health status, increased emotional support, and increased development of a trust relationship with the NCMr. The category of decreased hospital admissions was formed by collapsing statements that linked decreased hospital

admissions or the ability to be discharged from a long-term care facility to the intervention of an NCMr. The increased utilization of other health-care resources category was formed by collapsing statements that described NCMr actions that assisted the subjects to identify or obtain access to needed services and supplies for home use. The category of increased monitoring of health status was formed from statements that described NCMr actions related to assessment of health status and ongoing appraisal of progress, symptom stability, and treatment effectiveness. The increased understanding of health status category was formed by statements that described NCMrs' providing information about health problems, disease symptoms, and strategies for health management. The category of increased emotional support was formed by collapsing statements that described actions of the NCMrs that assisted subjects to accept their illness, reduce their stress and depression, and provided a sense of encouragement. The last category was formed by statements that indicated the clients' perceptions that they had developed a trusting relationship with their NCMrs. These statements described the association between the subject and the nurse case manager as one that exceeded their usual conceptions of the client-nurse relationship. The general themes of these statements indicated that the subjects sensed a friendship with the NCMrs and had developed feelings of affection and trust. Further, subjects described NCMr attitudes as demonstrating caring, personal involvement,

BOX 26-5

EXEMPLAR OF CLIENTS' STATEMENTS INDICATING INCREASED QUALITY OF LIFE

[In reference to her perception of how the NCMr made a difference in her life] "[my NCMr] is a pretty terrific person. And uh, I know I could never have gotten out of this without [my NCMr]. I know when [my NCMr] was coming and it was an uplift and after [my NCMr] was gone, it was 2 or 3 days before I was down and then [my NCMr] was back. Those first weeks after the hospital, I missed [my NCMr] a tremendous amount [between visits]. I don't know what people used to do when they got dumped out of the hospital and then nobody saw them. You know they go back home into the same thing that builds them up to what sent them to the hospital again, God. No [I] definitely feel, in fact I've started trying to figure out a new certain part of my life. . . . I want a job, I want to go out into the world again and I want to start a third part of my life. I've already had the first two parts. . . . I don't know, I'm trying to figure it out right now. . . . Because I have no intention sitting here arid turning into a dead old hulk. So even if it has to be volunteer work."

BOX 26-6

EXEMPLAR OF CLIENTS' STATEMENTS INDICATING INCREASED GENERAL SELF-EFFICACY

[In reference to her perception of how the NCMr made a difference in her life] "Well [my NCMr] has changed my outlook a lot. [Researcher asked, "How did the NCMr do that?"] All my life I have been a fighter. I did, I just, I gave up, I didn't care. [My NCMr] put some self-confidence back in my life."

genuine interest, and commitment. Clients also described feelings that the NCMr was as important to them as their family. Selected examples of these statements by category are presented in Box 26-8.

The findings of this qualitative analysis identifying additional outcome categories are consistent with the earlier findings of Lamb and Stempel (1991, 1994) who determined that clients viewed the NCMr as an expert who could assist in the assessment and stabilization of their physiological problems and facilitate access to needed health-care services. Further, they reported that clients viewed the NCMr as assisting them to learn improved self-care activities such as adherence

BOX 26-7

EXEMPLAR OF CLIENTS' STATEMENTS INDICATING DECREASED SEVERITY OF ILLNESS

"And my breathing is much better and my oxygen level is much, much better now. I can go short periods of time without oxygen. I have, my attitude is better toward people. I'm not as negative toward people, to criticize. I'm not as quick to criticize people as I was. My appetite is better and when I feel that I'm really getting into depression I'll get up and go some place instead of sitting, you know instead of sitting here [and] going and getting in bed."

to medication and other health-related regimens and an improved ability to recognize the signs of exacerbation of their symptoms and to seek early assistance.

The notion of the client and the NCMr forming a trusting relationship is also supported by other authors (Mound, et al., 1991; Rheaume, et al., 1994; Sowell & Meadows, 1994; Wadas, 1993; Wagner & Menke, 1992) who have commented on the nature and importance of the nurse-client relationship which develops when the nurse case manager works closely with the client across the health-care continuum. Among the important components identified were the personal quality and continuity of the nurse case manager/client relationship (Gibson et al., 1994; Mound et al., 1991; Rheaume et al., Wagner & Menke, 1992) and the formation of a partnership based on trust (Lamb & Stemple, 1991, 1994; Sowell & Meadows, 1994; Wadas, 1993).

CONCLUSION

The results of both quantitative and qualitative data analysis support the conclusion that focus of NCMr interventions practiced via the PNCM model is substantially different from that of acute care nursing. Central to this type of advanced nursing practice is the formation of a therapeutic nurse-client relationship from which mutually derived client outcomes emerge. The central aim of these outcomes is directed toward the restoration and maintenance of the clients' self-care abilities and the promotion of the most maximally possible state of health. The NCMr serves as the clients' advocate, resource manager, educator, monitor of ongoing health status, and as a source for emotional support and health information. Some of the cost benefits that were derived from the implementation of the PNCM model with high-risk chronically ill adults were realized because of the resultant client care outcomes of the experience. Clients reported increased

BOX 26-8
ADDITIONAL OUTCOME CATEGORIES

Decreased Hospital Admissions

". . . Also, where would I have been if it would not been for [my NCMr]? You know, I think about that." [Researcher asked, "What did you conclude?"] "That I would have been right back in the hospital , you know two or three times. Just not knowing, just not, you know with the chronic thing like this of course, my mind is slipping, I think it's the beginning of Alzheimer's. I'm pretty sure that I would be back in the hospital and giving me those high doses of steroids."

Increased Utilization of Other Health Care Resources

[In reference to the NCMr arranging for personal care, Meals on Wheels and house cleaning services] ". . . But [my NCMr] got me into that [community service for the homebound] organization. So, [my NCMr] got me my meals, and then [my NCMr] got me on personal care and also an hour and a half cleaning the house. So, how can you beat that?. . . That's what [my NCMr] has done for me. [My NCMr] is looking into finding a handicapped apartment where it might be less expensive. This one is $290.00 a month. And I only draw $487.00 Social Security. So when you $290.00 out of that, it don't do very far."

Increased Monitoring of Health Status

"Well, she [NCMr] came out here and took my blood pressure and weight, talks to me, finds out how I was doing at that time. [If my NCMr] didn't like what I was doing of [if] I didn't think that I was doing what I should. Well, [my NCMr would] call the doctor for me. . . [my NCMr] kept me in touch with the doctor, nearly every time [my NCMr] been here."

Increased Understanding of Health Status

[In reference to how the NCMr has made a difference in her ability to control symptoms]. "Well it directed my feelings, because I had no knowledge of anything, Okay? Medically or what was wrong with me or anything about it. It directed the right channels. I would ask questions and [my NCMr] would answer me. And [my NCMr] would watch me and we would talk and we would have marvelous conversations and it would enlighten me in what was happening to me."

Increased Emotional Support

". . . Of course I had talked to [my NCMr] about this son of mine. . . . How he was a constant burden to me, you know. And [my NCMr] counseled me on that and I took a 75 degree turn in dealing with my son. So I had a talk with him and my son said, ". . . Well what is [your NCMr] doing for you? Well, I said I don't know what [my NCMr] will do, right now [my NCMr] is my sole support in helping me to overcome my fears of having the chronic disease."

Increased Development of a Trust Relationship

". . . But I feel that [my NCMr] made a difference in my life. Knowing [my NCMr] has made a difference. You know, we have a relationship and, I know it's patient and client and a nurse, but there is a friendship there too. . . . "It's not cold blooded, just come in and do you and go out just like you were a number. I'm a human being to [my NCMr]. And [my NCMr] treats me that way. Even if I was old as Methussie [my NCMr] still treats me like a human being. But [my NCMr] is so caring that I just look forward to [my NCMr] coming, as much as any of my family.

---

stability in symptom distress and improved symptom management. They reported a lessening of their severity of illness and physical disability. These factors seem to be associated with decreased recidivism and decreased acuity and length of stay, if hospital admission were necessary, based on case-managed clients reported in studies concerned with fiscal outcomes (Gibson, et al., 1994; Hospital Reduces Admissions, 1992; Rogers et al., 1991).

A major challenge facing nursing professionals during this current reactive economic climate is to develop innovative clinical nursing intervention strategies which are cost sensitive and outcome efficacious. Current cost-effectiveness strategies, such as restraints on institutional length of stay and constrictions on the range of reimbursement for health-care services have altered the ability to provide holistic nursing care for chronically ill persons. This in turn has fostered the evolution of the role of the nurse case manager (NCMr) and the development of nurse case management (NCM) models which are cost effective, guided by client outcomes, and population specific. Most research studies have focused on the more tangible outcomes of NCM related to cost effectiveness, but limited research has explored the capacity of NCM interventions to promote positive changes in quality of care outcomes.

This study demonstrated that the less tangible, and often less valued, educative and supportive intervention strategies provided by NCMrs made an important difference in the self-care outcomes in clients who were chronically ill. It is conceivable that the focus of NCMr interventions on assessment-monitoring and teaching-informing increased the subjects' compliance with the therapeutic regimen, promoted the early identification and treatment of recurrent disease exacerbation, and assisted the subjects to understand and more effectively manage their chronic illnesses. Still, the relationships between fiscal results and quality care outcomes need further examination.

Paramount to the improvement in the client's self-care outcomes is the development of a therapeutic NCMr-client relationship based on trust and mutual respect. Further exploration of the antecedent events and qualities of the client-NCMr interaction which foster and promote the development of the trusting relationship is warranted.

Finally, there is justification to explore the use of this model with other fragile and high-risk populations such as children and young to middle adults with progressive, high-maintenance conditions. In the future, as NCMr interventions are refined a clearer understanding of both the outcomes and processes of NCMr practice via the PNCM model should emerge.

REFERENCES

American Nurses Association. (1988). *Nursing case management.* (Publication No. NS-32), Kansas City, MO: Author.

Bower, K. A. (1992). *Case management by nurses.* Kansas City, MO: American Nurses Publishing.

Brockopp, D. Y., Porter, M., Kinnaird, S., & Silberman, S. (1992). Fiscal and clinical evaluation of patient care: a case management model for the future. *Journal of Nursing Administration, 22* (9), 23-27.

Clough, J., & Thomas, K., (1992). Health promotion/illness prevention through wellness clinics and nursing case management. *Arizona Nurse, 45* (3), 1.

Cohen, E. L., & Cesta, T. G. (1993). *Nursing case management: from concept to evaluation.* St Louis: Mosby.

Ethridge, P. (1991). A nursing HMO: Carondelet St. Mary's experience. *Nursing Management, 22* (7), 22-27.

Ethridge, P., & Lamb, G. (1989). Professional nursing case management improves quality, access and costs. *Nursing Management, 20* (3), 30-35.

Fralic, M. F. (1992). The nurse case manager: Focus, selection, preparation and measurement. *Journal of Nursing Administration, 22* (11), 13-14, 46.

Gibson, S. J., Martin, S. M., Johnson, M. B., Blue, R., & Miller, D. S. (1994). CNS-directed case management: cost and quality in harmony. *Journal of Nursing Administration, 24* (6), 45-51.

Hicks, L., Stallmeyer, J., & Coleman, J. R. (1992). Nursing challenges in managed care. *Nursing Economics, 10,* 265-275.

Hinton-Walker, P. (1993). Care of the chronically ill: paradigm shifts and directions for the future. *Holistic Nursing Practice, 8* (1), 56-66.

Hospital reduces admissions, saves half a million dollars with community-based CM. (1992). *Case Management Advisor, 3,* 119-121.

Lamb, G. S. (1992). [Nursing case management satisfaction survey]. Unpublished raw data.

Lamb, G. S., Stempel, J. E. (1991, October). *Nursing case management: the patient's experience.* Paper presented at the meeting of the American Nurses' Association Council of Nurse

Researchers' International Nursing Research Conference, Los Angeles, CA.

Lamb, G. S., & Stempel, J. E. (1994). Nurse case management from the client's view: growing as insider-expert. *Nursing Outlook, 42* (1), 7-13.

Lynn-McHale, D. J., Fitzpatrick, E. R., & Shaffer, R. B. (1993). Case management: development of a model. *Clinical Nurse Specialist, 7,* 299-307.

Michaels, C. (1992). Carondelet St. Mary's experience. *Nursing Clinics of North America, 27,* 77-85.

Mound, B., Gyulay, R., Khan, P., & Goering, P. (1991). The expended role of nurse case managers. *Journal of Psychosocial Nursing, 29* (6), 18-22.

Newman, M. A., Lamb, G. S., & Michaels, C. (1991) Nurse case management: the coming together of theory and practice. *Nursing and Health Care, 12,* 404-408.

Olivas, G. S., Del Togno-Armanasco, V., Erickson, J. R., & Harter, S. (1989a). Case management: a bottom-line care delivery model Part I: the concept. *Journal of Nursing Administration, 19* (11), 16-20.

Olivas, G. S., Del Togno-Armanasco, V., Erickson, J. R., & Harter, S. (1989b). Case management: a bottom-line care delivery model Part II: adaption of the model. *Journal of Nursing Administration, 19* (12), 12-17.

Pegels, C. C. (1988). *Health care and the older citizen economic, demographic and financial aspects.* Rockville, MD: Aspen.

Petryshen, P. R., & Petryshen, P. M. (1992). The case management model: an innovative approach to delivery of patient care. *Journal of Advanced Nursing, 17,* 1188-1194.

Rheaume, A., Frisch, S., Smith, A., & Kennedy, C. (1994). Case management and nursing practice. *Journal of Nursing Administration, 24* (3), 30-36.

Rogers, M., Riordan, J., & Swindle, D. (1991). Community-based nursing case management pays off. *Nursing Management, 22* (3), 30-34.

Rusch, S. (1986). Continuity of care: from hospital unit to home. *Nursing Management, 17* (12), 38-41.

Sherman, J. J., & Johnson P. K. (1994). CNS as unit-based case manager. *Clinical Nurse Specialist, 8,* 76-80.

Sowell, R. L., & Meadows, T. M. (1994). An integrated case management model: developing standards, evaluation, and outcome criteria. *Nursing Administration Quarterly, 18* (2), 53-64.

Strumpf, N. E., & Knibbe, K. K. (1990). Long-term care, fulfilling promises to the elderly. In J. C. McCloskey & H. K. Grace (Eds.). *Current issues in nursing* (pp. 215-225). St Louis: Mosby.

Tahan, H. (1993). The nurse case manager in acute care settings. *Journal of Nursing Administration, 23* (10), 53-61.

Trinidad, E. A. (1993). Case management: a model of CNS practice. *Clinical Nurse Specialist, 7,* 221-223.

Wadas, T. M. (1993). Case management and caring behavior. *Nursing Management, 24* (9), 40-46.

Wagner, J. D., & Menke, E. M. (1992). Case management of homeless families. *Clinical Nurse Specialist, 6,* 65-71.

Watson, P. M., Lower, M. S., Wells, S. M., Farrah, S. J., & Jarrell, C. (1991). Discovering what nurses do and what it costs. *Nursing Management, 22* (5), 38-45.

Weyant, J. (1991, February). *St. Joseph Medical Center in Wichita, community-based nurse case management department report.* Paper presented at the meeting of third annual Nurse Case Management Exchange, Tucson, AZ.

Zander, K. (1988). Nursing case management: strategic management of cost and quality outcomes. *Journal of Nursing Administration, 18* (5), 23-29.

Zander, K. (1990a) Case management: a golden opportunity for whom? In J. C. McCloskey & H. K. Grace (Eds.). *Current Issues in Nursing,* 3rd ed. (pp. 199-204). St Louis: Mosby.

Zander, K. (1990b). Differentiating managed care and case management. *Definition, 5* (2), 1-2.

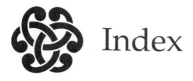

Index

Page numbers followed by (b) indicate a box. Page numbers followed by (f) indicate a figure. Page numbers followed by (t) indicate a table.

A

AACN, 33
Academia, involvement of in health-care redesign, 43-47
Academic health centers, 43-44; *see also* academic nursing centers
Academic institutions, inflexibility and, 46
Academic nursing centers, 68-76, 80; *see also* academic health centers
Accessibility to care, 29-30, 83, 163, 166
Accountability, 17, 35, 229
ACHIS, 76
Acute episode tool, clinical pathways as, 224-32
Adjustments, in pathway, 98, 100(f)
Administrative support, lack of, 183-84
Administrators, perspective of, 182
Advanced practice nurses, individual, accountability and, 17
Advanced practice nurses (APN), 10-20
   business relationships and, 17
   case management and, 56-62, 185
   core curriculum components for, 55-62
   education and preparation for, 38
   evolution of, 34
   goal of, 16
   new realities for, 17-18
   primary care and, 14-15
   quality of care and, 38
   role of, 7-8, 223-24
   technical skills of, 61(b)
Advanced primary caregiver, preparation of, 18
Advantages to implementation, 215, 216
Advocacy role, 31, 189, 192, 200
Age, as indicator of risk, 169
Agency mission, 190, 191(f)
AIDS, The Denver Nursing Education Project and, 63-67
American Association of Colleges of Nursing (AACN), 33
American Nurses Association (ANA), 33
American Organization of Nurse Executives (AONE), 33
ANA, 33
Analysis
   of interview data, 264-67
   qualitative, 265-68
   statistical, of quantitative data, 262-64
AONE, 33
Appraisal, of risk, 170
Assertiveness of nurse, primary-care services and, 16-17

B

Assessment
   of existing case management model, 216-17
   in MS study, 127
   summary, care pathway implementation and, 98, 99(f)
Associate nurse role, 223
Automated Community Health Information System (ACHIS), 76-78

Barriers, academia and, 45-46
Behavior of client
   change, readiness and, 126, 127
   illness and, 29
Benefit documentation, 188
Biomedical paradigm, eclipse of, as trend, 30
Block nurses, 22-24
Bonding, 106
Boyte, Harry, 22
Broker role, 189, 192, 201
Business relationships, advanced practice nurses and, 17

C

Capitation, 112, 247, 248
Care
   continuum of, 12-17, 19, 107
      nursing resource needs in, 33
   coordination of, 161, 163-67, 183
   delivery of, 8-9
   evaluation of, 16
   management of, 164(b), 92-94, 163-64
   orientations towards, 94
Care continuum, 107, 110
Care pathways, 96-102, 110
Career strategies, planning, 32
Caregiver role, 11, 189, 192, 198
Caring
   the art of nursing and, 106-7
   definition, 113
   as innovative delivery system, 105-16
   nursing process and, 121
Carondelet Community Health Services (Arizona), 82
   sample contract proposal, 249-56
Case associates, 213-18
Case management, 13-14, 21-23, 48-54
   nursing, 31, 56
   purpose, services and description of, 125
   types of, 203

Case manager, job description of, 217(b)
Case studies
   analysis of client base, 204
   at Silver Spring Community Nursing Center, 75
   client choices, community nurse case management and, 136
   collaboration of multiple case managers, 206
   collaboration with rural facility, 239
   collaborative outcomes, 109
   emergency department, frequent user of, 137
   environmental needs, addressing, 137
   fragmented delivery system, 109
   in integrated continuum of care, 103
   lack of integration of services, 89
   long-term care, 154
   Lutheran General Health System, 94-103
   Lutheran Health Care Network, 170-80
   mastectomy home care pathway, 235
   MS exacerbation, 127
   nurse case management and, 108
   political strategies, 23-27
   premature neonate, 237
   spouse of MS client, 130
   student nurse view, of community nurse case management, 138
   wellness promotion, in senior center, 138
CCN, 90
Change
   academia and, 46
   establishing a framework for, 31-33
   social, 31-32
   strategies for, 33-37
Change theory, 58
Chief Financial Officers, perspective of, 182
Child populations, risk identification in, 172-73
Chronic care, 87-104
Chronic care network (CCN), 90
Chronic complex illness model, 55
Chronically ill populations, 166-67
Churches, parish nurses and, 145-46
City support, for LAH/BNP, 24
Classification/intervention scheme, Omaha System, 77
Client
   care coordination, 164(b)
   as expert, 125, 128
   involvement, in clinical pathways, 228-29
   learning experiences, in curriculum design, 51-52

Client—cont'd
  life management skills, primary care
      provider and, 16
  outcomes, 71, 257-68
      responsibility for, 125
  perspective, 132
  populations, 163-65
  record, individual, Automated
      Community Health Information
      System and, 77
  report, 77, 78(t)
  satisfaction, 65, 112-13, 242-43
  as seen in life context, 18
  selection, 236
  transition through system, 28
Client-centered approach, 49
Client-nurse partnership, theory of, 119-23
Client-nurse relationship, 121
Climate creation, 56-57
Clinical database, Automated Community
    Health Information System, 76
Clinical documentation systems, 71-72,
    76-79
Clinical laboratories as teaching site, 72, 76
Clinical nurse specialists, 223
Clinical outcomes, clinical pathways
    and, 229
Clinical pathways as acute episode tool,
    224-32
Clinical reasoning process, 165
Collaboration, 50, 108, 223
  interdisciplinary, clinical pathways
      and, 228
  learning experiences in curriculum
      design, 52
  planning and management, need for, 94
  quality outcomes and, 107
Collaboration Project, Interregional
    Cardiovascular, 114(b)
Colleagues, nursing, 34
Committee for development of common
    protocols, 96
Common Wealth: A return to citizen politics, 22
Communication
  between providers, 93
  implementation of case management
      and, 187
  in pathways, importance of, 101
  strategies for, 213
  tool, care pathway implementation and,
      98, 99(f)
Communities, as clients, 24
Community
  health services in, 18
  importance of, in LAH/BNP, 24-25
Community centers, 85
Community health care
  nurses and, 23
  as thrust in new environment, 7
Community health practice, determinants
    of, 8
Community meetings, public relations
    and, 26
Community nurse case management,
    outcomes of, 138(b)
Community Nursing Center (CNC)
    model, 73
Community nursing centers, 69-70, 81-86
Community-based case management, 22
Community-based health-care programs,
    7(b)

Community-based nursing intervention
    models, 73
Community-based practice environment,
    5-6
Community-based supportive services,
    chronic illness and, 90
Competency programs, 190, 192, 197-201
Compliance, care pathways and, 102
Computerized clinical documentation
    systems, 71-72, 76-79
Conditions, type and number of, as
    indicator of risk, 169
Consciousness, theory of health and, 121
Consumer confidence, 39
Consumer involvement, 4
Continuing Care Pathways (CCP), 96, 97(t)
Continuing education, 45
Continuity of care, 232
Continuity of case manager-client
    relationship, 261
Continuum
  of care, 12-17, 19, 107
  case managers and, 184-85
  chronic care and, 87-104
  definition of, 87
  development of case management on, 236
  development of common protocols on, 96
  high-risk clients and, 232
  information system features and, 92(b)
  nursing resource needs in, 33
  objectives of, 236
  outcomes of, 238, 240-42
  role of nurse in, 15, 16
  standardization of care management
      and, 94
  team approach in managing, 15-16
  see also pathways
Continuum teams, in Lutheran General
    Health System, 103(b)
Continuum-based case management, 113,
    163-64
Contract proposal, sample, 249-56
Control, of variables, 13
Cooperation, 50
Coordination
  of care, 12-17, 49-50, 89
  of learning experiences in curriculum
      design, 52
  of services, 68-69
Coordinator role, 189, 192, 199
Cost-containment methods, 257
Cost-effectiveness
  in care, 23, 53
  community nursing centers and, 83
  as mandate, 112
  nursing care partnerships and, 65
  patient services and, 17
Costs
  control of, 77-78
  documentation of, 188
  excessive, as force driving change, 4
  issues of, 162-63
  management of, 166-67
  of nursing care, 11
  nursing practice and, 120
  outcomes, 112-13
  payment and, in new environment, 5
  reduction of, through case management,
      171
  savings, 154-55
  unnecessary, 12

Costs—cont'd
  vs quality, in new environment, 8
  see also resources
Counselor, parish nurse as health, 142
County support, for LAH/BNP, 24
Crisis intervention, 245-46
Critical paths, 163, 164(b)
Cross-training, of primary nurses, for
    home care pathway, 232
Curriculum
  altering for emerging roles, 16
  at professional schools, 35
  challenge to create ideal, 55
  components, for advanced practice
      nurses, 55-62
  design, values and, 51
  HIV/AIDS modular, at Denver Nursing
      Project in Human Caring, 65-67
  integration of case management into,
      50-53
  integration of key elements into, 53
  nursing case management in, 48-54
  teaching case management and, 53

D

Data
  analysis of interview, 264-67
  categories, selected, in Automated
      Community Health Information
      System, 77(t)
  collection, 214
  collection tools, development of, 153
  nursing, clinical documentation systems
      and, 71
Database, Automated Community Health
    Information System, 76
Delivery systems, building, 35
Deming philosophy of quality
    improvement, 60
Demonstration of case management, 188
Demonstration programs, acute and
    long-term care, 89-90
Demonstration projects, Silver Spring
    Community Nursing Center (SS
    CNC), 73
Denver Nursing Project in Human Caring,
    63-67
Design and implementation of case
    management, 181-88
Differentiated nursing practice, 222-44
Disciplines, values exploration across,
    50-51
Discounted fee for service, 246-47
Dissemination of knowledge, 60-61
District nurse, 24
Documentation
  implementation of care pathways and,
      98, 101(f)
  implementation of case management
      and, 188
  streamlined, clinical pathways and, 228
  systems, clinical, 71
Downsizing, nurses and, 13

E

"Economic and Quality of Care Issues with
    Implications on Scopes of Practice—
    Physicians and Nurses," 34
Economics, 59-60

Education, 72
    academia and, 44-45
    academic nursing centers and, 72-73
    case manager skills and, 219-20
    continuing, 45
    health, 35
    implementation of case management
        and, 187, 213
    in development of case manager, 192-94
    integration of key elements into, 53
    levels, at Denver Nursing Project in
        Human Caring, 64
    of nurse case managers, 258-59
    of nurses, 55-62
    nursing, approach to, 53
    nursing care partnership and, 65
    nursing case management and, 76
    of primary nurses, for home care
        pathway, 232
    reform of system of, 48-49
    requirements of, 72, 85, 234-35
    system, deconstruction of, 30-31
Educator, parish nurse as health, 142
Effective political action: Prescription for
    nurses, 23
Elected officials, 24, 25
Emerging health-care system, 5-6
Employment, 4, 32
Environment, new practice, 3-9
Episode-based case management, 163-64
Ethics and ideals, 58-59
Ethnic diversity, as trend, 29
Evaluation
    implementation of care pathways and,
        98, 101(f)
    of nurse case management, 215-16
    of risk, 170
Evolution, 64-65
    academia and, 46
    of case manager, 194, 195(f), 196(b)
Exacerbation triggers, 125-26
Expectations, higher, 15-17

F

Factoring, 213
Faith communities, nursing and, 140-48
Families of MS clients, 130-31
Family
    block nurse case management and, 22
    involvement, in clinical pathways,
        228-29
    satisfaction, 242-43
Fear, as inner city issue, 144-45
Fee for service, discounted, 246-47
Feedback, in integrated delivery system,
    58
Finance management, integrated, chronic
    care and, 90-91
Financial barriers, 183
Financing
    health care, 32
    integration of, 93
    population-based health care and, 83
Fiscal outcomes
    clinical pathways and, 229
    of professional nurse case management
        model, 259-60
Foundations, public relations and, 26
Framework, for change, establishing,
    31-33

Freedom
    the art of nursing and, 106, 107
    as innovative delivery system, 105-16
Frequency, of activities, 262
Funding, 73
    for community nursing centers, 82
    as obstacle, 135
    public relations and, 26

G

Geriatric issues, managing, 96
Global health agenda, 33
Goals
    of case management, 163
    in development of marketing plan,
        207-8, 210
Goldwater & Lloyd-Zusy, 23
Grass roots efforts, 21-27

H

Health
    determinants of, 44
    education, 35
    as focus of delivery system, 5
    as focus of health plan, 16
    perceived, as indicator of risk, 169
    redefinition of, 33, 36
Health agenda, national and global, 33
Health care
    accessing, in MS study, 128
    delivery model, Silver Spring
        Community Nursing Center, 74-75
    financing, 32
    labor force, 21st century, 32
    poor access to, 79
    programs, community-based, 7(b)
    providers, recent changes by, 5
    redesign, academia's involvement in,
        43-47
    reform, 3
    resources, effective and efficient use of, 78
    services, changes in move to primary
        care, 12-13
    spending, 112
    transformation, 19
        nursing's response to, 28-39
        trends and implications for, 29-31
Health-care system
    deconstruction of, 30-31
    emerging, characteristics of, 6(b)
    reconstruction of, 31
Health maintenance organization (HMO),
    59
Health model, 105-6
Health Needs Assessment tool, 172, 175-77
Health professionals
    decreased demand for, 30
    future roles and competencies, 44-45
Health promotion, at Silver Spring
    Neighborhood Center, 74
Health services, 18, 35
Health-systems change, complexity of, 4-5
High Risk Maternal Case Management
    Referral Form tool, 173, 178
High-risk clients, 84, 232
High-risk specialists, nurse case managers
    as, 84-85
HIV/AIDS, The Denver Nursing
    Education Project and, 63-67

HIV/AIDS education program, Living
    with HIV, 65
HMO, 59
Holism, as new paradigm, 4
Holistic focus of providers, 35
Holistic nursing model, 125
Holistic values, 36
Home care
    pathway, 232
    program, 247-48
Homelessness, church programs and, 145
Hospice model, 107
Hospital
    downsizing, nurses and, 11
    in rural community, 211-21
    services
        avoidance of, 17
        nurses and, 11
Hospital-based case management, 110-12,
    203
Hospitalization, home care pathways and,
    229, 232
Hospitals, recent changes by, 5
Human caring, Jean Watson's theory of, 63
Human resource management inequities,
    184-85
Human systems theory, 56, 58

I

Ideals and ethics, 58-59; see also values
Illness, as core of health services, 12
Illness service, in transition to primary
    care environment, 13
Immigrants, as inner city issue, 144
Implementation of case management, 110,
    150-54, 188, 212-14, 238
    at long-term care facility, 149-58
    design and, 181-88
    obstacles to, 135-36
Implications and trends, health-care
    transformation and, 29-31
Income distribution, 31
Independent case management, 203
Independent nursing services, 64
Independent Practice Association (IPA),
    59-60
Information, integration of, 93
Information systems
    integrated
        chronic care and, 91-92
        key to pathway growth and
            expansion, 102
    management, 72
        Automated Community Health
            Information System, 76-78
    for nursing practice and research, 76-79
    support, 186-87
Inner-city, parish nurses and, 144-47
Insurance companies, recent changes by, 5
Insurance-based case management, 203
Integrated care network, 85
Integrated clinical pathway (ICP), 224
Integrated delivery system, 56
Integrated information system, 102
Integrating services across continuum,
    chronic care and, 87-104
Integration
    keys to, 89-94
    lack of, 96
    of life and health services, 18

Integration—cont'd
   of linkages and relationships, 18, 19
   with service providers, 17
Intensity of activities, 262
Interdependence, in health care, 34
Interdisciplinary education, 52
Interdisciplinary perspective, values and
   curriculum in, 51
"Intermediate technology," 32-33
Internal analysis, in development of
   marketing plan, 206-7, 209
Interregional Cardiovascular
   Collaboration Project, 114(b)
Intervention models, community-based
   nursing, 73
Intervention strategies, 69, 70-71
Interventions
   case managers and, 85
   clients with MS, 131
   intensity and frequency, 262
Interview data, analysis of, 264-67
IPA, 59-60
Isolation, in MS study, 129-30

J

Job description
   case associate, 218(b)
   case manager, 217(b)
Jobs, in health care, 4
Joint Commission on Accreditation of
   Hospitals, 135-36

K

Key elements of case management, 48-54
Knowledge
   in Deming philosophy, 60
   dissemination of, 60-61

L

LAH/BNP, 22-27
Laws, implementation of, 26
Layoffs, workplace reconfiguration and, 11
Leadership, 58
   as component of nursing case
      management, 58
   intervention, nursing, 8-9
   nursing, 36-37, 110, 113
   in reform, 49
Learning experiences, development of,
   51-53
"Learning society," 32
Legal system, deconstruction of, 30-31
Lessons, learned by parish nurses, 146-47
Life management skills, of client, primary
   care provider and, 16
Linkages and relationships, integration of,
   18-19
Living at Home/Block Nurse Program
   (LAH/BNP), 22-27
Living with HIV educational program,
   65-67
Lobbying, 26-27
Loeb Center, 70
Long-term care, 149-58
LPN's, as case managers, 151, 152
Lutheran General Health System,
   continuing care at, 94-103

Lutheran Health Care Network, case
   study of, 170-80

M

Managed care
   community nursing centers and, 82
   economics and, 59-60
   environment, 11
Management information systems, 72, 76-78
Market audit, in development of
   marketing plan, 204-6, 209
Marketing plan
   development of, 207, 210
   for nurse case management services,
      203-10
Marketing of services, 202-8
Markets, expanded, multinationality and,
   29
Maternal populations, risk identification
   in, 172-73
Mediating systems, deconstruction of,
   30-31
Medical approaches to health service, 14
Medical dominance, 52
Medical education, traditional model of, 29
Medical model
   old, described, 12
   paradigm and, 3-4
Medically supportive nursing services, 64
Medicare Hospice Election, 107
Medications, number and type of, as
   indicator of risk, 169
Mental health population, 115(b)
Merger of facilities, 215
Mission statement in development of
   marketing plan, 203, 209
Mobility, adapting to MS, 130
Model and process, development of, 108-9
Modeling, client health and, 106
Models
   case management, 34
      cooperation and, 34
      hospital-based, 110-12
      revision of redefined, 220-21
   chronic complex illness, 55
   community health, 82
   Community Nursing Center (CNC), 73
   community nursing centers, 81-82, 85
   community-based nursing intervention,
      73
   development of community-based
      nursing intervention, 73
   holistic nursing, 125
   hospice, 107
   hospital-based case management, 110-12
   nurse case management, redefinition of,
      216-21
   nursing, community nurse case
      management, 134
   outreach, 82
   parish nursing, 140-48
   pathway, 94-103
   professional nurse case management,
      258-68
   professional nursing practice, 120
   Silver Spring Community Nursing
      Center, 74-75
   Sioux Valley Hospital, 223-43
   transition from illness to health, 105-6

Models of care, nursing, 70
Models of health-care delivery, team
   based, 70
MS clients, challenges of, 131
Multiculturalism, as trend, 29-30
Multinationality, as trend, 29-30
Multiple Sclerosis (MS) research study,
   126-32

N

National Chronic Care Consortium
   (NCCC), 96
National health agenda, 33
National League for Nursing (NLN), 33
Network, case management, 164-65
Night shift nurses, 153-54
Nightingale, Florence, 113
NLN, 33
Nurse assertiveness, primary-care services
   and, 16-17
Nurse managed centers; see nursing centers
Nurse manager as case manager, 151, 152
Nurse practitioners, 223
Nurse satisfaction, 212-13
Nurse-client partnership, theory of, 119-23
Nurse-client relationship, 121
Nurses
   new roles for, 6-9
   perspective of, case management and, 182
Nursing, redefinition of, 33-34
Nursing assistants, 153
Nursing care partnerships, 64-65
Nursing case management, 31, 56
Nursing centers, 69-70
   academic, challenges for, 80
   community, case management in, 81-86
Nursing clinics; see nursing centers
Nursing HMO, capitation and, 247-48
Nursing homes, 150
Nursing information systems, 76-80
Nursing leadership, 36-37, 49
Nursing model, community nurse case
   management and, 134
Nursing models of care, 70
Nursing organizations; see AACN; ANA;
   AONE; NLN; nursing centers
Nursing practice
   cost and, 120
   differentiated, 222-44
   evolution of, 214-15
   general facts about, 38
   model of professional, 120
Nursing process, nonoperational, 211-12
Nursing resources, changes required in
   use of, 15
Nursing services, 64
Nursing theory, 106, 119
Nursing's Agenda for Health Care
   Reform, 7

O

Objectives, 236
Obligations, of nurse, 18
Obstacles to implementation, 135, 183-88,
   215
Older Americans Act, 26-27
Omaha System, classification/intervention
   scheme, 69, 77

Organizational support of case managers, 194
Orientation to case manager role, 189
Outcome orientation
    as element of case management, 50
    learning experiences, in curriculum design, 52
    as mandate, 112
Outcomes
    of case management on continuum, 238, 240-42
    client
        of nurse case manager interventions, 261
        responsibilities, 125
        as result of intervention, 257-68
    clinical and fiscal, clinical pathways and, 229
    of community nurse case management, 136-39
    cost and quality, 112-13
    desired, in implementation, 216
    in development of marketing plan, 208, 210
    past, in community nursing centers, 82
    quality, 113
    research, 71
Outreach models, 82

P

Paradigm
    eclipse of biomedical, as trend, 30
    nursing, 120
    nursing vs medical, 119
    shift, 3-4
    shifting, needed changes and, 55-56
Parish nursing, 140-48
Partners, nursing, 34
Partnerships, 124-32, 260-66
    churches and health-care system, 146
    nursing care, 64-65
    plan of care reflecting, 126
Pathologies, type and number of, as indicator of risk, 169
Pathways
    care, implementation of, 96-102
    Continuing Care, at Lutheran General Health System, 96, 97(t), 98(t)
Patient; see client
Patriarchal influence, biomedical paradigm and, 30
Pattern, health as expression of, 120
Pattern recognition, 121-22
Payment and costs in new environment, 5
Payment environment, capitated, 11
Payment sources, in community nursing centers, 82
Pediatric Case Management Referral Form tool, 173, 180
Penal system, deconstruction of, 30-31
Per-diem reimbursement, 247
Perspectives of key players, 182-83
Philosophy, 75, 190, 191(f)
Physician satisfaction, 243
Physician-based case management, 203
Physicians
    community nurse case management and, 135

Physicians—cont'd
    perspective of, 182
    specialty, 12
Pilot project, community nurse case management and, 134-35
Plan of action
    development of, 217-19
    implementation of, 219-20
Planning process, clinical pathways and, 224, 228
Point-of-service structures, control and, 14
Policy development, 214
Political activism, nurses and, 6-7
Political process, nurse involvement in, 21-27
Political strategies, case study, 23-27
Population
    older adult, 21-23
    widely spread, as obstacle, 135
Population-based health care, financing of, 83
Population needs, development of case managers and, 190, 191(f)
Power structure, mediating systems and, 31
PPO, 60
Practice
    academia and, 45
    differentiated nursing, 222-44
    environment
        community-based, 5-6
        new, 3-9
    theory guiding, 120-21
Practitioners; see advanced practice nurses
Preferred Provider Organization (PPO), 60
Prenatal Health Assessment tool, 173, 179
Preventive care, primary, 30
Previous service utilization, as indicator of risk, 168-69
Primary block nurses; see block nurses
Primary care, 14-15
Primary care nurse, goal of, 16
Primary care providers, 10-20
Primary-care services, nurse assertiveness and, 16-17
Primary-care systems, changes in health care services and, 12-13
Primary caregiver, advanced, preparation of, 18
Primary health services, move toward, 11
Primary nurse role, 223
Primary Nursing Delivery System, 110
Primary nursing practice, preparation for, 18-19
Primary point of care, provider and, 12
Primary preventive care, 30
Primary services, resources and, 16
Principles, 163
Privatization, era of, 31
Process of interventions, 261
Professional accountability, clinical pathways and, 229
Professional associations, 37
Professional nurse case management (PNCM) model, 258-68
Professional nursing practice, model of, 120
Professional practice, evolution of, 214-15
Professional socialization, 35-36
Program, parish nurse, 141-48
Program management, 164(b)

Providers
    holistic focus, 35
    as managers of pathway, 101
    primary point of care and, 12
Psychology, knowledge of, in Deming philosophy, 60
Public, health practices of, 34
Public health, public policy and, 35
Public policy
    education and, 72-73
    nurses and, 6-7, 8
    public health and, 35
    Silver Spring Community Nursing Center success and, 79-80
Public relations, importance of good, 25-26

Q

Qualifications, 258-59
Qualitative analysis, activities, 265-68
Qualitative outcomes, 137, 139
Quality
    case management contribution to, 165-66
    as effect of change, 8
Quality care, 161-62
Quality of care issues, in reformed health-care system, 44
Quality of case manager-client relationship, 261
Quality, cost, and access imperatives, 161-67
Quality improvement, continuous, 60, 150
Quality of life, 154
Quality outcomes, 112-13
Quantitative data, statistical analysis of activities, 262-64

R

Rationale for implementing, 212
Readiness, behavioral change and, 126, 127, 131-32
Reasoning process, clinical, 165
Reconstruction of health-care system, 31
Redefinition of nurse case management model, 216-21
Referrals, parish nurses and, 142
Reform, health-care, 3
Refugees as inner-city issue, 144
Regulation, increased, multinationality and, 29-30
Reimbursement, 39
    capitation, 112
    for community nursing centers, 82
    influence on nurse case management, 245-56
Relationships
    building, 187-88, 260-66
    with elected officials, 24, 25
    linking and integrating services, 18, 19
Research, 60-61
    academia and, 45
    academic nursing centers and, 71-72
    case management issues and, 76
    as component of nursing case management, 60-61
    as related to interventions, 76

Research database, Automated Community
        Health Information System, 76
Resource efficiency, 50, 53
Resources
    limited, research by academia and, 45
    linkage, 18
    management of, 164(b)
    needs, in development of marketing
        plan, 207, 210
    parish nurses and, 142
    primary services and, 16
    shared, 45
Responsibilities, nursing, in restructuring
        effort, 33
Results, initial, 134-35
Retraining, for noninstitutional practice, 13
Revenue protection, 245-46
Risk identification, 168-80
Risk-adjusted capitated demonstration
        project, 248
Roles
    advanced practice nurse, 223-24
    advocacy, of nursing, 31
    associate nurse, 223
    of case manager, 236, 238
    clarification, case managers and, 185
    development of, 189, 258
    integration of, 12
    new
        for nurses, 6-9
        in primary-care environment, 13,
            14(b)
    of nurse in continuum of care, 15, 16
    nursing, in restructuring effort, 33
    of parish nurse, 142-44
    of primary nurse, 223
Rural community, 133-39, 211-21

S

Satisfaction, 242-43
    of families and nurses, 154
Schools, professional curriculum at, 35
Screening, for risk, 170
Self-assessments, health, as risk
        identification method, 170
Self-care in new paradigm, 4
Self-discovery, academia and, 47
Self-help groups, churches and, 140-41
Self-reliance in new paradigm, 4
Self-responsibility in new paradigm, 4
Service, goal of, 14
Service mobility, 17
Service population of Silver Spring
        Community Nursing Center, 74
Service providers, integration with, 17
Services
    in continuum of care, 88(b)
    coordination of, 68-69
    health, 35
    lack of integration of, chronic illness
        and, 89
Shared governance, 214, 224
Shared resources, 45
Sharing of client information, 91
Silver Spring Community Nursing Center,
        73-80
Silver Spring Community Nursing Center
        (SS CNC), 73-80

Silver Spring Neighborhood Center (SS
        NC), 74
Sioux Valley Hospital model, 223-43
Sites for teaching, 45
Skills
    needed by leader, 58
    technical, for Advanced Practice Nurse
        role, 61(b)
Social change, 31-32
Social issues as health-care issues, 30
Social-systems change, 4-5
Social workers, perspective of, 182
Socialization, professional, 35-36
Software, continuum's information
        system, 92
Staff
    changes, implementation and, 153
    development of, 189-201
    turnover, 154
Standardization
    of care, development of, 96
    of care management, 94
State government, relationships with
        elected officials, 24
Statistical analysis of quantitative data,
        262-64
Strategies
    of agency, development of case
        managers and, 190, 191(f)
    at Silver Spring Community Nursing
        Center, 74
    for change, 33-37
    intervention, 69
    for risk identification and assessment,
        173-74
    supplemental, 163
    to overcome obstacles, 187
Student participation, professional
        services and, 45
Subscriber-based system, 12
Support
    lack of, 183-84
    organizational, 194
Support services, community-based,
        chronic illness and, 90
Survey of community nurse case
        management facility, 135-36
System, knowledge of, in Deming
        philosophy, 60
Systems theory, 57-58

T

Talking points document exemplar, 38-39
Team approach in managing continuum of
        care, 15-16
Team-based models of health care
        delivery, 70
Team players, relationships between, 17
Technical skills, for Advanced Practice
        Nurse role, 61(b)
Technology, 17
Terminal illness, Medicare Hospice
        Election and, 107
Theory
    guiding practice, 120-21
    of knowledge, in Deming philosophy,
        60
Therapeutic relationship building, 260-66

Tools
    clinical pathways, 224-32
    communication, care pathway
        implementation and, 98, 99(f)
    data collection, development of, 153
    Health Needs Assessment, 172, 175-76,
        177
    High Risk Maternal Case Management
        Referral Form, 173, 178
    Pediatric Case Management Referral
        Form, 173, 180
    Prenatal Health Assessment, 173-79
    risk screening, presentation of, 173-74
Training of primary nurses, for home care
        pathway, 232
Transformation of health care
    academia and, 46
    nursing's response, 28-39
Trends and implications, health care
        transformation and, 29-31
Tri-council, 33
Triggers, exacerbation, 125-26
Trust, 75
    the art of nursing and, 106-107
    as innovative delivery system, 105-16
Turf battles, 135, 185-86

U

Underemployment, 32
Unemployment, chronic, 32
Uninsured population, as force driving
        change, 4
Unit nurse manager, as case manager,
        151-52
Universities, public relations and, 26
University schools of nursing, academic
        nursing centers and, 70
University of Wisconsin-Milwaukee
        (UWM), 73

V

Values
    core nursing, 36
    curriculum and, 50-51
    fundamental, shifts of, 32-33
    guiding collective work, 35-36
    nursing, 23
Variance record, in pathway, 98, 100(f)
Variation, knowledge of, in Deming
        philosophy, 60
Vendors, information systems and, 92
Vision, new, transformative change and,
        28
Vision of agency, development of case
        managers and, 190, 191(f)
Volunteerism, importance of, 25
Volunteers, parish nurses and, 143

W

Washington, D.C., relationships with
        elected officials, 24-25
Watson, Jean, theory of human caring, 63
Whole person focus, 19
Work, concept of, 32
Workplace reconfiguration, layoffs and, 11
World view, shift of, 32-33